Cases on Virtual Reality Modeling in Healthcare

Yuk Ming Tang
Hong Kong Polytechnic University, China

Ho Ho Lun
Hong Kong Polytechnic University, China

Ka Yin Chau
City University of Macau, China

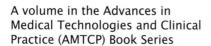
A volume in the Advances in
Medical Technologies and Clinical
Practice (AMTCP) Book Series

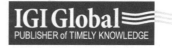

Published in the United States of America by
    IGI Global
    Medical Information Science Reference (an imprint of IGI Global)
    701 E. Chocolate Avenue
    Hershey PA, USA 17033
    Tel: 717-533-8845
    Fax: 717-533-8661
    E-mail: cust@igi-global.com
    Web site: http://www.igi-global.com

Library of Congress Cataloging-in-Publication Data

Names: Tang, Yuk Ming, 1978- editor. | Lun, Ho Ho, 1996- editor. | Chau, Ka
   Yin, editor.
Title: Cases on virtual reality modelling in healthcare / Yuk Ming Tang, Ho
   Ho Lun, Ka Yin Chau, editor.
Description: Hershey, PA : Medical Information Science Reference, [2022] |
   Includes bibliographical references and index. | Summary: "This book
   explores the application of virtual reality in healthcare settings,
   allowing readers to reference modelling and rendering techniques,
   dressing, and animation in healthcare applications"-- Provided by
   publisher.
Identifiers: LCCN 2021050588 (print) | LCCN 2021050589 (ebook) | ISBN
   9781799887904 (hardcover) | ISBN 9781799887911 (ebook)
Subjects: MESH: Virtual Reality | Delivery of Health Care
Classification: LCC R859.7.A78 (print) | LCC R859.7.A78 (ebook) | NLM W
   26.55.V6 | DDC 362.10285--dc23/eng/20211101
LC record available at https://lccn.loc.gov/2021050588
LC ebook record available at https://lccn.loc.gov/2021050589

This book is published in the IGI Global book series Advances in Medical Technologies and Clinical Practice (AMTCP) (ISSN: 2327-9354; eISSN: 2327-9370)

British Cataloguing in Publication Data
A Cataloguing in Publication record for this book is available from the British Library.

For electronic access to this publication, please contact: eresources@igi-global.com.

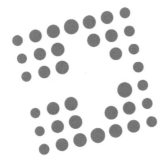

Advances in Medical Technologies and Clinical Practice (AMTCP) Book Series

ISSN:2327-9354
EISSN:2327-9370

Editor-in-Chief: Srikanta Patnaik, SOA University, India; Priti Das, S.C.B. Medical College, India

MISSION

Medical technological innovation continues to provide avenues of research for faster and safer diagnosis and treatments for patients. Practitioners must stay up to date with these latest advancements to provide the best care for nursing and clinical practices.

The **Advances in Medical Technologies and Clinical Practice (AMTCP) Book Series** brings together the most recent research on the latest technology used in areas of nursing informatics, clinical technology, biomedicine, diagnostic technologies, and more. Researchers, students, and practitioners in this field will benefit from this fundamental coverage on the use of technology in clinical practices.

COVERAGE

- Clinical Nutrition
- Clinical High-Performance Computing
- Nursing Informatics
- Biometrics
- Biomechanics
- Biomedical Applications
- Medical Informatics
- Clinical Data Mining
- Neural Engineering
- Patient-Centered Care

IGI Global is currently accepting manuscripts for publication within this series. To submit a proposal for a volume in this series, please contact our Acquisition Editors at Acquisitions@igi-global.com or visit: http://www.igi-global.com/publish/.

Titles in this Series

For a list of additional titles in this series, please visit: http://www.igi-global.com/book-series/

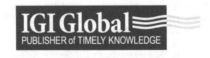

701 East Chocolate Avenue, Hershey, PA 17033, USA
Tel: 717-533-8845 x100 • Fax: 717-533-8661
E-Mail: cust@igi-global.com • www.igi-global.com

Editorial Advisory Board

Table of Contents

Detailed Table of Contents

Chapter 1

  Xiaoxiao Liu, City University of Macau, China
  Ka Yin Chau, City University of Macau, China
  Hoi Sze Chan, Hong Kong Polytechnic University, China
  Yan Wan, Faculty of Business, City University of Macau, China

Current virtual reality technology applications in healthcare perform potential
abilities in clinical and nursing practices. This review aims to analyse the use and
the development direction of virtual reality technology in the whole healthcare field.
Researchers searched (n = 5,209) English-language literature related to the application
of virtual reality in healthcare on the basis of the Web of Science online database
and used VOSviewer 1.6.17 to visualise and analyse the time trend co-authorship,
co-occurrence keywords, and country distribution of the literature. Furthermore,
they found that the application of virtual reality technology in healthcare shows
an overall fragmentation and a relatively concentrated trend, focusing on medical
education, rehabilitation therapy, and psychological interventions. Augmented reality
and COVID-19 are present research hotspots.

Chapter 2

A Review on Data-Driven Methods for Human Activity Recognition in
Smart Homes...21

Jiancong Ye, South China University of Technology, China
Junpei Zhong, The Hong Kong Polytechnic University, China

The smart home is one application of intelligent environments, where sensors are equipped to detect the status inside the domestic home. With the development of sensing technologies, more signals can be obtained with heterogenous statistical properties with faster processing speed. To make good use of the technical advantages, data-driven methods are becoming popular in intelligent environments. On the other hand, to recognize human activity is one essential target to understand the status inside a smart home. In this chapter, the authors focus on the human activity recognition (HAR) problem, which is the recognition of lower levels of activities, using data-driven models.

Chapter 3

The Implications of Virtual Reality (VR) for the Aged......................................41

Yui-yip Lau, Division of Business and Hospitality Management, The
Hong Kong Polytechnic University, Hong Kong, China
Ivy Chan, Division of Business and Hospitality Management, The Hong
Kong Polytechnic University, Hong Kong, China

As virtual reality (VR) technology continuously evolves in this century, the number of such applications have undoubtedly increased significantly. Nevertheless, the VR market for the aged is still in a blue ocean. The Hong Kong population is aging more quickly than ever before. This puts a huge stress to the healthcare systems in Hong Kong. In this chapter, the authors describe the updated VR technologies and their applications in a series of emerging healthcare services such as training and green burial for the aged. To this end, the chapter will provide management staff in homes for the aged, hospitals, healthcare service providers, and other health service professionals with the latest concepts and good practices in VR for the aged. The humanistic, holistic, and integrated care for the aged will be achieved in the future.

Chapter 4

Virtual Reality in Patient-Physician Relationships...63

Haoyu Liu, City University of Macau, China
Bowen Dong, City University of Macau, China
Pi-Ying Yen, Macau University of Science and Technology, China

The chapter examines the applications of virtual reality (VR) in patient-physician relationships. Specifically, this chapter focuses on three-dimensional medical imaging that facilitates explanation purposes. Though the literature on VR in medicine exists, the discussion of applying VR in patient-physician relationships, an immensely important topic of medicine, is sparse. The authors present a case of VR application in orthopedics to demonstrate how this technology promotes patient-physician relationships and, as a result, affects the medical industry. The opportunities and challenges of applying VR to medicine are also discussed. This chapter contributes to better incorporating VR into treatment and understanding the impact of emerging technologies on medicine.

Chapter 5

Karen Sie, Hong Kong Polytechnic University, China
Yuk Ming Tang, Hong Kong Polytechnic University, China
Kenneth Nai Kuen Fong, Hong Kong Polytechnic University, China

With the development of new technology, it is common that excessive use puts undue strain on the hands and finger tendons. This increases the risk of developing many forms of tendonitis. The objective in this project is to use the latest virtual reality (VR) technology to build a preventive rehabilitation game for raising public awareness of upper limb tendonitis. A survey of 141 respondents was first undertaken to find how much the general public knows about upper limb tendonitis. A virtual game is then created using the Unity3D game engine and 3Ds Max for 3D modeling. It is evaluated after being tested by five participants. The majority of respondents to the questionnaire did not know the cause or implications of tendon issues. Almost half of them spent 8.8 hours per day on computers and smartphones, with only 4 minutes per day spent exercising their hands and fingers. The participants gave positive comments towards the designed rehabilitation game and believe it can help to avoid fatigue caused by prolonged smartphone and computer use.

Chapter 6

N. Raghavendra Rao, FINAIT Consultancy Services, India

Many technologies tend to be applicable only in a specific industry or defined area of operation in business. The case of information and communication technology is different. The potential of information and communication technology in any sphere of activity in any discipline is more useful. Information and communication technology is a driving force in providing a good scope in making use of the various concepts in this discipline for designing models as per the requirements of a particular application. The concepts of cloud computing and virtual reality have proved to be significant particularly in the healthcare sector. This chapter gives an overview of the above concepts and related technology. Further, this chapter explains the case illustrations by adopting the above concepts for designing a virtual medical research initiative in the virtual reality environment.

Chapter 7

The authors proposed an anatomy-based methodology for human modeling to enhance the visual realism of human modeling by using the boundary element method (BEM) and axial deformation approach. To model muscle deformation, a BEM with linear boundary elements was used. The significance of tendons in determining skin layer deformation is also discussed. The axial deformation technique is used to allow for quick deformation. To control tendon deformation, the curve of the axial curve is changed. Each vertex of the skin layer is linked to the muscles, tendons, and skeletons beneath it. The skin layer deforms in response to changes in the underlying muscle, tendon, and skeleton layers. This chapter made use of human foot modeling as the case study. Results have illustrated that the visual realism of human models can be enhanced by considering the changes of tendons in the deformation of the skin layer. The lower computational complexity and enhanced visual realism of the proposed approaches can be applied in human modelling for virtual reality (VR) applications.

Cloud computing, big data, wearables, the internet of things, artificial intelligence, robotics, and virtual reality (VR), when seamlessly combined, will create the healthcare of the future. In the presented study, the authors aim to provide tools and methodologies to efficiently create 3D virtual learning environments (VLEs) to immerse participants in 3600, six degrees of freedom (6DoF) patient examination simulations. Furthermore, the authors will discuss specific methods and features to improve visual realism in VR, such as post-processing effects (ambient occlusion, bloom, depth of field, anti-aliasing), texturing (normal maps, transparent, and reflective materials), and realistic lighting (spotlights and custom lights). The presented VLE creation techniques will be used as a testbed for medical simulation, created using the Unity game engine.

Chapter 9

Mian Yan, School of Intelligent Systems Science and Engineering, Jinan University, China

Alex Pak Ki Kwok, School of Intelligent Systems Science and Engineering, Jinan University, Hong Kong, China

Cheng Yao Wang, Department of Electrical Engineering, City University of Hong Kong, Hong Kong, China

Xin Lian, School of Computer Science and Technology, Xi'an Jiaotong University, China

Can Biao Zhuang, School of Intelligent Systems Science and Engineering, Jinan University, China

Chang Gao, School of Intelligent Systems Science and Engineering, Jinan University, China

Ying Ting Huang, School of Intelligent Systems Science and Engineering, Jinan University, China

The continuous technological advancement of computer simulation, display technology, and the internet of things leads to the opportunities to use cross-reality (XR) technologies in crisis management. XR emphasizes the compositions of different concepts in reality-virtuality continuum under a shared online virtual world, including virtual reality (VR), augmented reality (AR), and mixed reality (MR). It is touted as a promising tool to facilitate crisis management strategies in different stages, including prevention, onsite management, and recovery. This research contributes to the field of research in VR, XR, and crisis management (an essential component of healthcare) in the following four ways: (1) It proposes an idea to apply XR in crisis management. (2) It proposes a framework to connect VR, AR, and MR serving one purpose. (3) It presents a qualitative study to examine the user perception of the XR-based crisis management method. (4) It brings out the challenges and opportunities of using XR in crisis management.

Chapter 10

Farzad Sabetzadeh, City University of Macau, China

Yusong Wang, City University of Macau, China

Augmented reality (AR) technology has been widely used in various business applications in the past five years. Since the beginning of 2020, with the COVID-19 pandemic and its impact on various industries, AR has become one of the technologies that have significantly reduced physical interactions between buyers and sellers. This chapter reflects its finding in fours areas: 1) eCommerce mobile AR apps can allow customers to better interact with products virtually. 2) AR facilitates customer shopping journey in three stages of purchasing, namely before-purchase, purchase, and after-purchase stages. 3) Design and develop mobile AR apps with two features of virtuality and interactivity to the extent that enables customers to favor AR apps to the offline shopping experience in a sustainable trend. 4) Online retailers can utilize their AR apps to predict target customers' preferences, hence giving them effective promotions to motivate them to buy their preferred products online.

Foreword

Today, AI (Artificial Intelligence), VR (Virtual Reality), AR (Augmented Reality) and MR (Mixed Reality) have found many applications in Information Science and Technology. They have been used in various platforms to develop virtual reality products and services such as product design, collaborative learning and training, 3D games, Building Information Management, etc. For example, in NASA and the Jet Propulsion laboratory, VR/AR is used to conduct various types of astronaut training and health assessment and evaluation. They are used to conduct simulations in deep space explorations, including spaceflight, International space station activity and spacewalk, on the moon and Mars. Recently, in China, the Chang'e-5 successfully returned the first Chinese acquired lunar regolith sample and Tiawen-1-Zhurong completed the first Chinese soft landing on Mars. Tiangong is a space station that the Chinese are now building in low Earth orbit. These developments are realized with the applications of Virtual Reality Digital Twin and VR in the Tiangong space stations to monitor the astronauts' daily activities and health conditions with the teams on earth. Other applications of VR/MR including the learning and training in Moon and Mars landing, the design of Lunar Surface Sample Acquisition and Packaging instrument for returning the lunar regolith, and the Mars Landing intelligent Surveillance Camera onboard the Mars lander are built with the 3D reconstruction of Moon and Mars surfaces with the robots and in the near future with the astronauts working together. We can see scientists and engineers are making benefits of the technology to accomplish many challenging tasks. We are happy to have this book which presents virtual reality in the healthcare environment. The book follows a very practical and interesting approach, dedicated to all readers who would like to understand all the insights of this interdisciplinary research area which integrates and innovates in VR/AR/MR. This book would also be a good choice for academics and industrialists who want to bring specific theory and case studies into their classrooms and working environment in an easy-to-understand way.

Andrew W. H. Ip
University of Saskatchewan, Canada & Warwick Manufacturing Group,
University of Warwick, UK & The Hong Kong Polytechnic University, Hong Kong

Preface

Virtual Reality (VR) has drawn much attention in the last few years, especially in healthcare applications. Unfortunately, very few medical professionals know what modelling tools can facilitate the construction of realistic 3D models and scenarios for a specific application of VR simulation in their workplace. The most popular tools used for 3D modellings include ZBrush, Blender, SketchUp, AutoCAD, SolidWorks, 3Ds Max, Maya, Rhino3D, CATIA, etc. However, these tools are more difficult to grasp at the application level, especially in a specific industry, such as the healthcare sector. Therefore, this book will help medical professionals understand and have a clear picture of the application of these tools.

Firstly, the chapter reviews the development and applications of VR technology and its related software and hardware. And then, this book used cases to illustrate the applications for the medical professionals interested in setting up the VR simulation at their workplaces, from 3D modelling to computer programming. The medical professionals could follow the methods in this book to create the VR simulations needed to improve their work efficiency.

UNIQUENESS OF THE BOOK

The uniqueness of this book demonstrates the application of virtual reality (VR) in the healthcare sector with cases. This book is suitable for medical professionals and professionals from different industries to understand how to set up VR simulations in their workplaces.

TARGET AUDIENCE

The potential target audience is medical professionals and professionals from computer sciences, computer engineering, product designers, etc. In addition, this book is also suitable for readers from other industries who may need to apply VR technology in their fields.

Here is the summary of the structure of the book and its 10 chapters.

Chapter 1: A Visualization Analysis Using the VOSviewer of Literature on Virtual Reality Technology Application in Healthcare

The first chapter analyzes the use and development direction of virtual reality (VR) technology in the healthcare field have potential abilities in clinical and nursing practices. The authors have identified the English-language literature related to the application of VR in healthcare based on the Web of Science online database. VOSviewer 1.6.17 is used to visualize and analyze the time trend co-authorship, co-occurrence keywords, and country distribution of the literature.

Chapter 2: A Review on Data-Driven Methods for Human Activity Recognition in Smart Home

The second chapter discusses the human activity recognition (HAR) problem, which is the recognition of lower levels of activities using data-driven models. Smart homes are an application of intelligent environments, where sensors are equipped to detect the status inside a domestic home. With the development of sensing technologies, an increasing number of signals can be obtained with heterogeneous statistical properties at a faster processing speed. Data-driven methods are becoming popular in intelligent environments to make good use of the technical advantages. However, recognizing human activity is an essential target for understanding a smart home's status.

Chapter 3: The Implications of Virtual Reality (VR) for the Aged

The third chapter describes the updated VR technologies and their applications in emerging healthcare services, such as training and green burial for the aged. As VR technology has continuously evolved in this century, such applications have undoubtedly increased significantly. The Hong Kong population is ageing more quickly than ever before and putting enormous stress on its healthcare systems. This chapter will also explain the latest concepts and good practices in VR for the aged. Humanistic, holistic, and integrated care for the elderly will be achieved in the future.

Chapter 4: Virtual Reality in Patient-Physician Relationships

The fourth chapter examines the applications of virtual reality (VR) in patient-physician relationships focusing on three-dimensional medical imaging. The authors present a case of VR application in orthopedics to demonstrate how this technology promotes patient-physician relationships to affect the medical industry. This chapter also contributes to better incorporating VR into treatment and understanding the impact of emerging technologies on medicine.

Chapter 5: Virtual Reality Scenes Development for Upper Limb Tendonitis Rehabilitation Game

This chapter aims to use the latest virtual reality (VR) technology to build a preventive rehabilitation game to raise public awareness of upper limb tendonitis. With the development of new technology, excessive use is expected to put undue strain on the hands and fingers' tendons, this increases the risk of developing many forms of tendonitis. A virtual game was then created using the Unity3D game engine and 3Ds Max for 3D modelling and evaluated after five participants' testing. The participants gave positive comments toward the designed rehabilitation game and believed it could help avoid fatigue caused by prolonged smartphone and computer use.

Chapter 6: Designing a Conceptual Virtual Medical Research Initiative in the Virtual Reality Environment

Many technologies tend to be applicable only to a specific industry or defined areas of business operations. The concepts of cloud computing and VR have proved to be significant, particularly in the healthcare sector. This chapter provides an overview of the above concepts and related technologies by explaining the case illustrated by adopting the above concepts for designing a virtual medical research initiative in a VR environment.

Chapter 7: Anatomy-Based Human Modeling for Virtual Reality (VR)

This chapter used human foot modelling as a case study to propose an anatomy-based methodology for human modelling to enhance the visual realism of human modelling using the boundary element method (BEM) and axial deformation approach. The significance of tendons in determining skin layer deformation is also discussed. The proposed approaches' lower computational complexity and enhanced visual realism can be applied in human modelling for VR applications.

Chapter 8: Prototyping VR Training Tools for Healthcare With Off-the-Shelf CGI – A Case Study

Cloud Computing, Big Data, Wearables, the Internet of Things, artificial intelligence, robotics, and virtual reality (VR), when these technologies are seamlessly combined, they will create future healthcare. In this chapter, the authors aim to provide tools and methodologies to efficiently create 3D virtual learning environments (VLEs) to immerse participants in 360°, six degrees of freedom (6DoF) patient examination simulations. Furthermore, the authors will discuss specific methods and features to improve visual realism in VR, such as post-processing effects (ambient occlusion, bloom, depth of field, anti-aliasing), texturing (normal maps, transparent and reflective materials), and realistic lighting (spotlights and custom lights).

Chapter 9: Cross Reality in Crisis Management

The continuous technological advancement of computer simulation, display technology, and the Internet of Things has led to opportunities to use cross-reality (XR) technologies in crisis management. This chapter contributes to the field of research in VR, XR, and crisis management (an essential component of healthcare) in the following four ways: (1) it proposes the application of XR in crisis management; (2) it proposes a framework to connect VR, AR, and MR serving one purpose; (3) it presents a qualitative study to examine user perceptions of the XR-based crisis management method; and (4) it brings out the challenges and opportunities for using XR in crisis management.

Chapter 10: Demystifying Augmented Reality (AR) in Marketing From the E-Commerce Perspective

Augmented reality (AR) technology has been widely used in various business applications over the past five years, such as AR has become a technology that has significantly reduced the physical interactions between buyers and sellers. This chapter attempts to reflect its findings in four areas: 1) eCommerce mobile AR apps can allow customers to better interact with products virtually; 2) AR facilitates customer shopping journey in three stages of purchasing, namely, before-purchase, purchase, and after-purchase stages; 3) Design and develop mobile AR apps with two features of virtuality and interactivity to the extent that enables customers to favour AR apps to the offline shopping experience in a sustainable trend; 4) Online retailers can utilize their AR apps to predict target customers' preferences, thus giving them effective promotions to motivate them to buy their preferred products online.

CONCLUSION

This book explores the application of VR technology in different healthcare contexts. It presents an easy-to-understand case study format for users at all levels and disciplines of modelling, textures, dressings, and animations in healthcare applications. The conclusions will help people in healthcare to better apply VR technology and help people in other fields understand and use VR technology.

Acknowledgment

We sincerely appreciate all the excellent scholars who contributed to this book, and with your help, this book was completed successfully. We are also thankful to those who participated in the double-blind review process and provided valuable comments on this book, and your comments have greatly helped the improvement of this book. The publication of this book was substantially supported by the Innovation and Technology Fund (ITF) of the Hong Kong Special Administrative Region, China (Project Ref.: PRP/071/20FX). Finally, we would like to acknowledge the Department of Industrial and Systems Engineering support from the Hong Kong Polytechnic University, Hong Kong. We also acknowledge support from the City University of Macau for the enhancement of this book publishing.

Chapter 1
A Visualisation Analysis Using the VOSviewer of Literature on Virtual Reality Technology Application in Healthcare

Xiaoxiao Liu
City University of Macau, China

Ka Yin Chau
https://orcid.org/0000-0002-0381-8401
City University of Macau, China

Hoi Sze Chan
Hong Kong Polytechnic University, China

Yan Wan
Faculty of Business, City University of Macau, China

EXECUTIVE SUMMARY

Current virtual reality technology applications in healthcare perform potential abilities in clinical and nursing practices. This review aims to analyse the use and the development direction of virtual reality technology in the whole healthcare field. Researchers searched (n = 5,209) English-language literature related to the application of virtual reality in healthcare on the basis of the Web of Science online database and used VOSviewer 1.6.17 to visualise and analyse the time trend co-authorship, co-occurrence keywords, and country distribution of the literature. Furthermore, they found that the application of virtual reality technology in healthcare shows an overall fragmentation and a relatively concentrated trend, focusing on medical education, rehabilitation therapy, and psychological interventions. Augmented reality and COVID-19 are present research hotspots.

DOI: 10.4018/978-1-7998-8790-4.ch001

INTRODUCTION

With the current burst of 5G communication technology, artificial intelligence and the Internet of Things a simple keyboard–mouse type of human–machine interaction technology can no longer meet the requirement of technological innovation (Krupitzer et al., 2020). Virtual reality (VR), which provides a sense of immersion, could be the high-tech technology that changes the way humans live (Zhan, Yin, Xiong, He, & Wu, 2020). Virtual reality technology is a fusion innovation of multiple technologies (Chen, Zou, & Wang, 2021). Moreover, it integrates computer technology, human–computer interaction technology and graphics technology to create a virtual and realistic three-dimensional visualisation environment using graphics technology, network technology and interpersonal sensing technology (Shao et al., 2020).

Virtual reality technology has the following features: 3-dimension visualisation, immersion, simulation, interactivity and presence (Servotte et al., 2020). It is increasingly employed in the military, education, industry, entertainment and health-care fields (Javaid & Haleem, 2020). In addition, virtual reality technology has been applied earlier to aviation and military training, which can simulate the operation and training of new weapons or aircraft. It has also replaced dangerous actual operations and has allowed large-scale military exercises in a simulated environment (Ahir, Govani, Gajera, & Shah, 2020). Loucks et al. (2019) affirmed the usefulness of virtual reality exposure therapy for the treatment of military traumatic stress disorder. VR application on military is considered as early research on virtual reality technology application in health care. Since then, it has been attracting considerable attention (Rizzo & Koenig, 2017). Given the clinical costs or risk aversions of treatment option factors, advances in virtual reality technology mean more efficient treatment options for doctors and better patient experiences (Aziz, 2018).

Many reviews on virtual reality technology applications in health care have performed potential abilities on clinical education, physical therapy, anxiety management, acute and chronic pain management and nursing (Rousseaux et al., 2020). Nonetheless, visualisation studies on the correlation or similarity of related literature across the whole health-care field have been neglected. Due to the wide virtual reality technology applications and highly comprehensive value, this may induce a lack of research, broadness and rigour. Compared with other similar reviews, the current study purposefully identified the relationships between the literature pieces examining healthcare-related fields. Virtual reality technology is still evolving, and there is still much room for the exploration and development of its application in the health-care field. Systematically combining the published academic literature pieces in a visualisation way can help us find the research trend and understand the research hotspots. Therefore, analysing the literature on the application of virtual reality technology in the whole health-care field is necessary to present relatively rigorous scientific research (Yu et al., 2020).

After overviewing the application and research progress of virtual reality technology, we identified 5,209 academic literature pieces, which are all related to virtual reality technology and health care, in the Web of Science from 2012 to 2021 and analysed them using VOSviewer software. We aimed to understand the following: (1) What are the main research themes of virtual reality technology in the health-care field? (2) What are the future research directions? Providing new perspectives and references for health-care professionals to make full use of virtual reality technology is expected.

The rest of the present paper is structured as follows: Section 2 deals with the development of virtual reality technology and application in the health-care field; Section 3 displays the methodology; Section 4 exhibits the visualisation analysis result of the literature; and Sections 5 and 6 present the discussion and conclusion.

LITERATURE REVIEW

Virtual Reality Technology Overview

VR is a computer-generated technology that immerses people in a virtual environment constructed from data (Mäkinen, Haavisto, Havola, & Koivisto, 2020). The user can interact with the virtual environment naturally by using specific equipment to simulate physical presence in the virtual environment, thereby gaining a sense of immersion in the corresponding real environment (Fertleman et al., 2018). VR has originated from computer graphics, which rely on three-dimensional (3D) head-tracking display technology to create a simulated multi-sensory experience (Pan & Hamilton, 2018).

The core of VR is a blend of immersion, interactivity and presence (Mandal, 2013). Specifically, immersion is related to the level of sensory stimulation and is influenced by the similarity of the simulated environment to reality (Snoswell & Snoswell, 2019), which is defined as the level of user engagement in the experience (Kim, Jeon, & Kim, 2017). Presence is the subjective psychological feeling of the behaviour of a user in a virtual environment. To some extent, presence feels like the result of immersion (Schäfer, Reis, & Stricker, 2021). Interactivity emphasises the fluid level of human–computer interactions between the user and the virtual environment, which enables the user to feel the feedback from his/her behaviour (Mütterlein, 2018). Increased sensory stimulation can increase user presence (Mütterlein & Hess, 2017). Thus, the better the integration of these three indicators, the more realistic the user experience will feel (Kim et al., 2017).

3

The idea of virtual reality technology first appeared in a 1935 science fiction novel. It described the strange experience of the protagonist of the novel, Pygmalion, who enters another world when he puts on special glasses. Additionally, it is the first description of a virtual reality sensory experience involving hearing, sight and touch (Weinbaum, 2016). In the 1950s, a simulator called 'sensorama' and a head-mounted display developed by Lvan Sutherland enabled the user to interact with the machine in more real time (Koroliov & Lapko, 2021). Until 1989, Jaron Lanier first introduced the term 'virtual reality'. The concept was clear and gradually accepted by the community (Faisal, 2017), and this also marked the development of VR from the 'budding' period of VR 1.0 to the 'technical exploration' period of VR 2.0 (Delaney, 2016; Moskaliuk, Kimmerle, & Cress, 2010). After entering the 21st century, because of the advances in graphics processing and motion capture-related technologies, virtual reality technology has entered a 'breakthrough development' period of VR 3.0 (Sirkkunen, Väätäjä, Uskali, & Rezaei, 2016). Since 2012, the industrialisation of virtual reality technology has moved towards a new stage, the VR 4.0 'industrial application' period (Liu & Yang, 2021).

Virtual Reality Technology Application in Health Care

Virtual reality technology is broadly used in clinical, medical, nursing and psychological applications, such as remote surgery, acute and chronic pain management, clinical education and traumatic management (Pourmand, Davis, Lee, Barber, & Sikka, 2017). In 1993, doctors utilized VR to assist in the treatment of mental health disorders, and this was considered as the early usage of virtual reality technology in the medical field (Rizzo & Koenig, 2017). The recreation of the Vietnam War with virtual reality technology is a well-known case in psychological applications. It also significantly reduces the post-traumatic stress disorder (PTSD) symptoms of patients (Maples-Keller, Yasinski, Manjin, & Rothbaum, 2017).

Virtual reality technology can integrate the senses of sight, sound and touch, which can help students understand abstract concepts through immersive experiences (Snoswell & Snoswell, 2019; Y.-M. Tang, Au, Lau, Ho, & Wu, 2020). A researcher has designed and developed a virtual reality learning system on the topic of 'eye', which allows students to observe pathological changes in the eye, determine the condition more accurately and develop a treatment plan. This enhances the hands-on effect and increases motivation greatly in clinical education (Shim et al., 2003).

In the rehabilitation field, it is generally inappropriate for patients to train in a realistic environment due to their own limb movement limitations. Virtual reality technology not only simulates realistic scenarios but also makes training safer and more fun (Howard, 2017). Llorens, Colomer-Font, Alcañiz, and Noé-Sebastián (2013) developed a virtual balance training system that improves the balance of patients with brain injury by completing training programs, such as trunk postural control.

Currently, more advanced virtual reality technology has been applied to more sophisticated areas of health care, such as remote medical (Gupta, Bagga, & Sharma, 2020). A surgeon operates on a virtual mannequin and transmitted to a robotic instrument that mimics the actions to complete the operation (Desselle et al., 2020). Virtual reality technology has already been moving from a diagnostic to a therapeutic tool (Cieślik et al., 2020).

METHODOLOGY

We searched the English-language literature related to the application of VR in health care on the basis of the Web of Science online database and used VOSviewer 1.6.17 to visualise and analyse the time trends, co-authorship, co-occurrence keywords, country distribution and theme trends.

Data Collection

The first step in completing a literature review is to systematically select and classify the literature (Torraco, 2016). We firstly identified the Web of Science as the database of article selection. Because it is one of the leading academic online databases for scientific papers and research, it provides built-in analysis tools to produce representative results. More importantly, the search results can be exported as a document from the Web of Science for further analysis with software, such as VOSviewer (Yu et al., 2020).

To conduct the data collecting process, the search criteria were topics on 'VR in health care' or 'VR in medical field'. According to Cronin, Ryan, and Coughlan (2008) that a review period of 5-10 years is usually placed to provide a more comprehensive coverage of research in a field. We need to know the decade about how others have mapped the field of VR in health care, and how research have developed from there. Therefore, we obtained 8,319 records from January 1, 2012, to August 8, 2021. Core collections that are not at the same level must not be employed to ensure searching the high-quality literature (Zhu, Jin, & He, 2019). Hence, we screened the Science Citation Index Expanded (SCI-EXPANDED), Social Sciences Citation Index (SSCI) and Emerging Sources Citation Index (ESCI) as journal source collections, which enabled us to select the high-value literature efficiently (Pop et al., 2018), and 6,702 records were obtained. Finally, we selected the document type on 'article' and language on 'English', and we acquired 5,209 records to ensure the quality and relevance of the research. Table 1 displays the document retrieval flow.

Table 1. Document retrieval flow

Filter Type	Description	Filter Records (Web of Science)
The search strings words identification	The filter fulfils the search topic on "virtual reality in health care" or "virtual reality in medical field".	12568
Timeline freezing	Publications from Jan 1st, 2012, to Aug 8th, 2021.	8319
Journal screening	Only selecting SCI, SSCI and ESCI as the journal source collection.	6702
Eligibility	1. Documents type on "article". 2. Language on "English".	5209

Visualisation Analysis

We could identify the time trend in virtual reality technology in health-care research, distribution in countries and publishing institutions by the intrinsic function of the Web of Science. Furthermore, we used VOSviewer software to perform the data mining, mapping and clustering of the 5,209 literature pieces. VOSviewer software was developed by Van Eck and Waltman (2010) from Leiden University, The Netherlands. It can be employed for most common bibliometric studies, such as co-citation analysis, co-occurrence analysis and literature coupling analysis, to reflect the characteristics of elements in terms of their distance and strength of association and to display the data graphically (Cavalcante, Coelho, & Bairrada, 2021). The analysis results were labelled with coloured circles. Each colour performs one cluster, and the size of the circles was positively correlated with the occurrence. The number and size of the coloured circles can be seen as the weight of each item. The greater the weight of an item, the larger the label and circle of it (Yu et al., 2020).

RESULTS

Annual Distribution of Literature

There is a clear overall trend of growth after the analysis of the literature on annual distribution of 5,209 literature pieces, which is related on the application of virtual reality technology to health care (Figure 2). Compared with later, the number of literature published each year grew relatively flat before 2016, but since 2016, the number of literature published each year has all exceeded 400, with a high growth trend. After 2018, the average annual increase is approximately 13%. By the date of the literature searched, the number of literature on the application of VR in health care reached its peak in 2020 with 986 articles. Moreover, the number of literature from January to July 2021 is 639, which is already more than the number of literature in the entire year of 2018.

Figure 1.

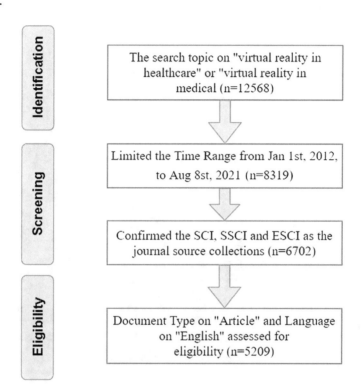

Co-Authorship Analysis

Organisation-Based Distribution Analysis

A visual analysis of the organisation-based distribution using VOSviewer exhibits that there are 5,624 research organisations engaged in research on VR in health care (Figure 3A). The name of the organisations is in the centre of the circle, the size of the circle represents the literature count by organisation, the distance between the circles represents the closeness of the collaboration between the organisations and the thickness of the connecting lines between the circles represents the strength of the association between the organisations. The top 10 organisations about the number of literature pieces issued are University Toronto, Stanford University,

University Washington, McGill University, Harvard Medical School, Tel Aviv University, University College London, Kings College London, Imperial College of Science, Technology and Medicine, University Illinois (Figure 3B). The results validate that the organisations with a higher number of literature have a stronger cooperation relationship and a stronger association. Moreover, the citations of the top 10 organisations are all bigger than 600, thereby indicating that their research has been recognised by scholars.

Figure 2. The analysis result of literature by year

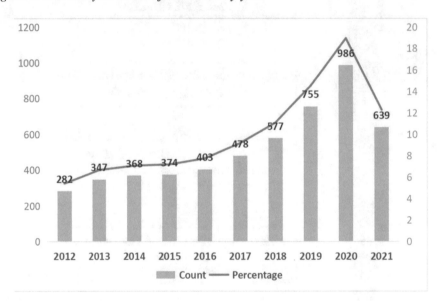

Country-Based Distribution Analysis

Figure 4A illustrates the results of the country-based distribution. The name of the countries is in the centre of the circle, the size of the circle represents the number of literature by country, the distance between the circles represents the closeness of the collaboration between the countries and the thickness of the connecting lines between the circles represents the strength of the association between the countries. The results verify that, with the USA as the centre, cooperation with countries, such as Canada, Australia, UK, Germany and China, is relatively strong and that the research association between the USA and these countries is strong. Figure 4B shows that the USA ranks first in terms of the number of literature, with 33.4% of the 5,209 publications, whilst the UK and China occupy the second and third places with 10.4% and 9%, respectively. They are closely followed by Germany (8.2%), Canada (8.1%), the Netherlands (6.6%), Italy (5.6%), Australia (5.4%), South Korea (4.8%) and Spain (3.8%).

Figure 3. The analysis result of top 10 organisation distribution

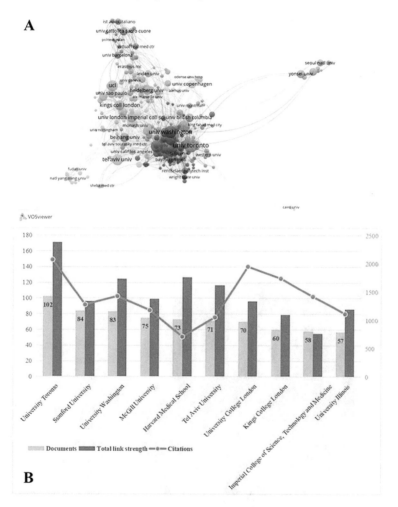

Co-Occurrence Author Analysis

The analysis of co-occurrence authors confirms that there are 23,005 authors for 5,209 documents and 429 authors with more than five publications. Amongst them, 89 authors have associations, and 314 links are divided into eight clusters. Each colour represents one cluster, and the total link strength is 1,203 (Figure 5). The result exhibits a trend of 'clustering concentration but the overall dispersion' about co-occurrence authors. Amongst them, Riva, Giuseppe, Wiederhold and Brenda K. have a relatively high number of literature and collaborate more closely.

Figure 4. The analysis result of top 10 country distribution

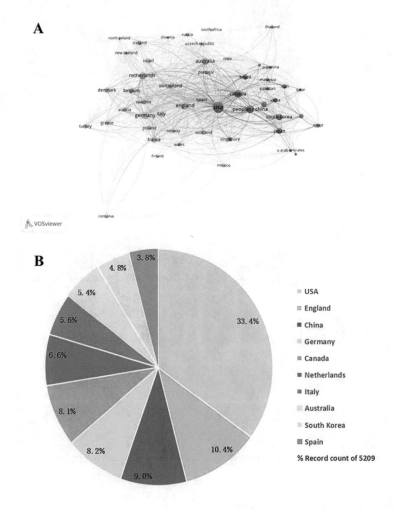

Co-Occurrence Keywords Analysis

The analysis of co-occurrence keywords affirms that there are 15,768 keywords for 5,209 documents. Figure 6A shows the network visualisation of 153 keywords, which have occurred more than 40 times. A total of 6,421 links are divided into four clusters. Each colour represents one cluster, and the total link strength is 39,844. According to the size of circles, which represents the weight of a keyword, 'virtual reality', 'simulation', 'education', 'performance', 'rehabilitation' and 'augmented reality' are the high-frequency keywords. This result illustrated that those words are the current research hotspots. The time-series mapping (Figure 6A) exhibits that the weight of 'augmented reality' and 'mixed reality', as research keywords, gradually increased around 2018. Notably, since the emergence of COVID-19 in December 2019, there have been nearly 50 research papers with virtual reality technology and COVID-19 as the subjects of studies in less than two years. This suggests that highly infectious diseases have given rise to the development and advancement of virtual reality technology.

Figure 5. The analysis result of co-occurrence authors

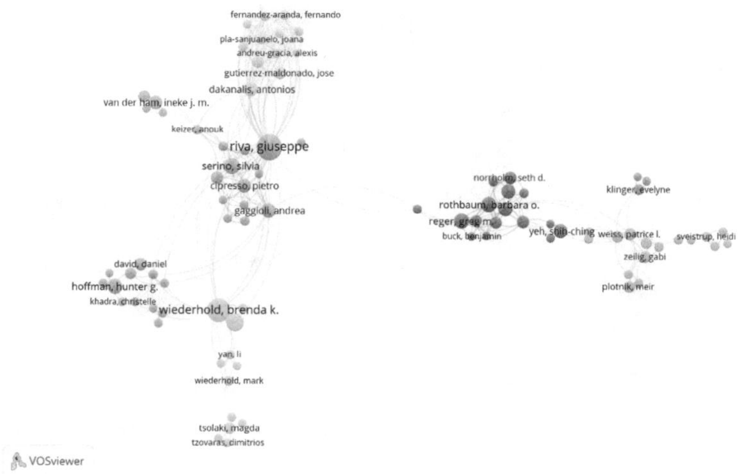

DISCUSSION

This section is a further discussion of the results of the 5,209 literature pieces, with the expectation that it will help scholars find more worthwhile topics for future research.

Figure 6. The analysis results of keyword co-occurrence

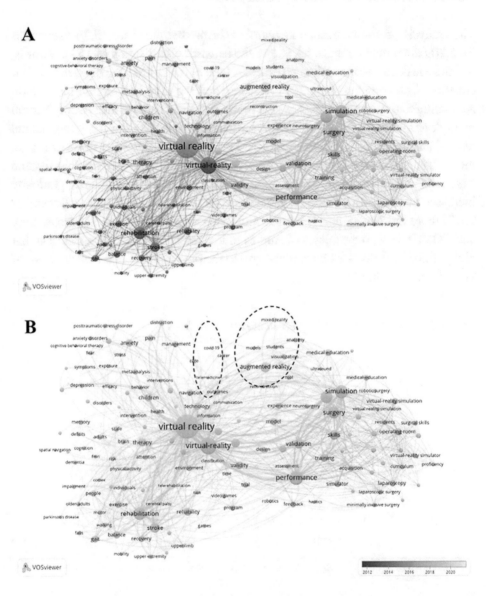

Current Situation of Virtual Reality in Health-Care Research

In the last decade, the literature on the application of virtual reality technology in health care has grown year by year, indicating that more and more scholars are concerned with the value of virtual reality technology. Meanwhile, they are also willing to explore the boundaries of its application in the medical field. The growing number of literature represents that the results of those scholars have been recognised (Xie, Chen, Wang, Zheng, & Jiang, 2020).

Virtual reality technology first originated in the USA, leading in hardware and software. The distribution of the top 10 authors and top 10 research organisations illustrates that the USA continues to be a leader in research on the health-care applications of virtual reality technology, which is consistent with the research outcome of Wang et al. (2020). Compared with the more technologically advanced European and American countries, China is a late beginner in the field of virtual reality technology, but the results of country distribution assert that China has quickly caught up and has only ranked third after the UK. This indicates that virtual reality technology has got highly valued in China and is particularly well practiced in areas such as simulated surgical operating environments (Yan et al., 2020). At the same time, the results can visually show the distribution of organisations and help them find teams to work with.

In addition to the distribution of the development on virtual reality technology applications in the medical field, the results also corroborate that the technology has applied a simulated environment in which medical interns can wear simulated equipment for clinical practice to obtain an in-depth learning effect. Our findings are also in accord with Y. M. Tang et al. (2021) that immersive virtual reality technology is effective and safe in medical education. Additionally, VR is realistic and vivid, interactive and immersive training, regardless of time, geographical, medical and teaching conditions. Medical interns can practice in a simulated hospital environment and avoid possible errors of judgements or medical errors in performing real operations.

The advances of virtual reality technology bring interactive experiences and a sense of presence to medical education through simulated environments, but they are not far enough. The simple stimulation of sight and sound is no longer sufficient for the demands of treatment or rehabilitation. It is similar to the study of Y. Tang, Au, and Leung (2018). To be more efficient, augmented reality technology is introduced to improve image recognition and feel haptic feedback, with all three feelings enhancing one another to create an immersive and scenic experience. Augmented reality technology has developed rapidly in recent years, and the virtual meeting system V-ROOMS is an application design for mixed reality technology that combines virtual reality and augmented reality technologies. Further, it processes information and data through a virtual environment whilst adding a role in summarising the minutes of meetings (Bao, Guo, Li, & Zhang, 2019). This is positively helpful for the observation and training of medical students and for the online discussion of experts.

In addition to helping in medical student training, virtual reality technology can also assist patients in improving their rehabilitation outcomes through high-resolution medical analysis programs. The visualisation provided by virtual reality technology can show patients what can be expected from rehabilitation training, thereby improving the efficiency of health-care professionals whilst giving them greater relief. Further, virtual reality technology is more effective than traditional rehabilitation programs for the development of physical outcomes, which include the application of motor control, balance, gait and strength. The upper limb rehabilitation robot researched at Stanford University is able to provide multiple forms of feedback during training (Miao et al., 2021), thereby giving timely and reasonable pieces of advice on the basis of the status of patients to give full play to their initiative. Therefore, virtual reality technology could remove the limitations of relying solely on the therapist for rehabilitation training. Aziz (2018) also confirmed similar results in his/her study.

Future Direction of Virtual Reality in Health-Care Research

The application of virtual reality simulation technology in health care was the main research trend from 2012 to 2021 The topics most associated with it are education and training, performance and efficiency and rehabilitation therapy and augmented reality.

According to our research, virtual reality technology is highly effective in the education sector, which enables medical students to practice more. The experience of human–computer interaction allows patients to complete rehabilitation training in a relaxed state through the visual presentation of virtual tasks, which can effectively enhance the dynamic stimulation from the treatment plan and truly improve the treatment outcome. The topics have all largely attracted the attention of scholars and have yielded considerable results in their research. Nevertheless, there is a relative lack of applied research in diagnosis and treatment compared with early education and late-stage rehabilitation. Just as our results of time-series mapping presented that COVID-19 is a current global health-care challenge. It has greatly contributed to the development and adoption of VR, augmented reality, and mixed reality. Because of the epidemic, telemedicine has become the focus technology of VR and augmented reality. It allows not only for remote technical training for health-care staff members but also for the effective risk avoidance of contracting diseases for them. Hence, the application of virtual reality technology in disaster emergency management is a topic worthy of study. When a sudden disaster occurs, real scenes are implanted into the system, using VR visualization technology, relying on three-dimensional electronic sand table, and a set of three-dimensional dynamic digital plans are deduced based on the analysis and assessment of the disaster situation. It can make emergency response more scientific and efficient. In addition, it can make sense to the design and development of a user platform, such as a self-health management system, which can combine with rehabilitation therapy. It also facilitates tracking and monitors patients after treatment and enables the reduction of the labour input and the increase of medical efficiency.

CONCLUSION

The current study extracted 5,209 literature pieces from the Web of Science from 2012 to 2021 related to the application of virtual reality technology in health care and presented an overview of scientific works in the medical domain. This study also used visualisation analysis to present the strength of the links between the literature pieces. Moreover, we believe that virtual reality technology is a sustainable industry to focus on disaster emergency management. In addition to the applications in medical education and rehabilitation training, platform development for self-health monitoring is a direction worthy of attention.

We considered the significance of this paper in three parts. Firstly, it provides the overall review of research on the application of virtual reality technology in health care to enhance the understanding of scholars. Secondly, we used VOSviewer software to obtain the visualisation results of publication count, co-occurring authors, organisations and countries to inform scholars seeking suitable collaborative teams. In addition, the analysis of co-occurring keywords not only reflects current research themes but also provides support for future worthwhile research directions of disaster emergency management and self-health monitoring. To some extent, VR can avoid clinical risks, improve the efficiency and science of treatment, the patient experience, even optimise the relationship of doctor-patient.

Literature selection bias may be a limitation of this study. It refers to the fact that all sample literature pieces were derived from only one database (Web of Science). This is because VOSviewer software can only handle multiple documents exported from one database at the same time. Therefore, there may be a possibility that the article selection is not comprehensive. Scholars can try to find more efficient tools in future studies.

REFERENCES

Ahir, K., Govani, K., Gajera, R., & Shah, M. (2020). Application on virtual reality for enhanced education learning, military training and sports. *Augmented Human Research*, *5*(1), 1–9. doi:10.100741133-019-0025-2

Aziz, H. A. (2018). Virtual reality programs applications in healthcare. *Journal of Health & Medical Informatics*, *9*(1), 305. doi:10.4172/2157-7420.1000305

Bao, J., Guo, D., Li, J., & Zhang, J. (2019). The modelling and operations for the digital twin in the context of manufacturing. *Enterprise Information Systems*, *13*(4), 534–556. doi:10.1080/17517575.2018.1526324

Cavalcante, W. Q. F., Coelho, A., & Bairrada, C. M. (2021). Sustainability and Tourism Marketing: A Bibliometric Analysis of Publications between 1997 and 2020 Using VOSviewer Software. *Sustainability*, *13*(9), 4987. doi:10.3390u13094987

Chen, H., Zou, Q., & Wang, Q. (2021). Clinical manifestations of ultrasonic virtual reality in the diagnosis and treatment of cardiovascular diseases. *Journal of Healthcare Engineering*, ●●●, 2021. PMID:34257848

Cieślik, B., Mazurek, J., Rutkowski, S., Kiper, P., Turolla, A., & Szczepańska-Gieracha, J. (2020). Virtual reality in psychiatric disorders: A systematic review of reviews. *Complementary Therapies in Medicine*, *52*, 102480. doi:10.1016/j.ctim.2020.102480 PMID:32951730

Cronin, P., Ryan, F., & Coughlan, M. (2008). Undertaking a literature review: A step-by-step approach. *British Journal of Nursing (Mark Allen Publishing)*, *17*(1), 38–43. doi:10.12968/bjon.2008.17.1.28059 PMID:18399395

Delaney, B. (2016). *Virtual Reality 1.0–The 90's: The Birth of VR in the pages of CyberEdge Journal*. CyberEdge Information Services.

Desselle, M. R., Brown, R. A., James, A. R., Midwinter, M. J., Powell, S. K., & Woodruff, M. A. (2020). Augmented and virtual reality in surgery. *Computing in Science & Engineering*, *22*(3), 18–26. doi:10.1109/MCSE.2020.2972822

Faisal, A. (2017). Computer science: Visionary of virtual reality. *Nature*, *551*(7680), 298–299. doi:10.1038/551298a

Fertleman, C., Aubugeau-Williams, P., Sher, C., Lim, A.-N., Lumley, S., Delacroix, S., & Pan, X. (2018). A discussion of virtual reality as a new tool for training healthcare professionals. *Frontiers in Public Health*, *6*, 44. doi:10.3389/fpubh.2018.00044 PMID:29535997

Gupta, S., Bagga, S., & Sharma, D. K. (2020). Hand Gesture Recognition for Human Computer Interaction and Its Applications in Virtual Reality. In *Advanced Computational Intelligence Techniques for Virtual Reality in Healthcare* (pp. 85–105). Springer. doi:10.1007/978-3-030-35252-3_5

Howard, M. C. (2017). A meta-analysis and systematic literature review of virtual reality rehabilitation programs. *Computers in Human Behavior*, *70*, 317–327. doi:10.1016/j.chb.2017.01.013

Javaid, M., & Haleem, A. (2020). Virtual reality applications toward medical field. *Clinical Epidemiology and Global Health*, *8*(2), 600–605. doi:10.1016/j.cegh.2019.12.010

Kim, M., Jeon, C., & Kim, J. (2017). A study on immersion and presence of a portable hand haptic system for immersive virtual reality. *Sensors (Basel)*, *17*(5), 1141. doi:10.339017051141 PMID:28513545

Koroliov, P., & Lapko, O. (2021). *Virtual Reality. Waltham Cross*.

Krupitzer, C., Müller, S., Lesch, V., Züfle, M., Edinger, J., Lemken, A., . . . Becker, C. (2020). *A Survey on Human Machine Interaction in Industry 4.0*. arXiv preprint arXiv.01025.

Liu, J., & Yang, T. (2021). *Word Frequency Data Analysis in Virtual Reality Technology Industrialization*. Paper presented at the Journal of Physics: Conference Series.

Llorens, R., Colomer-Font, C., Alcañiz, M., & Noé-Sebastián, E. (2013). BioTrak virtual reality system: Effectiveness and satisfaction analysis for balance rehabilitation in patients with brain injury. *Neurologia (Barcelona, Spain)*, *28*(5), 268–275. PMID:22727272

Loucks, L., Yasinski, C., Norrholm, S. D., Maples-Keller, J., Post, L., Zwiebach, L., ... Rizzo, A. A. (2019). You can do that?!: Feasibility of virtual reality exposure therapy in the treatment of PTSD due to military sexual trauma. *Journal of Anxiety Disorders*, *61*, 55–63. doi:10.1016/j.janxdis.2018.06.004 PMID:30005843

Mäkinen, H., Haavisto, E., Havola, S., & Koivisto, J.-M. (2020). User experiences of virtual reality technologies for healthcare in learning: An integrative review. *Behaviour & Information Technology*, 1–17. doi:10.1080/0144929X.2020.1788162

Mandal, S. (2013). Brief introduction of virtual reality & its challenges. *International Journal of Scientific and Engineering Research*, *4*(4), 304–309.

Maples-Keller, J. L., Yasinski, C., Manjin, N., & Rothbaum, B. O. (2017). Virtual reality-enhanced extinction of phobias and post-traumatic stress. *Neurotherapeutics; the Journal of the American Society for Experimental NeuroTherapeutics*, *14*(3), 554–563. doi:10.100713311-017-0534-y PMID:28512692

Miao, S., Shen, C., Feng, X., Zhu, Q., Shorfuzzaman, M., & Lv, Z. (2021). Upper limb rehabilitation system for stroke survivors based on multi-modal sensors and machine learning. *IEEE Access: Practical Innovations, Open Solutions*, *9*, 30283–30291. doi:10.1109/ACCESS.2021.3055960

Moskaliuk, J., Kimmerle, J., & Cress, U. (2010). Virtual Reality 2.0 and its Application in Knowledge building. In Handbook of research on Web 2.0, 3.0, and X. 0: Technologies, business, and social applications (pp. 573-592). IGI Global.

Mütterlein, J. (2018). The three pillars of virtual reality? Investigating the roles of immersion, presence, and interactivity. *Proceedings of the 51st Hawaii international conference on system sciences.* 10.24251/HICSS.2018.174

Mütterlein, J., & Hess, T. (2017). *Immersion, presence, interactivity: Towards a joint understanding of factors influencing virtual reality acceptance and use.* Paper presented at the Twenty-third Americas Conference on Information Systems, Boston, MA.

Pan, X., & Hamilton, A. F. C. (2018). Understanding dual realities and more in VR. *British Journal of Psychology, 109*(3), 437–441. doi:10.1111/bjop.12315 PMID:29851023

Pop, C., Cioara, T., Antal, M., Anghel, I., Salomie, I., & Bertoncini, M. J. S. (2018). *Blockchain based decentralized management of demand response programs in smart energy grids.* Academic Press.

Pourmand, A., Davis, S., Lee, D., Barber, S., & Sikka, N. (2017). Emerging utility of virtual reality as a multidisciplinary tool in clinical medicine. *Games for Health Journal, 6*(5), 263–270. doi:10.1089/g4h.2017.0046 PMID:28759254

Rizzo, A., & Koenig, S. T. (2017). Is clinical virtual reality ready for primetime? *Neuropsychology, 31*(8), 877–899. doi:10.1037/neu0000405 PMID:29376669

Rousseaux, F., Bicego, A., Ledoux, D., Massion, P., Nyssen, A.-S., Faymonville, M.-E., Laureys, S., & Vanhaudenhuyse, A. (2020). Hypnosis associated with 3D immersive virtual reality technology in the management of pain: A review of the literature. *Journal of Pain Research, 13*, 1129–1138. doi:10.2147/JPR.S231737 PMID:32547176

Schäfer, A., Reis, G., & Stricker, D. (2021). *Investigating the Sense of Presence Between Handcrafted and Panorama Based Virtual Environments.* arXiv preprint arXiv.03823.

Servotte, J.-C., Goosse, M., Campbell, S. H., Dardenne, N., Pilote, B., Simoneau, I. L., Guillaume, M., Bragard, I., & Ghuysen, A. (2020). Virtual reality experience: Immersion, sense of presence, and cybersickness. *Clinical Simulation in Nursing, 38*, 35–43. doi:10.1016/j.ecns.2019.09.006

Shao, X., Yuan, Q., Qian, D., Ye, Z., Chen, G., le Zhuang, K., Jiang, X., Jin, Y., & Qiang, D. (2020). Virtual reality technology for teaching neurosurgery of skull base tumor. *BMC Medical Education, 20*(1), 1–7. doi:10.118612909-019-1911-5 PMID:31900135

Shim, K.-C., Park, J.-S., Kim, H.-S., Kim, J.-H., Park, Y.-C., & Ryu, H.-I. (2003). Application of virtual reality technology in biology education. *Journal of Biological Education, 37*(2), 71–74. doi:10.1080/00219266.2003.9655854

Sirkkunen, E., Väätäjä, H., Uskali, T., & Rezaei, P. P. (2016). Journalism in virtual reality: Opportunities and future research challenges. *Proceedings of the 20th international academic mindtrek conference.* 10.1145/2994310.2994353

Snoswell, A. J., & Snoswell, C. L. (2019). Immersive virtual reality in health care: Systematic review of technology and disease states. *JMIR Biomedical Engineering, 4*(1), e15025. doi:10.2196/15025

Tang, Y., Au, K., & Leung, Y. (2018). Comprehending products with mixed reality: Geometric relationships and creativity. *International Journal of Engineering Business Management, 10.* doi:10.1177/1847979018809599

Tang, Y.-M., Au, K. M., Lau, H. C., Ho, G. T., & Wu, C.-H. (2020). Evaluating the effectiveness of learning design with mixed reality (MR) in higher education. *Virtual Reality (Waltham Cross), 24*(4), 797–807. doi:10.100710055-020-00427-9

Tang, Y. M., Ng, G. W. Y., Chia, N. H., So, E. H. K., Wu, C. H., & Ip, W. (2021). *Application of virtual reality (VR) technology for medical practitioners in type and screen (T&S) training.* Academic Press.

Torraco, R. J. (2016). Writing integrative literature reviews: Using the past and present to explore the future. *Human Resource Development Review, 15*(4), 404–428. doi:10.1177/1534484316671606

Van Eck, N. J., & Waltman, L. (2010). Software survey: VOSviewer, a computer program for bibliometric mapping. *Scientometrics, 84*(2), 523-538.

Wang, Q., Li, C., Xie, Z., Bu, Z., Shi, L., Wang, C., & Jiang, F. (2020). The development and application of virtual reality animation simulation technology: Take gastroscopy simulation system as an example. *Pathology Oncology Research, 26*(2), 765–769. doi:10.100712253-019-00590-8 PMID:30809768

Weinbaum, S. G. (2016). *Pygmalion's spectacles.* Simon and Schuster.

Xie, L., Chen, Z., Wang, H., Zheng, C., & Jiang, J. (2020). Bibliometric and visualized analysis of scientific publications on atlantoaxial spine surgery based on Web of Science and VOSviewer. *World Neurosurgery, 137*, 435-442.

Yan, C., Wu, T., Huang, K., He, J., Liu, H., Hong, Y., & Wang, B. (2020). The application of virtual reality in cervical spinal surgery: A review. *World Neurosurgery*. PMID:32931993

Yu, Y., Li, Y., Zhang, Z., Gu, Z., Zhong, H., Zha, Q., ... Chen, E. (2020). *A bibliometric analysis using VOSviewer of publications on COVID-19*. Academic Press.

Zhan, T., Yin, K., Xiong, J., He, Z., & Wu, S.-T. (2020). Augmented reality and virtual reality displays: Perspectives and challenges. *iScience, 23*(8), 101397. doi:10.1016/j.isci.2020.101397 PMID:32759057

Zhu, S., Jin, W., & He, C. (2019). On evolutionary economic geography: A literature review using bibliometric analysis. *European Planning Studies, 27*(4), 639–660. doi:10.1080/09654313.2019.1568395

Chapter 2
A Review on Data-Driven Methods for Human Activity Recognition in Smart Homes

Jiancong Ye
South China University of Technology, China

Junpei Zhong
The Hong Kong Polytechnic University, China

EXECUTIVE SUMMARY

The smart home is one application of intelligent environments, where sensors are equipped to detect the status inside the domestic home. With the development of sensing technologies, more signals can be obtained with heterogenous statistical properties with faster processing speed. To make good use of the technical advantages, data-driven methods are becoming popular in intelligent environments. On the other hand, to recognize human activity is one essential target to understand the status inside a smart home. In this chapter, the authors focus on the human activity recognition (HAR) problem, which is the recognition of lower levels of activities, using data-driven models.

INTRODUCTION

With the rapid development of intelligent technology, including sensing and communications, smart homes have obtained growing attention over the past few years, due to the demand of people in assisted living services. Smart home is a common term, defined as a house that integrates various digital devices and automation

DOI: 10.4018/978-1-7998-8790-4.ch002

systems to assist the users to live in a convenient and safe environment with a high quality of life. The concept of smart home has also evolved a lot, especially from the concept of "intelligent environment". With the information interaction and collaboration of multiple devices and systems, smart home aims to provide automatic assistance such as home appliance control, lighting control, telephone remote control, indoor and outdoor remote control, anti-theft alarm, environmental monitoring and programmable timing control, to improve home safety, convenience, and comfort (Galinina et al., 2015; Jiang, Liu, & Yang, 2004; Tsai, Wu, Sun, & Yang, 2000; Wilson, Hargreaves, & Hauxwell-Baldwin, 2017). It increases the quality of life of home inhabitant in term of security and safety, and takes care of the basic life of people with poor independence. This results on the study of smart home technology.

Overall, the current research on the field of smart home is extremely extensive, and mainly associated with Internet-of-Things (IoT) technology (El-Basioni, El-Kader, & Abdelmonim, 2013; Jie, Pei, Jun, Yun, & Wei, 2013; Malche & Maheshwary, 2017; Stojkoska & Trivodaliev, 2017) and artificial intelligence (AI) (Arriany & Musbah, 2016; Bakar, Ghayvat, Hasanm, Mukhopadhyay, & Systems, 2016; Do et al., 2018; Munir, Ehsan, Raza, & Mudassir, 2019; Zhong, Han, Lotfi, Cangelosi, & Liu, 2019). The IoT technology is a promising solution for advanced connectivity of anything in smart home to form a home network. It contains several communication schemes and interfaces to achieve smooth connection between devices. Using the speedy communication from IoT, AI, or data-driven methods, is the ability of a computer or computer-control machine to perform tasks by learning the model by the data the system previously got, which is similar human intelligence obtain experience (or prior). Smart-home-based data-driven technology including semantic understanding, human activity recognition (HAR) and smart robots, plays an important role to create a home with self-thinking and solving skills.

Depending on the needs of users, the smart home system is expected to perform some of the following tasks: perceiving, understanding and automatic assisting. In this chapter we will focus on the second part: understanding. In the smart home scenario, to recognize human activity, or HAR, is the key step to realize its basic functions. As an active research topic in machine learning areas, HAR is an important part of smart home. In order to develop the most appropriate and accurate methods and approaches of human activity, new approaches and algorithms based on advanced sensing technologies will be reviewed in this chapter. A perfect HAR system usually combines various hardware devices configured in the IoT and suitable algorithms in the smart home to predict the user's activities of daily living (ADL) like leaving house, cooking, toileting, showering, sleeping, etc., so that the home network can provide users with necessary services to avoid complicated operations. Specifically, the implementation of HAR can be subdivided into three subtasks. Firstly, to select the appropriate sensing devices and deploy them depending on the smart home environment; Secondly, because the data collected from the IoT devices is usually unstructured, filtering and preprocessing the data through appropriate feature extraction and processing technologies are needed; Finally, designing an algorithm model to predict activities. Although the focuses of this chapter will be the last step, the relevant basics of the previous steps will be also introduced.

This review will be organized as follows: In the second section, the background as well as its basic mathematical foundation of the HAR problems will be introduced. Since the data structures of different sensing techniques also result in different choices of learning methods, we will briefly introduce different sensors and their signals. Review of different data-driven machine learning methods, as well as the related papers, will be shown in section 3. At the end, we will point out some of the future research directions.

BACKGROUND

Human activity belongs to the lower level of understanding of human behavior. In the domestic environment, if equipped with proper sensors, the recognizable information can include the basic categories of activities, which belongs to the lower level of human behaviors. The recognizable information also includes higher level of personal information such as the identity of a person, their personality, and psychological state. On the other hand, the higher levels of human activities are difficult to recognize because two reasons: 1. They depend on the accuracy of lower-level recognition, and 2. The higher levels we are focusing on, the more contextual and domain knowledge is needed. Therefore, in this chapter we are mainly focusing on the lower levels of activities. For instance, attempting to recognize lower human activities, one must determine the kinetic states of a person, so that the computer can efficiently recognize this activity. Some of the human activities are referred to as lower levels of activities, such as "gestures" or "atomic actions" last short and not complicated, which are relatively easy to recognize. On the other hand, more higher levels of or more complex activities, such as "peeling an apple," may include a series of simple activities, are more difficult to identify. Therefore, the higher level of activities is usually decomposed into other simpler activities. The recognition of them also based on the results from lower levels. Besides, recognizing objects with the understanding of their affordance may also help to better understand human activities. Thus, as shown in Fig. 1, depending on their complexity, human activities are categorized into: (i) gestures; (ii) atomic actions; (iii) behaviors; (iv) biometric identity; (v) personality and (vi) psychological state.

Figure 1. Hierarchy of activity recognition

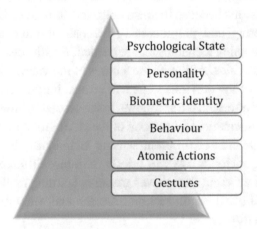

Also, the usage of activity recognition task in a smart home application aims to identify various actions which are performed throughout or during part of the entire duration based on one or many kinds of sensors. Therefore, the requirements of recognizing the well-trimmed signals and untrimmed signals are different. For instance, there are 5 different tasks in the well-known activity recognition challenge ActivityNet (Caba Heilbron, Escorcia, Ghanem, & Carlos Niebles, 2015)in which the recognition methods for trimmed and untrimmed videos can be quite different. Among the aforementioned methods, there are two main questions:

1. "What action?": this is the recognition problem which usually employ statistical methods such as Bayes' theorem or inference models, and,
2. "Whether the activity occurs?": this questions concerns the application of activity recognition since the meaningful activity usually sparsely distributes in the signals. Thus, we also need to detect the labelled data in the signals (Gupta & Davis, 2007).

The ultimate goal of human activity recognition is to detect, examine and recognize activities from sequences of signals. Motivated by this fact, the properties of such signals and the mathematical models should be suitable to each other. We will discuss these two parts in the following sections.

SENSING TECHNIQUES

In recent years, there are various kinds of sensor devices, including contact switch binary sensors, accelerometers, temperature and motion detectors, to name just a few, applying in numerous approaches for human activity recognition. According to the deployed way of sensors in behaviors monitoring, these sensors can be divided into two main categories in sensor-based activity recognition methods: ambient sensors and wearable sensors. In this section, we will describe the commonly used sensors in the advanced works that concentrate on monitoring diverse activities.

Depending on the selected devices and the data obtained from them, we can classify the HAR task into two categories. The first category is vision-based activity recognition, which uses visual sensing facilities to capture digital image or video, to monitor people's behavior. A visual object is separated from its background with different object segmentation techniques. Then, human activities are classified by the classifier with the extracted feature representations of the segmented visual object. The vision-based sensors usually provide unstructured data such as images, in the forms of pixels representing the spatial information using the lighting or temperature sensing components. Also it is possible that the vision-based sensors provide the video frames which are basically a temporal series of the images.

The second category is referred to as signal-based activity recognition, which use sensor network technologies for information gathering. Some sensors are distributed in the environment to monitor the interaction between the observer and environmental objects. Some sensors can be connected with the human body to directly collect the behavior information of the observer. The generated sensor information is usually processed through data fusion, feature extraction, classification algorithms to recognize activity. With the continuous increase of the population and the potential of smart home, the deployment of sensors in smart home and the work of sensor-based HAR have high scientific values.

ALGORITHMS

Data Preprocessing

Data preprocessing is the manipulation process for the raw data before we do any data processing. It transforms raw data into an understandable format and removes any outliners and noises. A good choice of data pre-processing method will improve the quality of the data and make the following data processing steps much easier. It is also an important step in data mining as we usually cannot work with raw data, and the pre-processing step can transform raw data into structured data.

In the HAR, data preprocessing is the processing of fixing or removing incorrect, corrupted, incorrectly formatted, duplicate, or incomplete data within a dataset. It usually includes the following steps:

1. Smoothing noisy data. Noisy data can affect the learned statistic parameters of the model, since the model cannot make use of data they cannot interpret. Therefore, noise should be cleaned to avoid the bias. The cleaning procedure is usually done after an examination of the noisy properties. The procedure includes binning, regression or other steps.
2. Ruling out abnormal data. Data inconsistencies can occur due to human errors (the information was stored in a wrong field) or measurement error. Similar as noisy data, the abnormal data should be also found out and be removed to avoid giving that data object an advantage.
3. Imputation of data. On the contrast to the previous two steps, the imputation deals with missing data by replacing it with substituted data.
4. Transformation of data. Considering we have a set of data with many dimensions. The processing of databases takes long time and challenging to properly store. Dimension reduction also aims to better present the high-dimensional set with a lower dimensional of data, which still keep their statistical properties.

Hidden Markov Model

The HMM is based on the assumption of Markov chain. A Markov chain is a stochastic process that moves through predefined states, with the probability of every transition being dependent only on the start and end state. The transition probabilities depict the chances of occurrences in sequences of random variables, states, each of which can take on values from some set. In the HAR, the sets can be signals or symbols but usually not include images. There are two assumptions about the HMM model: First, that the probability of a transition between contexts depends only on the current context, and second, that the probability of classifying an instance to a context depends only on the current context and the current setting. To use this model, both assumptions should hold, or it can be approximately hold in certain degrees. To build this model, we consider a sequence of stochastic state variables $\left(s_1, s_2, ..., s_t\right)$.

A Markov model embodies the Markov assumption, which states that the variable only depends on the transition probabilities of this sequence of the previous state (Figure 2):

$$s_1 P(s_t = a \mid s_1, s_2, ..., s_{t-1}) = P(s_t = a \mid s_{t-1})$$

Figure 2. Markov chain

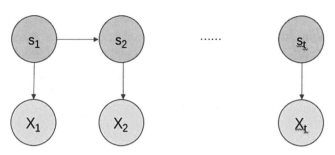

As mentioned, the HMM model usually deals with a single- or multi-channel signals when the two assumptions can be held. The HMM model is superior in giving a prediction given the current inputs and prior, which is suitable for alarming system. Such signals can be motion detector data. For instance, the system proposed by (Tim Van Kasteren, Noulas, Englebienne, & Kröse, 2008) constructs a dataset composed of 28 days of motion detector data as well as annotation with low installation cost. They first utilize Hidden Markov Model (HMM) and hidden semi-Markov model (HSMM) to map their binary data in divided time slices onto the hidden activity states successively. They discussed that, HMM only model the observation and transition probability between sensor events, while HSMM additionally model the duration of sensor events to predict human activity (TLM Van Kasteren, Englebienne, Kröse, & environments, 2010; Tim Van Kasteren et al., 2008). Meanwhile, they compared HMM and HSMM with another probabilistic models called Conditional Random Field (CRF) and semi-Markov Conditional Random Field (SMCRF) to show the effectiveness and potential of probability model. In (Viard, Fanti, Faraut, & Lesage, 2016), Viard et al. considered the activity discovery problem in sensor recorded dataset, and presented a HMM combined with a paradigm that build the association of relevant sensors to actions as a prior. The possible behavior decomposition of each activity was connected with the corresponding sensor. Then such approach was unnecessary to focus on the actions really performed in each activity in learning phase. By contrast, Kabir et al. considered the relationship between sensor position and activity, to combine position information with sensor activate data (Kabir, Hoque, Thapa, & Yang, 2016). Therefore, they proposed a two-layer HMM for activity recognition in Kasteren dataset. In the first layer, they predicted the activity range based on the position information of triggered sensors. In the second layer, they determined the exact activity from the sensor series and the selected activity range. In general, such two methods reasonably introduced additional knowledge-based information, to reduce the difficulty and complexity of direct mapping between low-level sensor data and high-level activities.

The work by (Sung-Hyun, Thapa, Kabir, & Hee-Chan, 2018) discussed the potential correlation between previous activities, present activities and current observation events, which was taken into account in recognition stage. They used a probabilistic log-Viterbi algorithm on second-order HMM. Separately, second-order HMM lead in the transition probability function of two previous states, with additional computational loss. The log-Viterbi algorithm provided assistance to simplify the operation through transforming frequent multiplication of probability into addition of sensor sequence by dynamic programming. Therefore, the proposed method was verified in the Kasteren dataset and achieved improvement in recognition accuracy and computational efficiency simultaneously.

Conditional Random Field Model

Similar as HMM model, the Conditional Random Field (CRF) is best suited to predict sequences where contextual information or state of the signals affect the current prediction, which specified the probability of possible labels for the undirected connection and given observations. Different from the HMM which is based on the Markov Chain, the CRF also considers the future observations while it is trying to learn a pattern. The CRF also uses contextual information from previous labels, but such kind of information is firstly used the extracted the common features through different time-steps, which are then further be used to train the sequences (Fig. 3). In the HAR applications, we can regard the contextual information as observations from the sensors with noise or other observed facts, while the posterior can be regarded as labels. CRF therefore can conditioning the probabilities to the observation sequences. They avoid computing the probabilities for every possible observation sequence. Rather than relying on joint probabilities $P(X,S)$, CRFs specify the probability of possible label sequences given the observation $P(X|S)$. The CRF has been used in activity recognition, activity monitoring in the intelligent environment contexts.

In the early days, (Tim Van Kasteren et al., 2008) and (Nazerfard, Das, Holder, & Cook, 2010) constructed two smart home case respectively. Compared with the former, the latter dataset added sensor events gathered by ambient temperature sensors node. Then Kasteren achieved a slight improvement through the modeling state duration by semi-Markov CRF (Nazerfard et al., 2010). In (Cook & Schmitter-Edgecombe, 2009), Latent-Dynamic CRF (LDCRF) was developed to recognize activities in smart homes, and verified its better performance in (Tim Van Kasteren et al., 2008) and WSU Apartment Testbed Dataset (L. Wang et al., 2011). These models assumed a set of middle vectors for representing possible hidden states for the activity labels, aiming to learn a more accurate potential sub-behaviors (uninterrupted actions) with significant differences of each activity label.

Figure 3. A Demonstration of CRF, where the features can be extracted from several states.

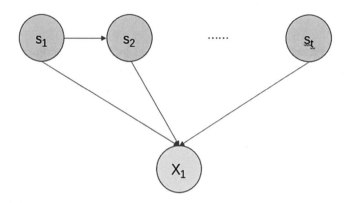

For the problem of multi-users activity recognition in smart home, (L. Wang et al., 2011) studied a temporal probabilistic model named Factorial Conditional Random Field (FCRF) to factory the basic linear-chained CRF by introducing co-temporal connections, which permitted multiple time slices generated by users to merge in the same time step. They generated a set of data by wearable accelerometer sensors and obtained a considerable recognition rate. However, the complexity of the model need to be optimized. With the inspiration of LDCRF, (Neogi & Dauwels, 2021) also introduced latent states describing sub-actions of activity labels into FCRF, to establish a model for the interaction between multi-users' latent dynamic. The experiment was conducted in the public dataset called UCI OPPORTUNITY (Roggen et al., 2010). Their provided FLDCRF-based variants can supply universal choice for different activity recognition tasks.

Naïve Bayes Classification

Bayesian theorem is a theory which can be used to estimate the probability of occurrence of events when certain (co-related) events occurred. And Naive Bayes classifiers are a family of "probabilistic classifiers" based on Bayes' theorem. Similar as HMM, it also holds assumptions, which we call them naïve independence assumptions between the features. Specifically, the naïve conditional independence assumption states:

$$P(x_i \mid y, x_1, ..., x_{i-1}, x_{i+1}, ..., x_n) = P(x_i \mid y)$$

Therefore, the Bayes' theorem (left) can be written as the following:

$$P\left(y \mid x_1,...,x_n\right) = \frac{P\left(y\right)P(x_1,...,x_n \mid y)}{P\left(x_1,...,x_n\right)} = \frac{P\left(y\right)\prod_{i=1}^{n}P(x_i \mid y)}{P\left(x_1,...,x_n\right)}$$

The Naïve Bayes Classifiers have been used in activity recognition. (Tim van Kasteren & Krose, 2007) introduced basic Bayesian framework for activity recognition in residence. (Sarkar, Lee, & Lee, 2010) applied Naïve Bayes Classification and integrate two famous smoothing strategies for settling the issue caused by sensor data sparsity. The two smoothing technologies used activity model and collective model as a prior to discount the probability of observable sensors in the activity and assign additional probability to non-observable ones in Bayesian updating process. (Yang, Lee, Choi, & Technology, 2011) used activity theory as the support to analyze the behavior logic and basic operation of daily activity. They designed a penalized Bayesian classifier, which parameters were refined by the mismatch evaluation function of both average time-consuming and theoretical operation process of behavior.

K Nearest Neighbors

The K Nearest Neighbors (KNN) algorithm is a supervised learning approach. The KNN firstly defines the distances between one specific focused point and all the other data points using different metrics. Then it selects specified number of examples (K) closest to the focused point, then it votes for the most frequent label. The selection of focused points runs in every iteration until every data point has assigned a label and the distances do not exceed a threshold. This approach can be used for both classification and regression, but in the HAR application, it is mainly used for solving classification problem. For example, a single tri-axial accelerometer sensor in mobile phone used in (X. Wang & Kim, 2015). They adopted K-Nearest Neighbor Classifier to work with online, real-time data for the classify tasks limited to activities related to the movement of devices. In (Fahad, Tahir, & Rajarajan, 2014), the authors hypothesize a serious of homogeneous activities in all activity categories, for aggregating those with less inter class variations by Lloyd's algorithm. Besides, multiple Evidence Theoretic K-Nearest Neighbors (ET-KNN) classifiers are used to classify the undivided activities in each cluster. (Fahad, Tahir, & Rajarajan, 2015) used Information Gain based on entropy to extract key features from all the features of pre-segmented classes, to improve performance for overlapping activities recognition. Then they applied ET-KNN with Dempster–Shafer theory (DST) evidence theory to treat each neighbor of a pattern as an item of evidence supporting to strengthen the classification effect of the data with uncertainty.

Support Vector Machine

Support Vector Machine (SVM) is a supervised learning method which usually achieves very high accuracy in classification with extracted features, compared with other classification methods. Using a kernel function, the SVM can map the data points in a high-dimensional space. Using the proper kernel function (i.e. "kernel trick"), SVM is good at performing a non-linear classification by implicitly mapping their inputs into high-dimensional feature spaces. In this space, we need to build a hyperplane that distinctly classifies the data points by maximizing the width of the gap between the data points and the hyperplane. New data examples are then mapped into the high-dimensional space and their labels can be predicted by the hyperplane.

Due to its excellence in prediction of labels, it has been used in many activities' classifications. (Z.-Y. He & Jin, 2008) presented an autoregressive (AR) model of time-series to establish feature representation of data, which are input to the Support Vector Machine (SVM) for classification task. The four-order AR coefficients had obvious distinction among different type of human activities. Soon afterwards, they are committed to the exploration of other feature representation methods, raising the efficient feature extraction method base on Discrete Cosine Transform (DCT) for remaining rich low-frequency information as well as Principal Component Analysis (PCA) for compressing main features (Z. He & Jin, 2009).

The works of (M'hamed Bilal Abidine) started with the problem of category imbalance in multiple public binary time series datasets, to propose several SVM-based method to tackle such issue. They chose the suitable regularization parameter C of the Soft-Support Vector Machines (C-SVM) method. The parameter C was adjusted dynamically with the number of category samples to avoid the overfitting problem in category with major samples. Later, they performed the Synthetic Minority Over-sampling Technique (SMOTE) to the categories with low number of samples in advance and provided a Cost Sensitive Support Vector Machine (CS-SVM) (Abidine, Fergani, Oussalah, & Fergani, 2014). These approaches utilized adjusting different penalty parameters for distinct classes of data to eliminate the imbalance effect. Moreover, the method named Optimized Cost-Sensitive Support Vector Machine (OCS-SVM) in (Fergani, Fergani, Fleury, & Communications, 2015) searched the best hyper-parameters rather than specifying ones in CS-SVM for cost sensitive criterion to adaptively achieve optimal result.

By considering the features in binary time series, Abidine also used PCA and Linear Discriminant Analysis (LDA) to transform origin binary data into energy like features or reduced dimension data. As a result, a modified Weighted SVM (mWSVM) combined with PCA and LDA based principle components were able to extract key feature representation from binary data and flexibly adjust the detection accuracy of SVM (Uddin & Uddiny, 2015).

Random Forest

Decision tree builds classification or regression models in the form of a tree structure. It breaks down a dataset into smaller and smaller subsets while at the same time an associated decision tree is incrementally developed. Nevertheless, Decision trees are prone to be overfitting, which stands for a situation that the model learns too much from the training set, but cannot describe the true situation of all the data. The small number of training data could result in such unwanted results. This could happen especially when a tree is too deep. To avoid the overfitting problem, random forest method is often used based on building several decision trees. Several decision trees are built based on different samples and takes their majority vote for classification. (Uddin & Uddiny, 2015) proposed a guided Random Forest (RF) for HAC. The origin RF can quantify the importance score of each feature regarding the prediction of the classes. As such, the guided RF algorithm ignored the features of low discrimination guided by importance score to reduce redundancy and had been examined among five datasets. However, (Dewi & Chen, 2019) selected important features by RF-based methods Varlmp, Borute, and Recursive Feature Elimination. Then a random forest classifier is generated from these features to identify activities. (Xu, Pan, Li, Nie, & Xu, 2019) exploited an improved RF algorithm combined with bagging parallel algorithm idea to generate original voting decisions. Then these results were corrected by activity similarity matrix, which can give assistance judgment according to considering external factors such as time and position. (ud din Tahir, Jalal, & Batool, 2020) extracted meaningful features from accelerometer and gyroscope data by 1-D Hadamard transform wavelet and 1-D LBP based extraction algorithm. The novel classifier SMO-RF was composed of Sequential minimal optimization method in pre-classification step and RF in re-classification for producing great result in accuracy.

Neural Networks and Deep Learning

While the previous methods attempt to extract features before doing the classification. This feature extraction step can reduce the number of features in a high-dimensional data points, such as images or wearable IMU sensors include 6-degree of freedoms. The extracted features are new features different from the existing ones (and then discarding the original features), and their number of dimensions is usually smaller than the previous one. These new reduced set of features should then be able to summarize most of the information contained in the original set of features using the previous methods.

A recent developed classification method called deep learning can skip this feature extraction step. The deep learning method (DNN) is developed from the artificial neural network (ANN) methods. ANN is a biologically inspired method by connecting a lot of simple computing units, called perceptron, together. A perceptron accepts input from the previous layer with a set of weights, which represents the significance of the input related to the task the perceptron is trying to learn. This simulates the neuron model which accepts electrical inputs from dendrites. But in our abstract model, these input-weight products are summed inside the perceptron and its output is calculated by the activation function. When the activation function decides the perceptron is to be activated, the signal can be seen to pass through and the perceptron fires.

Then the perceptrons are connected together, loosely like neurons are connected together in the human brain. The whole ANN or DNN is usually organized in a number of layers, in which each layer is made of perceptrons. The ANN or DNN then interprets sensory data through these layers and finds out the patterns it learned. Such patterns can be images, sound, text or time series (Naser, Lotfi, Zhong, & Applications, 2021). Thanks to the large number of layers in DNN, it can even skip the feature extraction.

The two popular schools of the successful deep learning methods for action recognition are based on either Two-Stream Convolutional Networks (TSN) (Simonyan & Zisserman, 2014) or 3D-convNet (C3D) (Tran, Bourdev, Fergus, Torresani, & Paluri, 2015) ideas. The TSN method is inspired by the findings in visual systems, where the ventral and dorsal pathways are separate to deal with the visual information for perception and action (Goodale & Milner, 1992). In the TSN model, the two-stream idea is used as two independent recognition streams (space and time). The spatial stream can perform motion recognition from static image frames. The temporal stream recognizes behavior from dense motion optical flows. Both of the two streams can be implemented by CNN. It has also been reported that the separation of the temporal stream and the spatial stream improves the generalization ability of the network. The C3D-related work describes a cube-like convolution kernel to be an effective video descriptor in three-dimension for the actions in videos. Particularly, the best size of the convolution kernel empirically should be $3 \times 3 \times 3$. The C3D method is easy to comprehensive because it owns the same principle of general 2D-CNN. In terms of architecture, the encoder-decoder architecture allows a sequence-to-sequence learning for prediction problems, where the sequences can have variable-lengths. These architectures are often used in natural language processing, but they have used in learning sensory signals in HAR too (Naser, Lotfi, & Zhong, 2020).

Figure 4. A sample of DNN

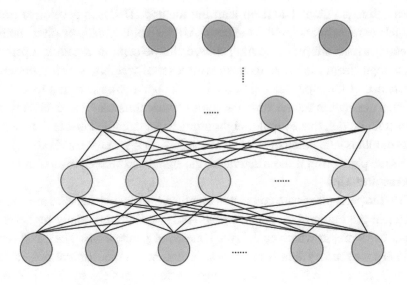

FUTURE RESEARCH DIRECTIONS

Multiple Sensor System

In terms of the real applications of activity recognition in a smart home, to design a system for recognize another person's activities is different from doing a classification with a data-set. In real applications both previously mentioned two research questions also hold the same assumption: the human activity recognition is based on a figure-centric scene of uncluttered background, where the actor is free to perform an activity. On the other hand, in a real application, the development of a fully automated human activity recognition system still faces challenges, such as extraction in background clutter, partial occlusion, changes in scale, viewpoint, lighting and appearance, and frame resolution. Besides, multiple sensors should be deployed to cover the whole area of the domestic environment. The multiple sensors also bring advantages and drawbacks in the aforementioned challenges.

To overcome these problems, a complete system of activity recognition should consist of three components, namely: (i) environment detection and subtraction (Elgammal, Duraiswami, Harwood, & Davis, 2002; Mumtaz, Zhang, & Chan, 2014), in which the multi-sensor system is able separate the invariants in the images, sounds or other signals which are invariant over time (background) from the dynamic objects or human (foreground); (ii) human tracking with multiple sensors, in which the sensors can fuse their information and their prior to locate human motion over time (Al-Qaness et al., 2019; Mohamed et al., 2017); and (iii) human action and object detection (Gao, Zhang, Xu, & Xue, 2015; Pirsiavash & Ramanan, 2012), in which the system is able to localize a human activity in an image.

Multimodal Recognition

Multi-modal means using the combination of information from a set of different types of sensors. Humans naturally understand each other and recognize others' intention by using not only reservation by also contexts and domain knowledge. In the applications of HAR, the benefit of using multi-modal recognition starts with the ability to improve the recognition in one type of modality (e.g., sound) and by using other modalities to assist (visual). This is particularly effective when the recognition capability is either impaired, needs clarification, or needs efficiency.

There has been increasing popularity to investigate the multimodal learning algorithms. For instance, (Aytar, Vondrick, & Torralba, 2017) used a shared representation to align three modalities. However, such a shared architecture is still doubtful whether it can handle heterogenous signals from different sensors. (Kaiser et al., 2017) proposed using a unified representation borrowed from natural language processing to solve this problem. But after all, how we can interpret different levels of activities is still an open question, some of which may relate to the grounding problem of human's own knowledge and mirroring. Using state-of-the-art deep learning (e.g. (Aytar et al., 2017)) which combines inputs from multimodal sources, will be more helpful to recognize the activities and meaning of the home environment. Also the deep learning architecture, which is similar to the behavior hierarchy (Fig. 1), may shed a light to extract a symbolic representation on a higher cognitive level.

CONCLUSION

In this chapter, different types of data-driven methods are introduced to process the signals from different sensors, in order to accomplish the task of human activity recognition. Using a large amount of data, developers and engineers do not need to manually design the program for recognize the activities. Besides, properly using these models also can achieve very accurate recognition results. Nevertheless, although the state-of-the-art learning methods achieve satisfaction recognition results in datasets. Real world sensors' deployment and integration in applications are still open questions.

ACKNOWLEDGMENT

The chapter is supported by the PolyU Start-up Fund (P0035417).

REFERENCES

Abidine, B. M. h., Fergani, B., Oussalah, M., & Fergani, L. J. K. (2014). *A new classification strategy for human activity recognition using cost sensitive support vector machines for imbalanced data*. Academic Press.

Al-Qaness, M. A., Abd Elaziz, M., Kim, S., Ewees, A. A., Abbasi, A. A., Alhaj, Y. A., & Hawbani, A. J. S. (2019). Channel state information from pure communication to sense and track human motion. *Survey (London, England)*, *19*(15), 3329. doi:10.339019153329 PMID:31362425

Arriany, A. A., & Musbah, M. S. (2016). *Applying voice recognition technology for smart home networks*. Paper presented at the 2016 International Conference on Engineering & MIS (ICEMIS). 10.1109/ICEMIS.2016.7745292

Aytar, Y., Vondrick, C., & Torralba, A. (2017). *See, hear, and read: Deep aligned representations*. Academic Press.

Bakar, U., Ghayvat, H., Hasanm, S., & Mukhopadhyay, S. C. J. N. G. S. (2016). Activity and anomaly detection in smart home. *Survey (London, England)*, *16*, 191–220. doi:10.1007/978-3-319-21671-3_9

Caba Heilbron, F., Escorcia, V., Ghanem, B., & Carlos Niebles, J. (2015). Activitynet: A large-scale video benchmark for human activity understanding. *Proceedings of the ieee conference on computer vision and pattern recognition*. 10.1109/CVPR.2015.7298698

Cook, D. J., & Schmitter-Edgecombe, M. (2009). *Assessing the quality of activities in a smart environment*. Academic Press.

Dewi, C., & Chen, R.-C. (2019). *Human activity recognition based on evolution of features selection and random Forest*. Paper presented at the 2019 IEEE international conference on systems, man and cybernetics (SMC). 10.1109/SMC.2019.8913868

Do, H. M., Pham, M., Sheng, W., Yang, D., & Liu, M. (2018). *RiSH: A robot-integrated smart home for elderly care*. Academic Press.

El-Basioni, B. M. M., El-Kader, S., & Abdelmonim, M. (2013). *Smart home design using wireless sensor network and biometric technologies*. Academic Press.

Elgammal, A., Duraiswami, R., Harwood, D., & Davis, L. (2002). *Background and foreground modeling using nonparametric kernel density estimation for visual surveillance*. Academic Press.

Fahad, L. G., Tahir, S. F., & Rajarajan, M. (2014). *Activity recognition in smart homes using clustering based classification.* Paper presented at the 2014 22nd International Conference on Pattern Recognition. 10.1109/ICPR.2014.241

Fahad, L. G., Tahir, S. F., & Rajarajan, M. (2015). *Feature selection and data balancing for activity recognition in smart homes.* Paper presented at the 2015 IEEE International Conference on Communications (ICC). 10.1109/ICC.2015.7248373

Fergani, L., Fergani, B., & Fleury, A. (2015). *Improving human activity recognition in smart homes*. Academic Press.

Galinina, O., Mikhaylov, K., Andreev, S., Turlikov, A., & Koucheryavy, Y. (2015). *Smart home gateway system over Bluetooth low energy with wireless energy transfer capability*. Academic Press.

Gao, Z., Zhang, H., Xu, G., & Xue, Y. (2015). *Multi-perspective and multi-modality joint representation and recognition model for 3D action recognition*. Academic Press.

Goodale, M. A., & Milner, A. (1992). *Separate visual pathways for perception and action*. Academic Press.

Gupta, A., & Davis, L. S. (2007). *Objects in action: An approach for combining action understanding and object perception.* Paper presented at the 2007 IEEE Conference on Computer Vision and Pattern Recognition. 10.1109/CVPR.2007.383331

He, Z., & Jin, L. (2009). *Activity recognition from acceleration data based on discrete consine transform and SVM.* Paper presented at the 2009 IEEE International Conference on Systems, Man and Cybernetics. 10.1109/ICSMC.2009.5346042

He, Z.-Y., & Jin, L.-W. (2008). *Activity recognition from acceleration data using AR model representation and SVM.* Paper presented at the 2008 international conference on machine learning and cybernetics.

Jiang, L., Liu, D.-Y., & Yang, B. (2004). Smart home research. *Proceedings of 2004 international conference on machine learning and cybernetics* (IEEE Cat. No. 04EX826). 10.1109/ICMLC.2004.1382266

Jie, Y., Pei, J. Y., Jun, L., Yun, G., & Wei, X. (2013). *Smart home system based on iot technologies.* Paper presented at the 2013 International conference on computational and information sciences. 10.1109/ICCIS.2013.468

Kabir, M. H., Hoque, M. R., Thapa, K., & Yang, S.-H. (2016). *Two-layer hidden Markov model for human activity recognition in home environments.* Academic Press.

Kaiser, L., Gomez, A. N., Shazeer, N., Vaswani, A., Parmar, N., Jones, L., & Uszkoreit, J. J. a. (2017). One model to learn them all. In Improving Supervised Classification of Daily Activities Living Using New Cost Sensitive Criterion For C-SVM. Academic Press.

Malche, T., & Maheshwary, P. (2017). *Internet of Things (IoT) for building smart home system.* Paper presented at the 2017 International Conference on I-SMAC (IoT in Social, Mobile, Analytics and Cloud)(I-SMAC).

Mohamed, R., Perumal, T., Sulaiman, M. N., Mustapha, N., & Manaf, S. (2017). *Tracking and recognizing the activity of multi resident in smart home environments.* Academic Press.

Mumtaz, A., Zhang, W., & Chan, A. B. (2014). Joint motion segmentation and background estimation in dynamic scenes. *Proceedings of the IEEE Conference on Computer Vision and Pattern Recognition.* 10.1109/CVPR.2014.54

Munir, A., Ehsan, S. K., Raza, S. M., & Mudassir, M. (2019). *Face and speech recognition based smart home.* Paper presented at the 2019 International Conference on Engineering and Emerging Technologies (ICEET). 10.1109/CEET1.2019.8711849

Naser, A., Lotfi, A., & Zhong, J. (2020). *Adaptive thermal sensor array placement for human segmentation and occupancy estimation.* Academic Press.

Naser, A., Lotfi, A., Zhong, J. (2021). *Towards human distance estimation using a thermal sensor array.* Academic Press.

Nazerfard, E., Das, B., Holder, L. B., & Cook, D. J. (2010). Conditional random fields for activity recognition in smart environments. *Proceedings of the 1st ACM International Health Informatics Symposium.* 10.1145/1882992.1883032

Neogi, S., & Dauwels, J. (2021). *Factored latent-dynamic conditional random fields for single and multi-label sequence modeling.* Academic Press.

Pirsiavash, H., & Ramanan, D. (2012). *Detecting activities of daily living in first-person camera views.* Paper presented at the 2012 IEEE conference on computer vision and pattern recognition. 10.1109/CVPR.2012.6248010

Roggen, D., Calatroni, A., Rossi, M., Holleczek, T., Förster, K., Tröster, G., . . . Ferscha, A. (2010). *Collecting complex activity datasets in highly rich networked sensor environments.* Paper presented at the 2010 Seventh international conference on networked sensing systems (INSS). 10.1109/INSS.2010.5573462

Sarkar, A. J., Lee, Y.-K., & Lee, S. (2010). *A smoothed naive bayes-based classifier for activity recognition.* Academic Press.

Simonyan, K., & Zisserman, A. (2014). *Two-stream convolutional networks for action recognition in videos.* Academic Press.

Stojkoska, B. L. R., & Trivodaliev, K. (2017). *A review of Internet of Things for smart home: Challenges and solutions.* Academic Press.

Sung-Hyun, Y., Thapa, K., Kabir, M. H., & Hee-Chan, L. (2018). *Log-Viterbi algorithm applied on second-order hidden Markov model for human activity recognition.* Academic Press.

Tran, D., Bourdev, L., Fergus, R., Torresani, L., & Paluri, M. (2015). Learning spatiotemporal features with 3d convolutional networks. *Proceedings of the IEEE international conference on computer vision.* 10.1109/ICCV.2015.510

Tsai, S.-M., Wu, S.-S., Sun, S.-S., & Yang, P.-C. (2000). *Integrated home service network on intelligent Intranet.* Academic Press.

ud din Tahir, S. B., Jalal, A., & Batool, M. (2020). *Wearable sensors for activity analysis using SMO-based random forest over smart home and sports datasets.* Paper presented at the 2020 3rd International Conference on Advancements in Computational Sciences (ICACS).

Uddin, M. T., & Uddiny, M. A. (2015). *A guided random forest based feature selection approach for activity recognition.* Paper presented at the 2015 International Conference on Electrical Engineering and Information Communication Technology (ICEEICT).

Van Kasteren, T., Englebienne, G., Kröse, B. (2010). *Activity recognition using semi-Markov models on real world smart home datasets.* Academic Press.

van Kasteren, T., & Krose, B. (2007). *Bayesian activity recognition in residence for elders.* Paper presented at the 2007 3rd IET international conference on intelligent environments.

Van Kasteren, T., Noulas, A., Englebienne, G., & Kröse, B. (2008). Accurate activity recognition in a home setting. *Proceedings of the 10th international conference on Ubiquitous computing.*

Viard, K., Fanti, M. P., Faraut, G., & Lesage, J.-J. (2016). *An event-based approach for discovering activities of daily living by hidden Markov models.* Paper presented at the 2016 15th International Conference on Ubiquitous Computing and Communications and 2016 International Symposium on Cyberspace and Security (IUCC-CSS).

Wang, L., Gu, T., Tao, X., Chen, H., & Lu, J. (2011). *Recognizing multi-user activities using wearable sensors in a smart home*. Academic Press.

Wang, X., & Kim, H. (2015). *Detecting User Activities with the Accelerometer on Android Smartphones*. Academic Press.

Wilson, C., Hargreaves, T., & Hauxwell-Baldwin, R. (2017). *Benefits and risks of smart home technologies*. Academic Press.

Xu, H., Pan, Y., Li, J., Nie, L., & Xu, X. (2019). *Activity recognition method for home-based elderly care service based on random forest and activity similarity*. Academic Press.

Yang, J., Lee, J., & Choi, J. (2011). *Activity recognition based on RFID object usage for smart mobile devices*. Academic Press.

Zhong, J., Han, T., Lotfi, A., Cangelosi, A., & Liu, X. (2019). *Bridging the Gap between Robotic Applications and Computational Intelligence in Domestic Robotics*. Paper presented at the 2019 IEEE Symposium Series on Computational Intelligence (SSCI).

ADDITIONAL READING

Ke, S. R., Thuc, H. L. U., Lee, Y. J., Hwang, J. N., Yoo, J. H., & Choi, K. H. (2013). A review on video-based human activity recognition. *Computers*, *2*(2), 88–131. doi:10.3390/computers2020088

Lara, O. D., & Labrador, M. A. (2012). A survey on human activity recognition using wearable sensors. *IEEE Communications Surveys and Tutorials*, *15*(3), 1192–1209. doi:10.1109/SURV.2012.110112.00192

Chapter 3
The Implications of Virtual Reality (VR) for the Aged

Yui-yip Lau
Division of Business and Hospitality Management, The Hong Kong Polytechnic University, Hong Kong, China

Ivy Chan
Division of Business and Hospitality Management, The Hong Kong Polytechnic University, Hong Kong, China

EXECUTIVE SUMMARY

As virtual reality (VR) technology continuously evolves in this century, the number of such applications have undoubtedly increased significantly. Nevertheless, the VR market for the aged is still in a blue ocean. The Hong Kong population is aging more quickly than ever before. This puts a huge stress to the healthcare systems in Hong Kong. In this chapter, the authors describe the updated VR technologies and their applications in a series of emerging healthcare services such as training and green burial for the aged. To this end, the chapter will provide management staff in homes for the aged, hospitals, healthcare service providers, and other health service professionals with the latest concepts and good practices in VR for the aged. The humanistic, holistic, and integrated care for the aged will be achieved in the future.

DOI: 10.4018/978-1-7998-8790-4.ch003

INTRODUCTION

The existing population has nearly reached 7.4 million. In the future, the population growth rate will be at 0.6%. As expected, the Hong Kong population will hit a peak of 8.22 million. There will be about 30% of elderly persons contribute to the overall Hong Kong population (Lau et al., 2020). Cheung and Yip (2010, pp. 257) addressed that "Hong Kong has one of the best life expectancy records in the world". On the one hand, the female life expectancy will dramatically increase from 75.3 years old in 1971 to 93.1 years old in 2066. On the other hand, the expectation for male life expectancy will also remarkably increase from 67.8 years old in 1971 to 87.1 years old in 2066 (Lau et al., 2020). Hong Kong has the longest life expectancy in the world as Hong Kong provides good quality healthcare, positive social factors, and excellent geographical location with subtropical climate (CUHK, 2021).

Hong Kong has finished the handover process of sovereignty since 1997. However, the rapid expansion of aging population brings a pressure of the existing elderly health care service and induces an extreme demand for cemetery space. The significant expansion of aging population is a serious challenge. Recently, there is a large wave of young generations plan to relocate from Hong Kong to other countries. A number of elderlies may need to take care of them without a proper care. As expected, social loneliness will be a serious problem of elderly in the future (Shao and Lee, 2020). This is a time to address how to provide a professional elderly health care service and educate the elderlies about engaging in death duties earlier in order to understand self-esteem in life via the use of virtual reality (VR). In doing so, an analysis of ageing population is critically eagerness for Hong Kong. In this chapter, the authors suggest the adoption of VR would maintain the sustainable development of homes for the aged and promote the concept of green burial. To date, none of research studies relevant with the implications of VR for the aged, notably in Hong Kong context.

This chapter is divided into three main sections. In Section 1, it mainly provides the research context and the overview of population ageing trend of Hong Kong. In Section 2, it identifies the deployment of VR for the aged through two illustrative case studies relevant with sustainability development of homes for the aged and green burial. Then, concluding remarks is given in Section 3.

THE DEPLOYMENT OF VR FOR THE AGED

Recently, the application of VR in the healthcare sector has showed an upward trend, notably simulating surgeries (Benferdia et al., 2018; Noghabaei et al., 2020) and rehabilitation training (Li, 2019). Farra et al. (2019, pp. 446) addressed that "virtual reality (VR) provides a productive medium for training, due to the ability to simulate, customize, and capture performance data for a wide variety of situations". Also, past research studies addressed that VR technologies have become a hot topic of healthcare industry because of their immersion abilities (Noghabaei et al., 2020). (Mosadeghi et al., 2016) carried out a case study with more than 500 hospital patients. Interestingly, a majority of hospital patients indicated that the VR experience was able to decrease anxiety and pain and was enjoyable. Noghabaei et al. (2020) indicated that academic scholars conducted a critical review the adoptions of VR in the healthcare industry from 2005 to 2015 and summarized that VR had performed three main promising areas including cognitive and motor rehabilitation, pain management, and eating disorders. Additionally, VR exhibits positive results of live disaster exercises or emergency training. To a certain extent, VR is relevant with user improvements and satisfaction of performance and knowledge (Farra et al., 2019). Clearly, the VR application for homes for the aged and green burial in the elderly discipline is under-researched.

In practice, implementing VR is a complicated exercise, and various adopters have deal with unfolded challenges to different stages. In doing so, the integration of an organized training curriculum into simulator training. Indeed, the professionals require to acquire a technical skill in using VR simulators (Benferdia et al., 2018). Li (2019) recognized the deployment of VR in healthcare may need to install the new or emerging technology with strong network support in the 5G period. In the 5G application, VR may need to integrate with cloud computing, self-determination medicine, and telemedicine so as to maintain instant response and produce an interactive or 'live' experience. Although the use of VR is a challenging task, the researchers pointed out that VR can motivate learners and improve their learning accomplishments (Noghabaei et al., 2020). As expected, it enables students and healthcare specialists to visualize and examine different designs (i.e., homes for the aged and green burial) via a VR context in this book chapter.

Sustainability Development of Homes for the Aged

Currently, there are 38,312 places (53%) in private homes; 19,874 subsidized places (27%) in subvented homes, self-financing homes and contract homes; 9,659 subsidized places (13%) under enhanced bought place scheme; and 5,209 non-subsidized places (7%) in non-profit making self-financing homes/contract homes. In other words, there are 49,552 places (68%) are offered by private sectors while 23,502 places (32%) are provided by non-governmental organizations (NGOs) (Social Welfare Department, HKSAR, 2021). In addition, the capacity of subsidized residential services for the elderly and the capacity of non-subsidized residential services for the elderly are given in Tables 1 and 2, respectively.

Table 1. The capacity of subsidized residential services for the elderly

	Hostel	Home for the Aged	Care-and-Attention Home				Nursing Home	Total
	Subvented Home Operated by NGO	Subvented Home Operated by NGO	Subvented Home Operated by NGO	Contract Home	Private Home Participating in "Enhanced Bought Place Scheme"	Subvented and Self-financing Home Operated by NGO	Contract Home	
Hong Kong	0	67	2,896	60	1,532	0	537	**5,092**
West Kowloon	0	0	1,459	81	2,862	112	734	**5,248**
East Kowloon	0	0	3,198	48	886	797	444	**5,373**
New Territories East	0	0	4,455	26	1,430	299	244	**6,454**
New Territories West	0	0	3,215	54	2,949	652	496	**7,366**

Source: Social Welfare Department, HKSAR (2021)

Table 2. The capacity of non-subsidized residential services for the elderly

	Hostel		Home for the Aged	Care-and-Attention Home			Nursing Home		Total
	Homes Operated by NGO	Private Home	Home Operated by NGO	Home Operated by NGO	Contract Home	Private Home	Home Operated by NGO	Contract Home	
Hong Kong	0	0	95	617	30	8.133	197	274	**9,346**
West Kowloon	0	0	96	455	50	10,291	0	449	**11,341**
East Kowloon	0	0	0	826	33	4,418	90	311	**5,679**
New Territories East	0	0	220	442	16	8,501	0	145	**9,324**
New Territories West	0	0	51	2,860	158	38,312	288	1,441	**43,521**

Source: Social Welfare Department, HKSAR (2021)

In Hong Kong, the existing population has almost accumulated at 7.4 million. The population is continuously increasing in the forthcoming years. By 2043, population in Hong Kong will be speculated to reach a peak of 8.22 million (Social Welfare Department, HKSAR, 2021). A Home for the Aged is a "must" for elderly to sustain their sound in body and mind. To the best of the authors' knowledge, Hong Kong private elderly home not only encounters stiff competition with different competitors, but also deals with external forces from government regulations, technological advancement, empowered customer and socio-cultural (Lau and Keung, 2018).

Basically, a Homes for the Aged is the suitable place to give meals, personal care, accommodation, and fundamental nursing and medical care to senior citizens (Lau et al., 2017). Due to the dramatic demand for Homes for the Aged in the forthcoming years and align with the HKSAR government policy master plan, the application of innovative technologies (e.g., VR, AI, IoT, blockchain, robotics, autonomous systems, and machine learning) play a vital role of strengthening the sustainability development of Homes for the Aged (Ho et al., 2021; Wong et al., 2021).

Recently, the concept of 'integrated care' has been arisen. Integrated care refers to the concern to improve a quality of care and patient satisfaction along with the efficiency and value from health delivery systems (Chan et al., 2019). He and Tang (2021, pp. 351) explained integrated care as "the organization and management of health services so that people get the care they need, when they need it, in ways that are user-friendly, achieve the desired results and provide value for money". The idea of integrated care is commonly appeared in Canada, England, Europe, and the United States. However, there is under-researched in Asian region (He and Tang, 2021). Boorsma et al. (2011) identified the improvement of residential care facilities (e.g., bathroom, washing machine, kitchenette, treatment) are crucial to sustain higher quality of care for elderly people. Indeed, garden setting with plant species provides elderly people with various levels of cognitive and physical disability foster the stimulus of sensory and exercise, enrich health condition, and diminish stress. The rationale behind is that there is an increasing trend of elderly people shifting from their homes to Homes for the Aged (Shi et al., 2019). However, a number of health care incidents addressed that some Homes for the Aged failed to deal with the rising incidence of chronic disease and to improve patient services with more harmonized and continuous care (Chan et al., 2019). Thus, the adoption of new, innovative technologies can improve the people perception of Homes for the Aged service delivery (Ruyter et al., 1997). As suggested by Shao and Lee (2020), the use of VR improves the users' performance expectancy, effort expectancy, and perceived enjoyment. In other words, it will positively influence user attitude and behavioral intention of homes for the aged service delivery. In the long-term, the deployment of VR could maintain sustainable development of homes for the aged in the future.

In the past few decades, most of the Homes for the Aged are facing a lack of health and medical professionals due to a high turnover rate and the young generations are not willing to join the Homes for the Aged sector. In doing so, it is expected that the integration of innovative technologies can motivate the existing professionals to retain their work at the industry and encourage the young generations to join the market. Furthermore, the development of innovative technologies can conduct a series of training to healthcare specialists to upgrade their relevant job skills. At the same time, it can increase the students' employability to contribute to the Homes for the Aged sector (Tang and Lau, 2020).

In the academic research studies, most of the Homes for the Aged studies were concentrated on the science and technology discipline. Clearly, there is a gap in exploring and identifying the problems of Homes for the Aged from business management discipline. In the book chapter, the study will illustrate a number of business management elements including logistics, marketing, accounting, hospitality management into the existing Homes for the Aged. To a certain extent, it definitely helps Homes for the Aged successfully change into a multi-functional and integrated one in the forthcoming years.

Accordingly, a series of VR scenarios will be developed to students and healthcare specialists. The VR scenarios will be integrated different business concepts (i.e., accounting, logistics, marketing and hospitality management) into practical Homes for the Aged. The developed VR programs will be interrelated to each other illustrating the training aspects of the students. Figure 1 illustrates the key performance areas of VR training. The health specialists and students can be identified as achieving the different proficiencies after they have completed the whole set of VR training.

Figure 1. The key performance area of VR training in elderly home caring proficiency

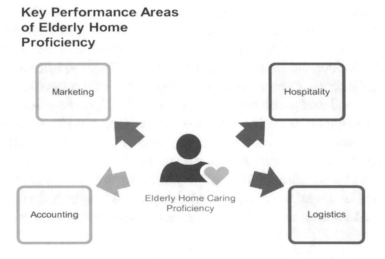

To a large extent, it can create the idea of integrated care to improve the health care service delivery. The design of VR scenario aim to create a new, innovative, and interactive learning environment in the digital era. The VR scenarios will focus on how to help healthcare specialists to upgrade their relevant job skills as well as increasing the students' employability. During the VR stimulation process, the researchers will conduct a mixed research approach to establish the research model and provide a constructive advice to the Homes for the Aged on how to transform into an a multi-functional and integrated one in the future.

After discussing with various healthcare specialists, four key performance areas (i.e., accounting, logistics, marketing and hospitality management) accounting for the core working processes of the elderly homes in Hong Kong. The design of these four scenarios will be used to train their fundamental problem handling and solving abilities. The scenarios include:

Accounting: In the accounting aspect, it is appropriate to develop a VR training scenarios of daily necessities (e.g., comb, shampoo, shower gel, diapers, nutritional milk, foley etc) and medicine stock taking. Apart from providing professional care for elderly, elderly home care service will also need to consider their daily and medical needs. However, inaccurate inventory record and stock replenishment are addressed by elderly homes. By simulating the daily necessitates and medication counting scenarios, students can investigate the procedures involved in the stock taking and recording in order to improve the accuracy of inventory record and stock replenishment. Inaccurate inventory record may create either stockout or overstock of daily necessities and medicine. The overstock may induce health hazards of medical waste and its disposal problem in the daily operations.

Marketing: In the marketing aspect, it only focuses on the customer relationship management relevant with the elderly and their family members. In order to attract the elderly to use the elderly home services, customer relationship management is very important. Improving customer service level fosters Homes for the Aged to sustain the community's good word-of-mouth, generate a favorable business image, reduce the potential risk for disputes, and increase the confidence from the elderly and their family members (Post-Acute Advisor, 2021). Therefore, this aspect will make use of the VR technology to mimics a number of problems and unfolded challenges (e.g., safety and health) encountered by the elderly. In particular, this is vital to improve health specialists' knowledge and skills due to COVID-19. In addition, the aspect will also train students to solve the problems directly.

Hospitality: Hospitality in elderly home refers to keeping the living place of elderly tidy, hygienic, and clean in order to increase their level of satisfaction. The hospitality in elderly home is unique among other industries in both its breadth and pervasiveness throughout everyday life from accommodation. In this aspect, it will simulate the tidy up the dormitory scenarios which is one of the most common and essential training required for each elderly home career. This is crucial to minimize the spread of virus in response to COVID-19 pandemic. To the best of the authors' knowledge, a number of confirmed COVID-19 cases have been identified in elderly home. As such, the public perceived that elderly home is a source of virus and provides an effective way to transmit the virus. The desirable living place of elderly home will rebuild the confidence in elderly and their family members. This VR training can also help to train students' positive behavior support towards the elderly and their self-caring ability.

Logistics: Logistics is a vital part of the elderly home caring service. Catering in logistics service is essential to each elderly. It is also vital to each student learning elderly home caring as it requires understanding the unique requirements of individual elderly. It is also challenging to provide a high quality and satisfaction catering service. In the VR training program, students will learn the procedures involved in providing catering service to the elderly. Preparing meals is main concern for the Homes for the Aged. To a certain extent, the elderly grows stronger and stronger due to the regular balanced and healthy meal plan. In general, the types of meals are determined by the elderly smell and taste, dental health condition, appetite, depression, and disease (Van De Walle, 2019).

In Table 3, it summarizes the examples, responsible parties and its' action taking or caring service needed in elderly homes.

Table 3. Key performance area of elderly home in action taking/caring service and responsible party

Kea Performance Areas	Examples	Action Taking / Caring Service	Responsible to:
Accounting	Stocktake of medicine	Nursing Team	Nurse-in-Charge / Registered Nurse
	Stocktake of daily necessities (comb, shampoo, shower gel etc.)	Social Work Team	Assistant Superintendent / Superintendent
	Stocktake of daily necessities (diapers, nutritional milk, foley etc.)	Nursing Team	Nurse-in-Charge / Registered Nurse
Marketing	Handle client's problem	Social Work Team	Superintendent
Hospitality	Tidy up the dormitory	Workman	Social Worker / Supportive Service Team Leader
Logistics	To prepare meals	Kitchen Team (Cook)	Social Worker / Nurse-in-Charge / Assistant Superintendent

Green Burial

In view of the land scarcity, aging population, and limited supply of columbarium, the Food and Environmental Hygiene Department (hereafter called "FEHD") has been promoting green burial to public since 2007. In the last few decades, the number of deaths in Hong Kong has steadily increased while the number of cemeteries in Hong Kong has kept the same for now. To a certain extent, the amounts of cemeteries are not sufficient to fulfil the demand except the completion of Sandy Ridge project in northern Hong Kong in the forthcoming years. The circumstance of handling the decreased has showed up at a bottleneck. In Table 4, it summarizes the number of cemeteries and deaths in Hong Kong.

Table 4. Number of cemeteries and deaths in Hong Kong

	2014	2015	2016	2017	2018	2019	2020
Private cemeteries	27	27	27	27	27	27	27
Public cemeteries	10	10	10	10	10	10	10
Number of deaths	45710	46757	46662	45883	47478	48706	50653

Source: Food and Environmental Hygiene Department, HKSAR (2021);
Centre for Health Protection, Department of Health, HKSAR (2021)

At present, FEHD monitors 13 Gardens of Remembrance and three designated Hong Kong water for the public to scatter cremated ashes of the deceased. The gardens of remembrance are located: Cape Collinson, Diamond Hill, Wo Hop Shek, Fu Shan, Kwai Chung, Tsang Tsui, Junk Bay, Cheung Chau, Peng Chau, and Lamma Island. The gardens of remembrance photos are provided in Figures 2, 3, and 4. The designated sea areas for the scattering of cremated human ashes include: East of Tap Mun, East of Tung Lung Chau and South of West Lamma Channel. The government provides support to the family members of the deceased with the free ferry service every Saturday. Figures 5 and 6 are given supplement information. In addition, FEHD arranges four memorial sailings each year, including two before the Ching Ming Festival and two before the Chung Yeung Festival so that the family members could perform tribute to the deceased.

To promote sustainable and eco- friendly method to handle the ashes of deceased, seminars in schools or elderly centers, and propagation through an online website accessible by public (https://www.greenburial.gov.hk/en/intro/index.html). People can search for key information about the principle of green burial, static photos of memorial gardens and application procedures are provided by FEHD.

Figure 2. The gardens of remembrance
Source: St James' Settlement

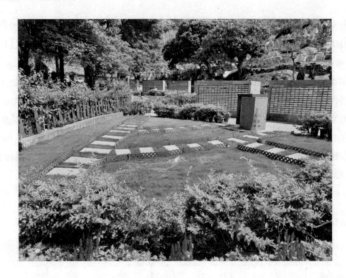

Figure 3. The gardens of remembrance
Source: St James' Settlement

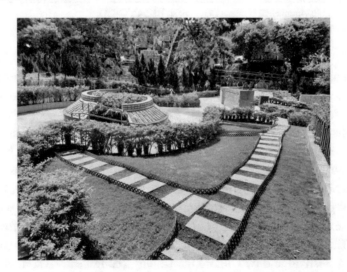

According to the discussion paper (https://www.legco.gov.hk/yr19-20/english/ panels/fseh/papers/fseh20200114cb2-482-5-e.pdf) of Legislative Council Panel on Food Safety and Environmental Hygiene Promotion of Green Burial on 14 January 2020, it showed that public awareness towards the concept of green burial is rising. In 2019, FEHD organized for 3200 visitors with 110 visits to different green burial facilities and services. However, conventions to bury deceased in traditional way as a kind of respect is more prevailing and hard to be retracted. The government statistics showed that the take-up rate for green burials remains low.

Figure 4. The gardens of remembrance
Source: St James' Settlement

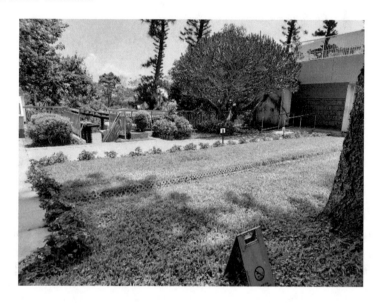

Figure 5. The scattering of cremated human ashes in the designated sea areas
Source: St James' Settlement

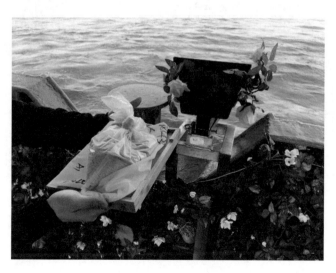

Figure 6. The Family members of the deceased with the free ferry service
Source: St James' Settlement

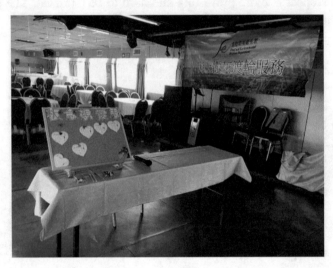

In 2019, the number of green burial cases in Hong Kong (including the scattering of ashes in Gardens of Remembrance ("GoRs") or at sea) reached 7,909, which represents an increase of over 2,500 cases (or around 47%) as compared with the figure in 2016. The relevant figures in the past four years are set out in Table 5.

Table 5. The usage of green burial service in hong kong

Year	Scattering of Ashes in GoRs		Scattering of Ashes at Sea (C)	Number of Green Burial Cases (A)+(B)+(C)	Percentage of Total Number of Deaths
	Food and Environmental Hygiene Department (A)	Private Cemeteries (B)			
2016	4 004	462	900	5 366	11.5%
2017	4 966	607	966	6 539	14.3%
2018	5 352	722	972	7 046	14.8%
2019 (up to November)	5 730	676	828	7 234	16.3%

Remarks: GoRs managed by private cemeteries include the GoR in the Junk Bay Chinese Permanent Cemetery and the GoR in the Pokfulam Chinese Christian Cemetery.

The decline of physical and mental health present different constraints to the active aging groups, such as loss of functional capabilities, mobility, social ties with others. Different studies show that the application of VR for older adults can improve the quality of their lives, reduce loneliness, promote positive emotions through geotechnology gaming or assistive exercises (Mascret et al., 2020; Syed-Abdul et al. 2019). For example, 23 elderly people underwent 30-day "Xbox 360 Kinect" VR training. The results showed that VR has positive impacts on their static and dynamic balance, improve motor impairment and reduce the risk of falls (Kamińska et al. 2018). Syed-Abdul et al. (2019) conducted a pilot study with 30 elderly aged 60 to 95 years old to use VR applications that facilitate physical movement and entertainment for six weeks. The survey results indicated the elderly perceived VR to be useful and using VR is an enjoyable experience to promote active aging life. Another experimental study was conducted on 20 stroke patients to play Serious Games. After six-week play, the patients had positive improvement for their cognitive rehabilitation of memory (e.g., buying several items) and attention (e.g., finding a specific virtual character) (Gamito et al., 2017). Therefore, adoption of immersive technology, virtual reality that enables the elderly to experience immersive process and life-like environment as an alternative promotional method might change their perception and attitudes towards green burial.

The theme of Green Burial centers on "returning to nature" after dead. The burial approach by disposing or scattering the ashes at dedicated gardens or seas is relatively eco-friendly, sustainable and brings a positive impact on ecosystems when comparing with the conventional burial approach. Howe (2019) cited the figures from Green Burial Council, conventional burial produces pollutants from 3 million gallons of toxic embalming chemicals fluid to underground water; conserves precious resources such as 20 million feet of wood and 17,000 tons of copper and bronze for coffins. It implies that if we take the choice of green burial, we can directly reduce the carbon footprint such as removing the steps in embalming chemicals, using biodegradable materials for casket. It is estimated that each cremation consumes as much energy, in the form of natural gas and electricity, as a 500-mile (800 kilometer) car trip (Vatomsky 2018). It is the ultimate legacy with the protected land for future generations. Despite the government advocates to green burial in Hong Kong, the traditional or religious beliefs to venerate the dead and preserve the deceased such as putting the ancestors' ashes in ceramic urns, or laying the cadaver in cemetery or burial plot, is hard to upend (Zheng 2018). In the absence of dialogue or communication of life planning, the family members of the deceased follow the convention, choose traditional funeral, and arrange of niches to express their respect and filial piety. Lau et al. (2020) summarized reasons for a low awareness of the idea of green burial in the public because of (1) insufficient communication between children and parents relevant with death; (2) a minority of colleagues, relatives, and friends discuss the main advantages of green burial service; and (3) ineffectual promotional channels and tools. In addition, funeral service providers, funeral logistics firms identified that the emergence of green burial will influence the profit of coffins and cemetery. Such as, the family of the decreased usually choose fragrant wood coffin or solid wood coffin. The price is available in a range between HKD 2 million and 3 million. However, eco-coffin will be charged between HKD 6,000 and HKD 0.2 million. Indeed, some additional exhumation services will progressively decrease and ultimately induce unemployment problem in the forthcoming years (Lau et al., 2020). In this vein, government or policy makers can adopt VR, one of the emerging technology-enabled media in elderly community for socializing, brain activity and positive mood, to promote the concept of green burial. VR can address the doubts or debunk the misconception of the elderly about green burial through well-thought design in physical fidelity and psychology fidelity.

VR is extensively used in business training that benefits employees to experience hands-on practice in a safe, controlled immersive environment. Fidelity can be primarily categorized into physical and psychological fidelity. Physical fidelity is defined as the degree of realism including surrounding environment, entities, artifacts that replicate the authentic physical setting of real-world contexts. Psychological fidelity refers to the extent of resemblance including the life-like feeling, sense of presence and emotional stances that mirror the cognitive and mental process undertaken by the users with their endeavors in actual tasks (Marini et al. 2012).

At present, the government provides 13 gardens of remembrance (GoR) and three designated regions for sea burial. Basic information about the green burial, static photos of the GoR and application procedures could be found from the official website in FEHD https://www.greenburial.gov.hk/en/home/index.html. To enhance the elderly to visualize the environment of those designated green burial places, promotion materials should be enhanced, such as more dynamic images, and thematic videos with audio effect.

The elderly people first choose their preferred companions for the GoR journey, such as son, grandchildren or a dog. Start from the nearest public transportation stops, such as MTR station or taxi stand, the elderly people can emulate the time spent, commuting route to be transported and access to the selected GoR. In terms of psychological aspect, the design of companion help decreases loneliness in the virtual environment (Graf, et al, 2020). The companions, as a type of social entity in the visit to GoR should be familiarized by the elderly as it can reduce their anxiety in this end-of-life planning journey. In addition, the elderly people find the true-like and genuine transportation process believable. In doing so, they would develop a positive sense of convenience to access GoR.

Walking slowly under the guidance of signage, the elderly people are led to the highland of GoR where they could enjoy 360-degree view of scenic environment, including the blue sky, boundless sea and green vegetation. The dynamic and panoramic views can stimulate the visual senses of the elderly. In addition, the VR could stimulate the auditory sense by the provision of different types of sound such as gentle splashing waves, sea-gull-screams, mild wind on swaying trees that replicate the natural environment in the GoR. Under the tranquil scene, the elderly people could feel the sustained beauty, relaxation and quietness as if they enjoy hiking.

After enjoying the captivating view in the GoR, the elderly people are led to the reception counter at GoR office. Taking an observer role, the elderly can attend to the conversation between a family and the officer, gain an understanding of the processes how the officers at the GoR handle cremated ashes. The officers check and verify the identity and registration details of the bereaved family, then, lead them to the scattering area and explain the operation. The elderly could follow the family, witness how the staff help pour the ashes of the deceased into the scattering device.

Before the ashes scattering, the family members conduct memorial rituals, for example making a group pray and express condolence message to each other. The pre-scattering processes help the elderly people to debunk their misconception about green burial that the family members ignored the dignified preparation of remains. Then, the family members take turn to hold the ash scattering device, release gradually, let the cremated ashes spread onto the lawn along the stone pavement. In the GoR journey, the elderly people are provided an option whether to hold the device and try to scatter part of the ashes intimately. The elderly could see the ashes lay on the soil where different vegetation or flowers are planted. The close observation and involvement in the scattering process allow the elderly people to mimic the feeling how their family members take care of their ashes in the blessed environment.

When the scattering of ash is completed, the family members return the device to the staff. The memorial process does not stop. The family members walk towards the stone pavement where they have scattered the ash, they can take a close look at the flourishing plants, butterflies performing spiral dance on flowers. Moreover, the elderly can watch how the front-line staff do the gardening prudently in other stone pavements where no ash scattering is carried out at that meanwhile. Accompanied the bereaved family in the scattering process, the elderly people could share the heartfelt grief and emotional pain due to their loss, and demystify the genuine emotional bonding is sustained in the green burial.

The VR journey is continued with the passage to the wall for plaques where the name plates are mounted on the memorial wall to honour the dead. The elderly people can realize the well-thought design that the plaques are perpendicular to the main road or not directly visible from the street (e.g., design in Diamond Hill Columbarium). Moreover, the natural ventilation is applied to the area of memorial wall that can minimize the negative impacts to mourners from smoke generated from incense burning. In terms of psychological fidelity, the elderly people can sense how the idea of green burial can alleviate the negative affect of the scary ash scattering structure or smoke to the neighborhood. The main workflow of the deployment framework of the VR for green burial is exhibited in Figure 7.

Based on Lau et al. (2020) suggestion, the study suggests to use VR in the area of green burial because of (I) the VR programme will enable the public to participate in the environment under controllable situation and will create a safe environment for them to comprehend green burial; (II) The VR programme allow to use regularly without the need to exhibit the actual scenario that may perhaps unacceptable to the public; (III) The VR programme minimizes wasting of resources engaged in actual cases that fulfill the concepts of green; and (IV) The VR programme encourages the stimulated context to give a natural sentiment and support the health education.

In essence, with the aid of VR, the elderly people are closely involved and engaged in the whole GoR journey. Being the companion in the GoR journey with the sadden family in the replicated scene, the elderly people could capture the highly resembled scenes and experience the emotional upset in a safe and controlled environment, while their anxiety is taken into account with the visit of the death-related place (forbidden area by tradition). Instead of comprehending the text-based information in web site or printed leaflets, the elderly people are enabled to visualize and comprehend a life-like process of green burial through their portable VR headsets and earbuds. The step-by-step episodes reproduced in the VR GoR journey organize the after-life planning information into digestible and relevant mode. Coupled with the animated images and vivid sounds from different parties provide a more concrete idea about green burial, the elderly people can gain their personal experience and recognize their realistic preferences when they have to decide after-life planning.

It is suggested that a face-to-face seminar about after-life planning could be conducted before deployment of VR to pay a visit to the GoR. As such, the elderly can prepare and plan their own funeral arrangement. Also, it fosters to promote an open-mindedness and positive attitude towards deploying VR to accept the idea of green burial. In addition, the practice of VR for the journey of GoR could be implemented on group-base instead of single elderly as the sense of collective presence towards a common task can alleviate their fear and anxiety towards aging and death (Shao and Lee, 2020). After the journey, a stress-free sharing or debriefing among the elderly participants is valuable as they could share views about the technology-enabled simulation such as hardware and duration. Most important of all, they could show mutual support, sense of open-mindedness to the long-term taboo of discussing and planning options of death arrangement.

Figure 7. The workflow of the VR framework – green burial

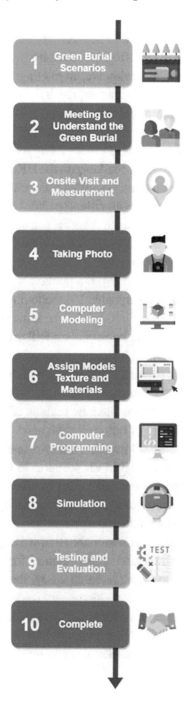

CONCLUSION

As VR technology continuously evolve in this century, the number of such applications have undoubtedly increased significantly. Despite VR are commonly applied in a number of applications in healthcare, marketing, entertainment, education, manufacturing, training, to name but a few, the VR market for the aged is still in a blue ocean. The Hong Kong population is aging more rapidly than ever before. In accordance with the population projections conducted by Census and Statistics Department, one in every three people in Hong Kong is expected to be older than 65 in 2066. This change not only poses challenge to the HKSAR governments, but also puts a huge stress to the healthcare systems. Aged care VR technologies not only revolutionising the aged care sector with virtual specific training, but also can provide innovative service or product to the aged. The VR can also be used to promote green burial to the elderly. To a certain extent, the enhancement of physical fidelity and psychological fidelity of VR debunk public's misconception of green burial. Also, such simulation experience can improve the public acceptance of green burial. In this book chapter, we describe the updated VR technologies and its applications in a series of emerging healthcare services such as training in elderly home and green burial for the aged. To this end, the book chapter will provide management staff in Homes for the Aged, hospitals, healthcare service providers, and other health service professionals with the latest concepts and good practices in VR for the aged. The humanistic, holistic, and integrated care for the aged will be achieved in the future.

In the book chapter, it addresses the new notions of elderly research, namely, green burial and integrated care of homes for the aged. Nevertheless, these issues are hot and urgent demand. Such topics are under-researched. Indeed, the authors proposed new, innovative, and feasible VR scenario to improve health specialists, public, and other stakeholders' understanding of the demand for the elderlies. Such interdisciplinary research provides a groundbreaking study between science, technology, and healthcare disciplines. Due to integrated care of homes for the aged and green burial are new idea, it is reasonable that we require time to improve the public progressively accept integrated care of homes for the aged and green burial by the VR deployment. In the next research study, the researchers could design and implement VR stimulations for elderly applications. As expected, the VR stimulations may need to undergo various trails and error stage. At a later stage, the new, innovative VR technologies fundamentally improve the personalized service delivery for the elderly and cultivate the caring culture among the aged care sector.

REFERENCES

Benferdia, Y., Ahmad, M. N., Mustapha, M., Baharin, H., & Bajuri, M. Y. (2018). Critical success factors for virtual reality-based training in ophthalmology domain. *Journal of Health & Medical Informatics, 9*(3), 1–14. doi:10.4172/2157-7420.1000318

Boorsma, M., Frijters, D. H. K., Knol, D. L., Ribbe, M. E., Nijpels, G., & van Hout, H. P. J. (2011). Effects of multidisciplinary integrated care on quality of care in residential care facilities for elderly people: A cluster randomized trial. *Canadian Medical Association Journal, 183*(11), E724–E732. doi:10.1503/cmaj.101498 PMID:21708967

Centre for Health Protection, Department of Health, HKSAR. (2021). Available at https://www.chp.gov.hk/en/statistics/data/10/27/380.html

Chan, K. H., Chan, H. H., Wong, C. W., & Lau, Y. Y. (2019). Strengthening STEM and Arduino to foster integrated cares in Hong Kong. *CPCE Health Conference 2019.*

Cheung, K. S. L., & Yip, P. S. F. (2010). Trends in healthy life expectancy in Hong Kong SAR 1996-2008. *European Journal of Ageing, 7*(4), 257–269. doi:10.100710433-010-0171-3 PMID:21212818

CUHK. (2021). *Why Hong Kong has the Longest Life Expectancy in the World.* Available at https://www.oal.cuhk.edu.hk/cuhkenews_202101_life_expectancy/

Farra, S. L., Gneuhs, M., Hodgson, E., Kawosa, B., Miller, E. T., Simon, A., Timm, N., & Hausfeld, J. (2019). Comparative cost of virtual reality training and live exercises for training hospital workers for evacuation. *Computers, Informatics, Nursing, 37*(9), 446–454. doi:10.1097/CIN.0000000000000540 PMID:31166203

Food and Environmental Hygiene Department. HKSAR. (2021). Available at https://www.fehd.gov.hk/english/

Gamito, P., Oliveira, J., Coelho, C., Morais, D., Lopes, P., Pacheco, J., Brito, R., Soares, F., Santos, N., & Barata, A. F. (2017). Cognitive training on stroke patients via virtual reality-based serious games. *Disability and Rehabilitation, 39*(4), 385–388. doi:10.3109/09638288.2014.934925 PMID:25739412

Graf, L., Liszio, S., & Masuch, M. (2020). Playing in virtual nature: improving mood of elderly people using VR technology. In *Proceedings of the Conference on Mensch und Computer (MuC '20).* Association for Computing Machinery. 10.1145/3404983.3405507

He, A. J., & Tang, V. F. Y. (2021). Integration of health services for the elderly in Asia: A scoping review of Hong Kong, Singapore, Malaysia, Indonesia. *Health Policy (Amsterdam)*, *125*(3), 351–362. doi:10.1016/j.healthpol.2020.12.020 PMID:33422336

Ho, T. S. G., Tang, Y. M., Tsang, K. Y., Tang, V., & Chau, K. Y. (2021). A blockchain-based system to enhance aircraft parts traceability and trackability for inventory management. *Expert Systems with Applications*, *179*, 115101. doi:10.1016/j.eswa.2021.115101

Howe, K. (2019). *Green Burials Benefit the Environment, But They Also Provide Opportunities for Fraud.* Retrieved on 2 July 2021 from https://absolutetrustcounsel.com/green-burials-benefit-the-environment-but-they-also-provide-opportunities-for-fraud/

Kamińska, M. S., Miller, A., Rotter, I., Szylińska, A., & Grochans, E. (2018). The effectiveness of virtual reality training in reducing the risk of falls among elderly people. *Clinical Interventions in Aging*, *13*, 2329–2338. doi:10.2147/CIA.S183502 PMID:30532523

Lau, Y. Y., Chiu, W. K., & Chan, G. H. H. (2017). Procurement management in the private elderly home. *CPCE Health Conference 2017*.

Lau, Y. Y., & Keung, K. L. (2018). An application of balanced scorecard in the private elderly home: A case study of Hong Kong. *CPCE Health Conference 2018*.

Lau, Y. Y., Tang, Y. M., Chan, I., Ng, A. K. Y., & Leung, A. (2020). The deployment of virtual reality (VR) to promote green burial. *Asia-Pacific Journal of Health Management*, *15*(2), 53–60. doi:10.24083/apjhm.v15i2.403

Li, D. (2019). 5G and intelligence medicine – how the next generation of wireless technology will reconstruct healthcare? *Precision Clinical Medicine*, *2*(4), 205–208. doi:10.1093/pcmedi/pbz020 PMID:31886033

Marini, D., Folgieri, R., Gadia, D., & Rizzi, A. (2012). Virtual reality as a communication process. *Virtual Reality (Waltham Cross)*, *16*(3), 233–241. doi:10.100710055-011-0200-3

Mascret, N., Delbes, L., Voron, A., Temprado, J., & Montagne, G. (2020). Acceptance of a Virtual Reality Headset Designed for Fall Prevention in Older Adults: Questionnaire Study. *Journal of Medical Internet Research*, *22*(12), e20691. Advance online publication. doi:10.2196/20691 PMID:33315019

Mosadeghi, S., Reid, M. W., Martinez, B., Rosen, B. T., & Spiegel, B. M. R. (2016). Feasibility of an Immersive Virtual Reality Intervention for Hospitalized Patients: An Observational Cohort Study. *JMIR Mental Health*, *3*(2), e28. doi:10.2196/mental.5801 PMID:27349654

Noghabaei, M., Heydarian, A., Balali, V., & Han, K. (2020). Trend analysis on adoption of virtual and augmented reality in the architecture, engineering, and construction industry. *Data*, *5*(1), 26–43. doi:10.3390/data5010026

Post-Acute Advisor. (2021). *Why Customer Service is the Key to Success for Assisted Living Facilities.* Available at https://postacuteadvisor.blr.com/2017/03/08/why-customer-service-is-the-key-to-success-for-assisted-living-facilities/

Ruyter, K. D., Wetzels, M., Lemmink, J., & Mattsson, J. (1997). The dynamics of the service delivery process: A value-based approach. *International Journal of Research in Marketing*, *14*(3), 231–243. doi:10.1016/S0167-8116(97)00004-9

Seifert, A., & Schlomann, A. (2021). The Use of Virtual and Augmented Reality by Older Adults: Potentials and Challenges. *Frontiers in Virtual Reality*, *2*, 1–5. doi:10.3389/frvir.2021.639718

Shao, D., & Lee, I. J. (2020). Acceptance and Influencing Factors of Social Virtual Reality in the Urban Elderly. *Sustainability*, *12*(22), 9345–9363. doi:10.3390u12229345

Shi, S. L., Tong, C. M., & Marcus, C. C. (2019). What makes a garden in the elderly care facility well used. *Landscape Research*, *44*(2), 256–269. doi:10.1080/01426397.2018.1457143

Social Welfare Department. HKSAR. (2021). Available at https://www.swd.gov.hk/en/index/site_pubsvc/page_elderly/sub_residentia/id_overviewon/

Syed-Abdul, S., Malwade, S., Nursetyo, A. A., Sood, M., Bhatia, M., Barsasella, D., Liu, M. F., Chang, C.-C., Srinivasan, K., Raja, M., & Li, Y.-C. J. (2019). Virtual reality among the elderly: A usefulness and acceptance study from Taiwan. *BMC Geriatrics*, *19*(1), 223–232. doi:10.118612877-019-1218-8 PMID:31426766

Tang, Y. M., & Lau, Y. Y. (2020). Medical training with virtual reality (VR) for the aged. *CPCE Health Conference 2020*.

Van De Walle, G. (2019). *9 Factors Affecting Nutrition in Older Adults.* Available at https://dakotadietitians.com/factors-affecting-nutrition/

Vatomsky, S. (2018). Thinking About Having a 'Green' Funeral? Here's What to Know. *The New York Times*. Retrieved on 2 July 2021 from https://www.nytimes.com/2018/03/22/smarter-living/green-funeral-burial-environment.html

Wong, S., Yeung, J. K. W., Lau, Y. Y., & So, J. (2021). Technical sustainability of cloud-based blockchain integrated with machine learning for supply chain management. *Sustainability*, *13*(15), 8270–8291. doi:10.3390u13158270

Zheng, M. (2018). *Green Burials: Why Hongkongers remain reluctant about alternative funerals*. Coconuts Hong Kong. Retrieved on 2 July 2021 from https://coconuts.co/hongkong/features/green-burials-hongkongers-remain-reluctant-alternative-funerals/

Chapter 4
Virtual Reality in Patient–Physician Relationships

Haoyu Liu
City University of Macau, China

Bowen Dong
City University of Macau, China

Pi-Ying Yen
Macau University of Science and Technology, China

EXECUTIVE SUMMARY

The chapter examines the applications of virtual reality (VR) in patient-physician relationships. Specifically, this chapter focuses on three-dimensional medical imaging that facilitates explanation purposes. Though the literature on VR in medicine exists, the discussion of applying VR in patient-physician relationships, an immensely important topic of medicine, is sparse. The authors present a case of VR application in orthopedics to demonstrate how this technology promotes patient-physician relationships and, as a result, affects the medical industry. The opportunities and challenges of applying VR to medicine are also discussed. This chapter contributes to better incorporating VR into treatment and understanding the impact of emerging technologies on medicine.

INTRODUCTION

The patient-physician relationship has been a hot topic in medicine for a long time. It ranks second in importance only to family relationships and is considered more important than relationships with colleagues or advisers (Pincock, 2003). Doctors

DOI: 10.4018/978-1-7998-8790-4.ch004

are also seen as the most trusted source of health information. This trust between doctors and patients sets up the foundation for their further collaboration and affects the treatment outcome directly (Baron and Berinsky, 2019). For example, a high-quality patient-physician relationship improves patient engagement in Human Immunodeficiency Virus (HIV) care (Flickinger et al., 2013). Specifically, HIV patients keep more appointments if providers treat them with respect, know them as people, listen carefully, and explain so that they can understand. Moreover, improving doctors' communication and relationship-building skills may increase patient retention in HIV care.

Many factors may affect the relationship between doctors and patients, and an essential one is communication between the two parties. According to Persaud (2005), effective communication is at the heart of the physician-patient relationship. Doctors have to be, in a sense, bilingual: They must learn the technical terminology to start a medical dialogue with colleagues; simultaneously, they must also learn to communicate with patients. However, it is sometimes unavoidable for doctors to employ technical terms in communication with patients. Doctors are trained for years and equipped with expert knowledge, but patients usually lack this expertise. As a result, patients have a tough time understanding the message that doctors try to deliver, and they also have difficulty expressing their feelings.

Poor patient-physician relationships can cause losses for both patients and doctors. On the patients' side, delayed diagnosis and treatment of conditions can endanger health and life, while unnecessary monetary costs may be incurred. On the doctors' side, the reputation of them and their hospitals may be damaged, and the daily operations of the hospitals can be affected.

Even worse, violence against doctors due to mistrust or conflicts has been an increasing issue in China (The Lancet, 2010, 2012), and these incidents can happen at different stages of treatment. The case of Wenbin Sun, for example, happened during the treatment process. Sun's mother was taken to Civil Aviation General Hospital on 4 December 2019 because of dysphagia. His mother did not get better during the treatment and had to stay in the hospital for observation. Sun did not correctly understand his mother's state at that moment, blamed the doctor for the lack of improvement in her condition, and attacked the doctor with a knife publicly in the hospital's emergency department. The example of Mingjun Yuan, by contrast, happened after the treatment process. Yuan went to Lanzhou Wuzhou Psoriasis Hospital for a course of pigmentation treatment. When the effect of the treatment did not meet Yuan's expectations, he did not consider it rationally. Hence, he became angry with the doctor and murdered him.

All the above examples suggest that medicine is a sophisticated science, and at the same time, it is not a panacea. This complexity characteristic of medicine produces problems in the patient-physician relationship (Beck, 2004). In current times, the management of patient-physician relationships is becoming increasingly challenging. First, due to the COVID-19 pandemic, the interaction between doctors and patients has increased, which creates more chances of misunderstandings and disputes. Due to the scarcity of medical resources, medical-related suit surges (World Health Organization, 2020). Second, the internet has brought a new information source to patients (Kilbride and Joffe, 2018). Diseases are a thing that everyone wants to keep away from. After diagnosis, a patient and their family members feel fear, and they may seek any alternative information sources and try to be their own doctors. However, such information may be unverified, and sometimes it can be misleading, but patients have difficulty distinguishing it from professional advice, leading to a lack of trust in doctors' decisions. Third, coverage of doctor-patient disputes on social media makes these events a public focus, potentially exacerbating the conflict between doctors and patients. Therefore, efficient and effective communication between doctors and patients has become crucial for overcoming these new forces that can undermine patient-physician relationships. The current chapter explains how VR, often used to demonstrate complex concepts, can play a unique role in enhancing doctor-patient communication in medicine.

The emerging technology of VR has stood out for use in various domains, including education, engineering, entertainment, and marketing. This technology simulates sensory experiences (such as sight, sound, smell, and touch) to provide users with an immersive feeling of being physically present in a situation. The contemporary concept of VR was first introduced in the 1960s and adopted in astronaut training in the 1970s. With the acceleration of related fields (such as computer graphics, computer vision, and artificial intelligence), VR started to show great market potential and business prospects during later decades. The acquisition of Oculus by Facebook for two trillion dollars pushed this technology to another peak (BBC, 2014).

The application of VR in medicine is not new. It was first witnessed in the 1990s when Hunter Hoffman at the University of Washington began to use VR to reduce pain perception among patients who had suffered severe burns (Arnaldi et al., 2018). In 1996, Stephane Cotin and his colleagues proposed a simulation system with force feedback for hepatic surgery (Cotin et al., 1996). Nowadays, VR is being utilized in various aspects of medicine due to its fast development.

This chapter focuses on introducing the use of VR to explain complex medical concepts to patients before surgery. A salient feature of VR is that it allows users to observe three-dimensional images in real-time without limit. This feature fits well in a typical type of communication in medicine, i.e., explaining surgery details to patients. As a pioneer of VR in medicine, Stanford Medicine uses a novel simulation system to create three-dimensional models that doctors and patients can observe and manipulate (Sandford Medicine, 2017). Traditional medical imaging is not friendly from patients' perspective, as a vast amount of knowledge is required to understand the images. This difficulty undoubtedly exacerbates the anxiety and panic of patients. VR provides patients with a more intuitive sense of surgery details and helps them better understand the risks that they face. Therefore, using VR to improve communication between doctors and patients before surgery should improve patient-physician relationships.

VR can also benefit patient-physician relationships by improving various aspects of the surgery itself. Remote surgery allows inexperienced doctors to acquire advice from experienced experts regardless of geographic location; virtual navigation prevents errors due to blind areas by providing doctors a comprehensive view of patients' bodies from both front and back; and live streaming surgery enabled by VR makes it possible for family members of the patients to witness the whole surgical procedure from the doctors' perspective. In the appendix, the authors will also briefly analyze how VR impacts surgical operations in some of the above aspects.

The remainder of this chapter is organized as follows. The authors review relevant literature in the next section. Sections 3 and 4 narrate a case study in orthopedics. Section 5 points out future research directions, and Section 6 concludes this chapter. Appendix 1 presents the interview protocol, and Appendix 2 provides additional analysis of VR's application during surgeries.

BACKGROUND

Patient-physician relationships have been extensively studied in the medical literature. Szasz and Hollender (1956) propose three basic models of patient-physician relationships: In the activity-passivity model, doctors directly do something to patients (like parent to infant); in the guidance-cooperation model, doctors tell patients what to do, and patients follow (like parent to child); and in the mutual participation model, doctors provide expert advice, and patients make use of that advice (like adult to adult).

In the first two models, the decision depends entirely on doctors, while in the third, the decision-making is shared, which is the more common relationship nowadays. Charles et al. (1997) summarize four features of shared decision-making in the medical encounter: (1) both doctors and patients are involved, (2) both share information, (3) both take steps to reach an agreement on the treatment, and (4) an agreement is eventually reached on implementation.

Emanuel and Emanuel (1992) propose four models describing patient-physician relationships in shared decision-making. In the paternalistic model, doctors present patients with selected information to convince patients of the treatment that doctors consider best. In contrast, in the informative model, doctors present patients with full information to let patients decide the treatment. The two models in between are the deliberative model, where doctors persuade patients of proper health values and let patients decide the treatment, and the interpretive model, where doctors help patients select the treatment based on patients' health values.

Mead and Bower (2000) summarize the factors influencing patient-physician relationships into five dimensions: patient factors (such as personality, gender, and age), doctor factors (such as ethnicity, knowledge, and attitudes), consultation-level influences (such as time and presence of third parties), professional-context influences (such as accreditation and government policy), and shapers (such as cultural norms and social expectations). Yedida (2007), on the other hand, suggests five different factors that affect patient-physician relationships: need (the extent to which patients' needs are solved), source of authority, establishment and maintenance of trust, emotional involvement of doctors with patients, and authenticity (the extent to which doctors and patients treat each other as individuals).

In both narratives, communication significantly affects the patient-physician relationship (see consultation-level influences in Mead and Bower (2000) and authenticity in Yedida (2007)), and it has been extensively studied from various aspects, such as narrative competence (Charon, 2001), out-of-pocket costs (Alexander, 2003), and legislative interference (Weinberger et al., 2012). Recently, Manalastas et al. (2021) proposed a novel method for visualizing the structure of patient-physician communication. Notably, patient-centered communication, which refers to the approach that doctors treat patients as unique individuals (Balint, 1969), try to see things from the patients' perspective (Stewart & Roter, 1990), and guide them using their education and experience (Byrne & Long, 1976), has attracted a lot of attention in recent years (Roter & Hall, 2004).

Other aspects of patient-physician relationships have also been studied. For example, Otani et al. (2012) find that doctor (staff) care becomes more (less) important with more severe medical conditions. In terms of patient experience, Doyle et al. (2013) find positive correlations between patient experience and patient safety / clinical effectiveness, but Snow et al. (2013) argue that though patient experience can give patients confidence, it cannot solve the power imbalance.

Notably, to the best of the authors' knowledge, the authors are among the pioneers in examining the impact of emerging technology on patient-physician communication and hence patient-physician relationships. Prominently, VR, as an emerging technology, has shown promise in recent years. Its application has been observed in diverse disciplines, including medicine. The application of VR in medicine can serve as a potent tool to enhance patient-physician communication and relationships. However, to date this new phenomenon has not received adequate attention. The authors thus take the lead on this cutting-edge topic. In particular, the current chapter looks at a case of applying VR in preoperative talks in orthopedics, which will be described in detail in the next section.

METHOD

This chapter intends to answer the question of how VR influences patient-physician communication (and hence relationships) and why this influence exists. As was noted in the previous section, there is a vacuum in the literature with respect to this topic. Most extant papers on the patient-physician relationship only describe its general underlying mechanisms, while research on the application of VR to patient-physician communication (and hence relationships) is at a very preliminary stage. Therefore, the authors adopt an explorative theory-building case study method. This method is considered an adequate approach to reflect respondents' experience, provide insights into this new phenomenon, and develop a testable theory for future studies (Eisenhardt, 1989). Through multiple data collection methods, including interviews and observation, the authors examine the process of doctors applying VR for preoperative talks. After describing the process, the impact of VR application on patient-physician communication (and hence relationships) is investigated.

Because VR is an advanced but expensive technology and only top hospitals with rich medical resources and financial support can embrace it, a single-case design was chosen as an accessible and inductive method for the authors to explore this novel phenomenon (Yin, 2008). The study was conducted in a provincial comprehensive grade-3 class-A hospital in a major city in northern China. The authors selected the current hospital as the source of informants for the theoretical purpose (theoretical sampling). The hospital has been on the Top 100 Hospitals List in China for four consecutive years, and its outpatient and emergency medical care ranks first in its province. The hospital jointly established the Institute of Digital Medicine and Computer Assisted Surgery with a Chinese multinational major appliances and electronics conglomerate and has developed an effective "industry-teaching-research" model. Notably, the hospital was one of the earliest in China to carry out digital medicine and computer-assisted surgery research and application. After years of growth, it has created an advantage in combining the research and development of digital medical equipment with clinical applications. Therefore, the choice of this hospital as our sample fits well with our research questions.

The authors primarily used in-depth interviews to collect data. Moreover, the authors utilized information from different sources (e.g., observation and archival documents) to triangulate and avoid bias. A convergence of information enhances credibility and gives more detailed insights into the targeted phenomenon (Carter et al., 2014; Yin, 2014). From 10 July 2021 to 1 August 2021, the authors conducted two waves of in-depth interviews involving three informants. The first informant is a distinguished expert in orthopedics, whose clinical direction is spinal deformity and spinal tumors. The second and third informants are young doctors who have just graduated from an accredited medical school and hold a medical degree. Table 1 presents a summary of the three informants.

Table 1. Summary of the informants

	Informant A (IA)	**Informant B (IB)**	**Informant C (IC)**
Position	Chief Physician	Residency	Residency
Length of Service (Years)	28	8	8
Gender	Male	Male	Female
Age	50-59	20-29	20-29
Race	Asian	Asian	Asian
Data Collection Method	Phone interview	Phone Interview	Phone Interview

Based on previous studies on VR and patient-physician relationships, the authors initially developed an interview protocol with a series of questions centering on (1) their perception of VR, (2) how to use VR in communication with patients or their family members, and (3) the feedback from physicians, patients, and their family members after using VR. The interview protocol is presented in Appendix 1. Because of the impact of the COVID-19 pandemic, the authors chose to collect data from each informant by semi-structured phone interviews (about thirty minutes), and the interview transcripts were then reviewed within two days. After two days, the authors conducted follow-up queries (about thirty minutes) to enhance the richness of the data. This process continued until no new information was derived from the interview (i.e., theoretical saturation).

With the informants' permission, all interview content was recorded. Then the authors transformed the content into transcripts and carefully checked the raw data within twelve hours to alleviate memory bias. The authors then categorized the raw data into first-order codes and aggregated them into more abstract second-order codes. After the coding process was finished, the authors jointly checked their first-order and second-order codes and determined the flow and relationships among these coherent categories with support from the literature (i.e., the third-order codes). A draft of this chapter was subsequently sent to the informants for confirmation of its accuracy and suggestion of minor modifications.

Specifically, the steps of data coding are as follows: (1) Interview transcript and informant coding - The authors transferred all phone interviews into scripts and provided an identifier for each informant (IA, IB, and IC, respectively). (2) First-order codes (open coding) - The authors obtained twelve first-order codes based on the raw materials. These themes include decision support, decision aid, enhancing cognition, reducing technical terminology, reducing complicated definitions, transferring knowledge, constructing complex concepts, conveying complex concepts, uncertain situations, unknown situations, ambiguity, and degree of threat. (3) Second-order codes (axial coding) - The authors abstracted four second-order codes from the twelve first-order codes. These constructs are information visualization (from decision support, decision aid, and enhancing cognition), information transfer (from reducing technical terminology and reducing complicated definitions), knowledge visualization (from transferring knowledge, constructing complex concepts, and conveying complex concepts), and uncertainty reduction (from uncertain situations, unknown situations, ambiguity, and degree of threat). Note that there are differences between information visualization and knowledge visualization (Tergan & Keller, 2005). Information visualization uses computer-aided applications to gain new insights, while knowledge visualization uses visual representations to improve knowledge transfer. Although both of them utilize the fact that human beings process visual information more quickly, their objectives, contents, and tools are different. Table 2 summarizes the data coding. (4) Third-order codes (selective coding) - Based on previous studies, the authors identify the possible relationship between these themes and develop an inductive model explaining how VR influences patient-physician relationships.

Table 2. Data coding process

Example Statements	First-order Coding (Themes)	Second-order Coding (Constructs)
Chief physicians, who are experienced, have an in-depth understanding of the disease. Although young physicians also understand the disease, the understanding is not as thorough. The anatomy is not as clear for young physicians, while VR makes it clearer.	Decision support Decision aid Enhancing cognition	Information visualization
Based on the patient's anatomy, for example, we will explain to the patient that there is a deformity in his/her body: The normal human body is like this, but your body is different from the normal one. The deformity compresses nearby blood vessels, as well as organs, which causes a series of symptoms.	Reducing technical terminology Reducing complicated definitions	Information transfer
What we have to do is place pedicle screws at some specific vertebrae. The screws are linked by a rod. By the twisting force of the rod, your spine can be returned to a normal condition, reducing the compression of blood vessels and relieving your symptoms.	Transferring knowledge Constructing complex concepts Conveying complex concepts	Knowledge visualization
When we do this step, it is possible to damage the nearby blood vessels and nerves. If patients look at animation and images, then they understand more clearly, and the communication efficiency is higher.	Uncertain situations Unknown situations Ambiguity Degree of threat	Uncertainty reduction

NARRATIVES AND ANALYSIS

Preoperative talks usually include three steps: First, doctors examine patients' conditions and plan the treatment (surgeries); second, doctors introduce the condition to patients; third, doctors communicate with patients on the treatment plan, of which the associated risk is an important part. Ideally, a consensus is reached between doctors and patients after preoperative talks. Figure 1 illustrates the process of preoperative talks, and the authors will give an account of how the process is impacted by VR's application in the following passage. Preoperative talks are critical in establishing trust, but at the same time, are a challenging task for doctors. Doctors need to patiently explain the treatment plan with well-understood terms, making patients fully aware of the effects and risks. Therefore, doctors are continuously looking for better ways to conduct preoperative talks.

Figure 1. The process of preoperative talks

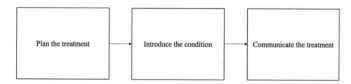

Both IA and IB used VR in medicine in August 2019 for the first time. As IA recalled, *"I met a VR person at a conference. He showed me some VR images of surgeries, and I was very interested. Since I happened to have a serious kyphosis patient, I invited him to build a VR model for me."* (A1). This technology immediately impressed IA and IB because it could help to understand the degree of deformity of a patient and the relationships among nearby blood vessels and nerves, which is impossible for traditional X-ray images. IB suggested that he was shocked by the power of VR. The hospital that IA and IB serve started to collaborate with the company to apply VR to a serious kyphosis case. After that time, IA continued working on related research and clinical applications with other companies. IC first heard about VR's application to medicine in 2019 but did not use it until 2021, and she also showed a positive attitude toward VR's application to medicine. Although accepted by doctors, VR applications in medicine have a long way to go; as IC commented, *"though VR applications grow fast and have a promising prospect, they are not yet prevalently used in medicine."* (C1).

Preoperative Talks

Before formal preoperative talks with patients and their family members, doctors need to totally understand the medical condition of patients. This requires rich surgical experience and a thorough understanding of the disease, which hinders young doctors. As IB stated,

Chief physicians, who are experienced, have an in-depth understanding of the disease. Although young physicians also understand the disease, the understanding is not as thorough. The anatomy is not as clear for young physicians, while VR makes it clearer. (B1).

At this pre-talk stage, VR can serve as a decision support system, which enhances the cognition of doctors (especially inexperienced doctors) by helping them visualize the condition of patients better to make better treatment decisions.

In the initial stage of a preoperative talk, it is usually very hard for patients and their family members to understand the condition and cause of the disease because they are not equipped with medical education and have no understanding of medical terminology. They have to form a concept of the problem based only on doctors' descriptions and X-ray images, which is time-consuming and emotionally exhausting. VR, as a visual aid, provides an effective communication device for transferring medical information. With VR, it is easier for doctors to explain the condition to patients, which significantly reduces the information barrier between doctors and patients. As IC commented,

Patients may not know the location and extent of spinal disc herniation, and they may not know their bone structure very well. When we use virtual reality, they will be better able to convince themselves how they are different from others and where they need to improve, and they usually pay more attention. (C2).

IB provided a detailed description of how to explain a condition.

Based on the patient's anatomy, for example, we will explain to the patient that there is a deformity in his/her body: The normal human body is like this, but your body is different from the normal one. The deformity compresses nearby blood vessels, as well as organs, which causes a series of symptoms. (B2).

Figure 2. An illustration of virtual reality modeling

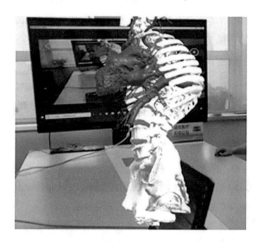

After coming to terms with their condition, understanding how the treatment, especially surgery, will be conducted is a further concern for patients. Doctors are often faced with difficulty in imparting their knowledge to patients due to the complexity of the concepts. In orthopedics, it is difficult for doctors to describe the surgical procedure through traditional X-ray images, as they are only two-dimensional rather than three-dimensional. However, VR can help patients better picture the whole surgical procedure. IB recalled how he explained a surgery to a patient through VR:

What we have to do is place pedicle screws at some specific vertebrae. The screws are linked by a rod. By the twisting force of the rod, your spine can be returned to a normal condition, reducing the compression of blood vessels and relieving your symptoms. (B3).

A critical component of describing a surgery is to describe the risk associated with it. People feel uncomfortable with uncertain situations. In the past, patients were not clearly informed about the risks they faced during surgeries (Bourquin et al., 2015), and this ambiguity made them nervous and anxious. The anxiety of patients led many of them to behave aggressively, hence deteriorating the patient-physician relationship. While a list of possible risks during surgery is provided in preoperative talks, patients and their family members may still form only a blurred view of the risks, and they remain uncertain about the exact consequences behind the risks. Through VR's application, doctors can explicitly explain the risks and thus reduce this uncertainty. IA recalled how he explained a surgery's risks to patients and their family members:

When we do this step, it is possible to damage the nearby blood vessels and nerves. If patients look at animation and images, then they understand more clearly, and the communication efficiency is higher. (A2).

He also added,

With VR, patients understand better; they understand better the consequences they need to undergo. (A3).

That is, patients learn that the treatment effect may not be as expected. Thus, if patients face unexpected outcomes after the treatment, they will consider it rationally and not blame doctors for the outcomes.

Overall, VR applications play a positive part in patient-physician communication and improve their relationships. IA mentioned,

VR makes communication more straightforward, and patients understand the surgical procedure and its risk more easily. (A4).

Moreover, by better understanding what doctors do and perceiving the difficulty and uncertainty during the treatment, patients will better accept unexpected results, significantly reducing disputes between the two sides.

Discussion

As previously discussed, preoperative talks have a tremendous influence on patient-physician relationships. Nervous patients seek treatment that provides an optimal balance between benefits and risks, and preoperative talks are the communication channel for doctors to persuade patients that the planned treatment is what they are looking for. However, doctors are in a quandary as to how to meet the high expectations of patients. In the past, physicians holistically explained diseases and treatments using technical terms, which is time-consuming and emotionally exhausting for patients. Otherwise, patients may lose trust in doctors and take withdrawal behaviors such as non-cooperation or complaint with the treatment.

In this chapter, VR is recognized as a powerful tool to relieve the tension between doctors and patients in preoperative talks. More specifically, VR with three-dimensional images and animations makes information visualization, information transfer, knowledge visualization, and uncertainty reduction easier, promoting patient-physician cooperation in the treatment process. Information visualization reinforces doctors' cognition when examining patients' conditions and planning their treatment; information transfer avoids the use of technical terminology that confuses patients; knowledge visualization enhances communication efficiency when complex concepts are involved; and uncertainty reduction soothes patients' anxiety when they are faced with unknown situations. Figure 2 shows an inductive process model of the way in which VR influences the patient-physician relationship in preoperative talks.

Figure 3. An inductive process model of VR's impact on patient-physician relationships in preoperative talks

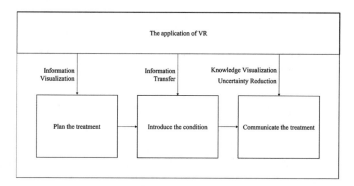

In addition to its impact on preoperative talks, the informants also discussed during the interview how they apply VR during surgeries, which provides insights into VR's potential impact in this realm. Specifically, remote surgery allows inexperienced doctors to obtain expert advice without constraints of geographic location, while virtual navigation provides doctors a comprehensive view of patients' bodies so that errors due to blind areas are avoided. A rise in the success probability of surgeries thanks to these benefits of VR would indirectly influence patient-physician relationships. Since the analysis of the use of VR during surgeries is not the focus of this chapter, it is postponed until Appendix 2.

Nevertheless, though VR applications work well in preoperative talks, they have not yet become widely popular for technical reasons; the preparation is time-consuming. To be specific, images of patients are created by radiologists, and these images have to be processed using software for optimal visualization and manipulation in three dimensions. In other words, it is not that convenient for hospitals to utilize VR every time. IC mentioned, *"we only use VR in special situations rather than ordinary cases."* (C3). She added, *"the technology is not mature enough. It cannot build models directly; it requires X-ray images to model. If this technology is better developed and builds models directly, it will be more convenient."* IB stated: *"We have to input data of patients to output models. The data are not in our department; they are in other departments. We have to copy data from them."* (C4).

FUTURE RESEARCH DIRECTIONS

In addition to the application of VR before surgery, which is the focus of this chapter, it is also interesting to examine the application of VR during surgery, i.e., computer-assisted surgery. In the past, the only devices available in operating rooms were laparoscopic cameras that allowed doctors to view the surface of the organs. As a direct application, VR (AR, augmented reality, to be exact) allows additional invisible information to be overlaid onto a doctor's vision, such as blood vessels or anatomical structures so that the doctor can operate with less uncertainty. This application should increase the success probability of surgeries and hence improve patient-physician relationships. In Appendix 2, the authors include a brief discussion of how computer-assisted surgery (or virtual navigation) may affect patient-physician relationships. A more rigorous examination, however, is beyond the scope of this chapter.

Second, VR also permits live streaming surgeries, where the family members of the patients can witness surgical procedures from the doctors' perspective. A patient undergoing cancer surgery at the Royal London Hospital is believed to be the first to have had his operation streamed live (BBC, 2016). In the past, the surgical procedures were not transparent from the family members' perspective. With the help of VR, family members can now see what the doctors see and sense the tremendous efforts they are making. By removing the opacity of operating rooms, the trust between doctors and patients (and patients' family members) is enhanced. This transparency also eliminates possible disputes during the surgery and is as well worth studying in the future.

Third, there are also general challenges of applying VR in medicine: (1) How to train doctors to appropriately adopt VR - Specialized training is necessary given the limited field and the absence of tactile information for some surgeries; (2) How to better plan surgeries using VR to reduce the duration and risk of surgeries - The three-dimensional models may offer a better-adapted solution to surgical planning, and by manipulating the models from all angles, doctors can plan the gestures to perform with a high degree of precision. Only when these challenges are overcome can VR release its full potential in medicine.

Fourth, managed care is another area worthy of attention. Managed care refers to a series of actions intended to reduce the cost and improve the quality of health care in the United States. Several studies look at patient-physician relationships in the context of managed care. For example, Emanuel and Dubler (1995) discuss how to preserve the patient-physician relationship in the age of managed care, while Mechanic and Schlesinger (1996) find that managed care changes patients' trust toward their doctors by eliminating choices and communications. Goold and Lipkin (1999) summarize opportunities and challenges in patient-physician relationships under managed care. However, these challenges have not been overcome, as shown in recent years when Kit et al. (2017) discovered again a predominantly negative correlation between managed care and patient-physician relationships.

CONCLUSION

This chapter discusses the applications of VR in medicine, primarily focusing on examining the process of doctors applying VR for preoperative talks and the impact of VR's application on patient-physician communication and hence their relationships. The authors adopt a case study approach and use in-depth interviews to collect data from three informants working in a top-ranked hospital in China. The authors obtained twelve first-order codes based on raw materials and abstracted them into four second-order codes.

The impact of VR's application on preoperative talks can be classified into four aspects: (1) Information visualization - VR helps doctors cognize the condition of patients, which facilitates better treatment decision-making; (2) Information transfer - With VR, it is easier for doctors to avoid technical terminology when they explain a condition to patients, which significantly reduces the communication barrier between doctors and patients; (3) Knowledge visualization - VR helps patients better picture the whole surgical procedure; (4) Uncertainty reduction - Through the application of VR, doctors can easily explain the risks of a surgery and ensure patients understand that the treatment effect may not be as expected. Overall, VR applications play a positive role in patient-physician communication and improve their relationships. The authors also discuss VR applications in remote surgery and virtual navigation in Appendix 2.

The contribution of this chapter is as follows. First, though there are papers examining the impact of emerging technologies on patient-physician relationships in general (Khanra et al, 2020; Lam et al., 2021), the authors are among the pioneers to focus on a specific technology in a specific stage of operations, i.e., preoperative talks. Notably, preoperative talks are critical in patient-physician relationships and are also one of the most challenging steps. Second, despite the fact that some researchers observe a positive impact of emerging technologies on patient-physician relationships, the mechanism behind this observation remains unclear. Figuring out the underlying mechanism can help (1) doctors to better utilize virtual reality, (2) companies to better design products, and (3) the government to better make public policy.

REFERENCES

Alexander, G. (2003). Patient-physician communication about out-of-pocket costs. *Journal of the American Medical Association*, *290*(7), 953–958. doi:10.1001/jama.290.7.953 PMID:12928475

Arnaldi, B., Guitton, P., & Moreau, G. (2018). *Virtual reality and augmented reality: myths and realities*. Wiley. doi:10.1002/9781119341031

Balint, E. (1969). The possibilities of patient-centered medicine. *The Journal of the Royal College of General Practitioners*, (17), 269–276. PMID:5770926

Baron, R. J., & Berinsky, A. J. (2019). Mistrust in science— A threat to the patient–physician relationship. *The New England Journal of Medicine*, *381*(2), 182–185. doi:10.1056/NEJMms1813043 PMID:31291524

BBC. (2014, March 26). *Facebook buys virtual reality headset start-up for $2 billion*. https://www.bbc.com/news/business-26742625

BBC. (2016, April 14). *Cancer surgery broadcast live in virtual reality*. https://www.bbc.com/news/av/technology-36046948

Beck, A. (2004). The Flexner report and the standardization of American medical education. *Journal of the American Medical Association*, *291*(17), 2139–2140. doi:10.1001/jama.291.17.2139 PMID:15126445

Bourquin, C., Stiefel, F., Mast, M., Bonvin, R., & Berney, A. (2015). Well, you have hepatic metastases: Use of technical language by medical students in simulated patient interviews. *Patient Education and Counseling*, *98*(3), 323–330. doi:10.1016/j.pec.2014.11.017 PMID:25535013

Byrne, P., & Long, B. (1976). *Doctors talking to patients*. HMSO.

Carter, N., Bryant-Lukosius, D., DiCenso, A., Blythe, J., & Neville, A. J. (2014). The use of triangulation in qualitative research. *Oncology Nursing Forum*, *41*(5), 545–547. doi:10.1188/14.ONF.545-547 PMID:25158659

Charles, C., Gafni, A., & Whelan, T. (1997). Shared decision-making in the medical encounter: What does it mean? (or it takes at least two to tango). *Social Science & Medicine*, *44*(5), 681–692. doi:10.1016/S0277-9536(96)00221-3 PMID:9032835

Charon, R. (2001). Narrative medicine. *Journal of the American Medical Association*, *286*(15), 1897–1902. doi:10.1001/jama.286.15.1897 PMID:11597295

Cotin, S., Delingette, H., Bro-Nielsen, M., Ayache, N., Clement, J., Tassetti, V., & Marescaux, J. (1996). Geometric and physical representations for a simulator of hepatic surgery. *Studies in Health Technology and Informatics*, *1*(29), 139–151. PMID:10163746

Doyle, C., Lennox, L., & Bell, D. (2013). A systematic review of evidence on the links between patient experience and clinical safety and effectiveness. *BMJ Open*, *3*(1), e001570. Advance online publication. doi:10.1136/bmjopen-2012-001570 PMID:23293244

Eisenhardt, K. (1989). Building theories from case study research. *Academy of Management Review*, *14*(4), 532–550. doi:10.5465/amr.1989.4308385

Emanuel, E., & Dubler, N. (1995). Preserving the physician-patient relationship in the era of managed care. *Journal of the American Medical Association*, *273*(4), 323–329. doi:10.1001/jama.1995.03520280069043 PMID:7815662

Emanuel, E., & Emanuel, L. (1992). Four models of the physician-patient relationship. *Journal of the American Medical Association*, *267*(16), 2221–2226. doi:10.1001/jama.1992.03480160079038 PMID:1556799

Flickinger, T., Saha, S., Moore, R., & Beach, M. (2013). Higher quality communication and relationships are associated with improved patient engagement in HIV care. *JAIDS Journal of Acquired Immune Deficiency Syndromes*, *63*(3), 362–366. doi:10.1097/QAI.0b013e318295b86a PMID:23591637

Goold, S., & Lipkin, M. (1999). The doctor-patient relationship. *Journal of General Internal Medicine*, *14*(S1), S26–S33. Advance online publication. doi:10.1046/j.1525-1497.1999.00267.x PMID:9933492

Khanra, S., Dhir, A., Islam, A., & Mäntymäki, M. (2020). Big Data Analytics in Healthcare: A systematic literature review. *Enterprise Information Systems*, *14*(7), 878–912. doi:10.1080/17517575.2020.1812005

Kilbride, M., & Joffe, S. (2018). The new age of patient autonomy. *Journal of the American Medical Association*, *320*(19), 1973–1974. doi:10.1001/jama.2018.14382 PMID:30326026

Kit, P., Rasid, S., Ismail, W., & Mokhber, M. (2017). Can managed care really improve doctor–patient relationship? *Journal of Health Management*, *19*(1), 192–202. doi:10.1177/0972063416682895

Lam, H. Y., Ho, G. T. S., Mo, D. Y., & Tang, V. (2021). Enhancing data-driven elderly appointment services in domestic care communities under COVID-19. *Industrial Management & Data Systems, 121*(7), 1552–1576. doi:10.1108/IMDS-07-2020-0392

Manalastas, G., Noble, L., Viney, R., & Griffin, A. E. (2021). What does the structure of a medical consultation look like? A new method for visualizing doctor-patient communication. *Patient Education and Counseling, 104*(6), 1387–1397. doi:10.1016/j.pec.2020.11.026 PMID:33272747

Mead, N., & Bower, P. (2000). Patient-centredness: A conceptual framework and review of the empirical literature. *Social Science & Medicine, 51*(7), 1087–1110. doi:10.1016/S0277-9536(00)00098-8 PMID:11005395

Mechanic, D., & Schlesinger, M. (1996). The impact of managed care on Patients' trust in medical care and their physicians. *Journal of the American Medical Association, 275*(21), 1693–1697. doi:10.1001/jama.1996.03530450083048 PMID:8637148

Otani, K., Waterman, B., & Dunagan, W. (2012). Patient satisfaction: How patient health conditions influence their satisfaction. *Journal of Healthcare Management, 57*(4), 276–293. doi:10.1097/00115514-201207000-00009 PMID:22905606

Persaud, R. (2005). How to improve communication with patients. *BMJ (Clinical Research Ed.), 330*(7494), s136–s137. Advance online publication. doi:10.1136/bmj.330.7494.s136

Pincock, S. (2003). Patients put their relationship with their doctors as second only to that with their families. *BMJ (Clinical Research Ed.), 327*(7415), 581-c–581. Advance online publication. doi:10.1136/bmj.327.7415.581-c PMID:12969915

Roter, D., & Hall, J. (2004). Physician gender and patient-centered communication: A critical review of empirical research. *Annual Review of Public Health, 25*(1), 497–519. doi:10.1146/annurev.publhealth.25.101802.123134 PMID:15015932

Snow, R., Humphrey, C., & Sandall, J. (2013). What happens when patients know more than their doctors? Experiences of health interactions after diabetes patient education: A qualitative patient-led study: Table 1. *BMJ Open, 3*(11), e003583. Advance online publication. doi:10.1136/bmjopen-2013-003583 PMID:24231459

Stanford Medicine. (2017, July 11). *Virtual reality system helps surgeons, reassures patients.* https://med.stanford.edu/news/all-news/2017/07/virtual-reality-system-helps-surgeons-reassures-patients.html

Stewart, M., & Roter, D. (1990). Communicating with medical patients. *Sage (Atlanta, Ga.).*

Szasz, T., & Hollender, M. (1956). A contribution to the philosophy of medicine. *A.M.A. Archives of Internal Medicine*, *97*(5), 585–592. doi:10.1001/archinte.1956.00250230079008 PMID:13312700

Tergan, S.-O., & Keller, T. (2005). *Knowledge and information visualization: Searching for synergies*. Springer. doi:10.1007/b138081

The Lancet. (2012). Ending violence against doctors in China. *Lancet*, *379*(9828), 1764. Advance online publication. doi:10.1016/S0140-6736(12)60729-6

The Lancet. (2010). Chinese doctors are under threat. *The Lancet, 376*(9742), 657. doi:10.1016/S0140-6736(10)61315-3

Weinberger, S., Lawrence, H. III, Henley, D., Alden, E., & Hoyt, D. (2012). Legislative interference with the patient–physician relationship. *The New England Journal of Medicine*, *367*(16), 1557–1559. doi:10.1056/NEJMsb1209858 PMID:23075183

World Health Organization. (2020, March 3). *Shortage of personal protective equipment endangering health workers worldwide*. https://www.who.int/news/item/03-03-2020-shortage-of-personal-protective-equipment-endangering-health-workers-worldwide

Yedidia, M. (2007). Transforming doctor-patient relationships to promote patient-centered care: Lessons from palliative care. *Journal of Pain and Symptom Management*, *33*(1), 40–57. doi:10.1016/j.jpainsymman.2006.06.007 PMID:17196906

Yin, R. K. (2014). Case study research: Design and methods. *Sage (Atlanta, Ga.).*

KEY TERMS AND DEFINITIONS

Comprehension: VR can offer support through its interaction to let users better understand certain complex concepts. This complexity can result from difficulty or even impossibility in accessing information.

Computer-Assisted Surgery: VR and other computer software are adopted for the training, planning, and operating of surgeries.

Orthopedics: The branch of medicine concerned with the skeletal system. Orthopedic doctors use both surgical and nonsurgical means to treat skeletal diseases, such as bone trauma, bone tumors, and spine diseases.

Patient-Physician Communication: Communication between doctors and patients is an essential element of patient-physician relationships. Efficient and effective communication facilitates accurate diagnosis, provides precise treatment instructions, and establishes trust with patients.

Patient-Physician Relationship: The relationship between doctors and patients is formed because of medical needs. This relationship is highly dependent on communication between doctors and patients.

Preoperative Talk: The patient-physician communication before a surgery usually includes explaining the disease, the procedure of the surgery, and the risk of the surgery. Proper preoperative talks increase the probability of successful surgery.

Virtual Reality: The system lets users carry out real tasks in a virtual environment through immersion in this environment or interaction with the system.

Visualization: Visualization adopts images, charts, and animations to convey messages. Visualization is a helpful way to communicate both abstract and concrete information.

APPENDIX 1: INTERVIEW PROTOCOL

General questions:

1. Could you please briefly introduce your background and work experience?
2. When was the first time you used VR?
3. What is your perception of VR?

Detailed questions:

4. How did you use VR when you communicated with patients or their family members?
5. How did VR affect your communication with patients or their family members?

Additional questions:

6. In which situation do you prefer to use VR?
7. Do you think it is a challenge for you to use VR?

APPENDIX 2: VR DURING SURGERIES

Besides preoperative talks, the informants also mentioned other VR applications in medicine, such as remote surgery and virtual navigation, which can also help patient-physician relationships.

Remote surgery solves geographical problems. In China, the distribution of medical experts is not balanced. There may be a lack of experts in hospitals in rural areas, and experts in major cities like Shanghai and Beijing may help to show-how via VR. The hospital that the authors studied in this chapter has remotely guided another hospital to perform surgery. IA said: *"We advise them remotely, for example, when to place screws, where to place screws, and in which direction. We will operate with pen and paper, and they can see because our visions overlap."* (A5). IB added, *"we are able to teach them in real-time, where is this part, what you need to do, and what you need to pay attention to. Because our visions overlap, they can know where we refer to, which helps them perform surgery."* (B4). IC commented, *"VR makes it possible to receive satisfactory treatment in one's hometown and helps a wider range of people resolve their medical conditions."* (C5).

Another VR application in medicine is virtual navigation. As stated in the chapter, there are some risks during the surgical process, some of which result from doctors' blind areas. With VR, doctors can have a comprehensive view of patients' bodies and improve performance accuracy in surgeries, especially complicated surgeries. IB gave an example in orthopedics, *"patients' spines are not as regular as normal people's; some spines are seriously deformed. Because patients face down during the surgery, you can only see from the back but not from the front. An experienced doctor may perform based on experience, while an inexperienced one may employ VR to increase accuracy."* (B5).

To summarize, VR also influences patient-physician relationships during surgeries by improving the success probability of surgical operations. First, VR resolves the geographic problem and helps patients in rural areas acquire advice from experts in major cities. Second, VR increases the performance accuracy during the surgery because blind areas of doctors are eliminated.

Chapter 5
Virtual Reality Scene Development for Upper Limb Tendonitis Rehabilitation Game

Karen Sie
Hong Kong Polytechnic University, China

Yuk Ming Tang
🆔 https://orcid.org/0000-0001-8215-4190
Hong Kong Polytechnic University, China

Kenneth Nai Kuen Fong
Hong Kong Polytechnic University, China

EXECUTIVE SUMMARY

With the development of new technology, it is common that excessive use puts undue strain on the hands and finger tendons. This increases the risk of developing many forms of tendonitis. The objective in this project is to use the latest virtual reality (VR) technology to build a preventive rehabilitation game for raising public awareness of upper limb tendonitis. A survey of 141 respondents was first undertaken to find how much the general public knows about upper limb tendonitis. A virtual game is then created using the Unity3D game engine and 3Ds Max for 3D modeling. It is evaluated after being tested by five participants. The majority of respondents to the questionnaire did not know the cause or implications of tendon issues. Almost half of them spent 8.8 hours per day on computers and smartphones, with only 4 minutes per day spent exercising their hands and fingers. The participants gave positive comments towards the designed rehabilitation game and believe it can help to avoid fatigue caused by prolonged smartphone and computer use.

DOI: 10.4018/978-1-7998-8790-4.ch005

INTRODUCTION

Virtual Reality (VR) technology was first developed in the mid-1960s and has become increasingly popular over time (Wilson, 1992). The first uses of virtual reality were in military and space-related research (Freitas et. al, 2014). According to Olasky et al. (2015), VR technology was then used in engineering, entertainment, education, and even medical settings. Rizzo and Kim (2005) found that both the therapist and the patient benefit from the use of virtual reality technology in rehabilitation. Therapists can utilize virtual reality surgical simulation to improve performance in real surgery by planning ahead of time. Patients with psychological issues, on the other hand, can be treated in secure virtual rehabilitation settings. Copyright © 2017, IGI Global. Copying or distributing in print or electronic forms without written permission of IGI Global is prohibited.

VR technology not only provides a safe environment for patients to do exercises, but also increases their physical and mental fidelity to do so (Lau et al., 2020). The VR environment enables real-time data collection and analysis, allowing therapists to alter and monitor patient development in order to improve rehabilitation efficiency and effectiveness (De Mauro, 2011). Celinder and Peoples (2012) strongly supported VR now being used on patients with psychosocial issues, neuromotor diseases, and cognitive issues. Moreover, VR has been applied for educational and training purposes in the medical field (Lau et al., 2021). The most common illnesses treated in VR rehabilitation include stroke (Fong et al., 2021), Post-Traumatic Stress Disorder (PTSD), and Parkinson's disease (Laver et al., 2015). Currently, there are only a few occupational disease applications. According to Liu and Chiang (2020), De Quervain's Tenosynovitis - a kind of tendonitis over the thumb and wrist, is due to tendon sheath inflammation. For the past twelve years, De Quervain's Tenosynovitis of the hand or forearm has ranked first among occupational disorders. Tendinosis is more common since there is a lack of public awareness of tendon problems. Rehabilitation also emphasizes on both the prevention and treatment of tendonitis.

VR has been used in other types of sickness rehabilitation, and it has been shown to increase patient or user motivation and promote a safe virtual environment (VE) (De Mauro, 2011). There have been numerous studies on the feasibility and escalation of patient motivation through the use of virtual reality in rehabilitation (Fidopiasti et al., 2006). However, existing VR rehabilitation technology is primarily aimed towards patients with psychosocial issues, neuromotor disorders, and cognitive issues. Although there are some VR rehabilitation games for stroke or PTSD patients, there is little research or application for occupational disorders, particularly De Quervain's Tendinosis. It is perceived that the main favorable advantage of employing VR is to increase patient motivation. Weiss et al. (2006) stressed that motivation is essential for efficient rehabilitation, so VR can be used to treat occupational disorders encouragingly.

The objective of this project is to develop preventive VR scenarios that focus on finger and wrist exercises. The VR game not only allows patients or users to be treated more engagingly, but also raises public awareness of repetitive cumulative trauma disorders and thereby reduces the risk of tendonitis. The intended audience for the game is individuals who have not been diagnosed with De Quervain's Tendinosis or any other tendon problems in their arms or shoulders. The game allows players to be treated more interactively while also raising public awareness of tendon problems. To develop a VR game, an idea is produced and tweaked several times in order to deliver the most user-friendly VR game environment at a reasonable cost. A non-immersive VR game is developed at the end of the project. The Leap Motion Controller (LMC) is employed as a gesture sensor device to regulate the software's feedback. A thorough and well-researched examination of VR and its applications, as well as tendon diseases, is completed afterward. Evaluation of the developed game, followed by testing results and questions from testers is done at the end.

LITERATURE REVIEW

Virtual Reality (VR) Technologies

VR is a technology that provides users immersive and interactive experience. Although there are many different definitions of virtual reality, they all share similar descriptions. Rield (2004) defined VR as an immersive, interactive, and three-dimensional computer-based experience that happens in real-time.

Non-immersive VR, semi-immersive VR, and fully immersive VR are the three categories of VR systems (Mujber et al., 2004). A computer with an advanced graphics card, software, a tracking device, and an image display system are the four main components of a VR system (Wang et al., 2018). Earphones, gesture-sensing gloves, and head-mounted displays (HMDs), and haptic-feedback devices were employed as examples of the gadgets that were utilized (Schultheis & Rizzo, 2001). VR has a distinct outstanding feature that allows the user to have a sense of belonging and presence in the VE (Grajewski et al., 2013). VR provides users with real-time data that can be used in complex interactions, behavioral tracking, and performance recording. Sherman and Craig (2019) mentioned that there are four key elements in experiencing virtual reality: virtual world, immersion, sensory feedback, and interactivity. These key elements can be presented to players with hardware devices and technologies mentioned.

Figure 1. System architecture of VRS and its VR-based extension
(Steinicke et al., 2005)

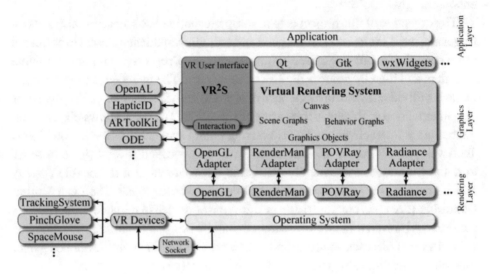

VR2S, the graphic layer of a VR system, is made up of three layers: application, graphics, and rendering (Steinicke et al., 2005), as shown in Figure 1. The VR engine, input and output devices, software and database, user, and task are the five basic aspects of VR. A canvas defines the drawing area for VE. Hierarchical scene graphs specify orientations with static and dynamic features of virtual objects. Behavior graphs represent the event and time-dependent behavior of the virtual scene, and graphic objects indicate its physical attributes. Steinicke et al. (2005) state that there are four key components to deal with during the development of a 3D application. Input and output devices make up user interfaces (UI). Input devices use mechanical, magnetic, ultrasonic, or optical mechanisms to check the user's location and movements. For example, trackers can use gloves, Head-Mounted Displays (HMDs), and Kinect to trace head, hand, and body position and orientation.

Regarding the review done by Guzsvinecz et al. (2019), the Leap Motion controller (LMC) is a hand tracker that has a one-meter hemispherical view area with a 150° field of view. It can be used to track a user's finger movement with a rate of over 200 frames per second such that the screen display keeps on changing with the user's every movement. LMC uses the right-handed Cartesian coordinate system and the axes. The accuracy of fingertip position tracking is precise to approximately 0.01 millimeters which allows accurate finger and hand gesture tracking.

LMC comprises three Infrared Light (IR) emitters and two cameras that belong to optical tracking systems. As analyzed by Weichert et al. (2013), LMC uses structured IR light to create a 3D depth map. LMC provides information about all fingers joints, even if they are not all visible, by estimating with an anatomical model of hand in Leap Motion software (Ebert et al., 2014). Certain hands and fingers movements can be recognized by the software. The movements are then linked to different command sets by the programmer.

VR in Healthcare and Medical Applications

In 1993, the first application of VR in medicine was for the treatment of mental health diseases (Rizzo & Kim, 2005). VR allows significant improvements in both time and quality (De Mauro, 2011). VR users can be divided into two categories: therapists and patients. VR is used by therapists for diagnosis and surgery rehearsal. The patient's rehabilitation is aided by VR technology, resulting in a faster recovery time and a more enjoyable treatment procedure. The next two sections describe the specifics of how VR is utilized and its benefits.

VR surgical simulation has already matured and is primarily employed in minimally invasive surgery. Organs in the virtual surgical environment not only look like genuine organs, but they also act like real organs. A study done by Wiederhold (2006) investigated if there is a way to complement smell in VR surgery. One of the most exciting developments in the use of virtual reality to treat patients with psychological disorders. Clinical anxiety disorders employ relaxation techniques to control their reactions when confronted with threatening situations (Wiederhold, 2006). VR allows for safe simulation, which in this situation allows for more effective and efficient therapy (Tang et al., 2021).

VR has the potential to divert patients from the discomfort of an injury, disease, or medical procedure (Malloy & Milling, 2010). VR is currently considered distraction therapy for acute labor and delivery pain. The discomfort of patients with serious burn wounds can be decreased by 30%-50%, according to researchers (Wiederhold, 2006). Gershon et al. (2004) researched youngsters with cancer and found that utilizing a virtual tool can reduce pain and anxiety. It is a revolutionary application of VR for vocational training and rehabilitation of brain-damaged people. Many studies have been conducted on stroke patients, demonstrating the usefulness of VR and affirmative progress (Cho et al., 2014).

Simulating 3D reconstruction of radiological cross-sections can provide a clear-cut perspective for therapists, and VR is becoming an important diagnostic tool (Wiederhold, 2006). Medical personnel can examine the simulated data to validate the diagnosis (Djukic et al., 2013). A plethora of studies and experiments demonstrate the benefits of using VR in rehabilitation. Both therapists and patients gain from VR. Because the tendency is higher than non-VR rehabilitation, medical personnel can increase treatment abilities and operation performance, while patients' recovery training becomes more effective.

Upper Limb Tendonitis and VR Rehabilitation

Many businesses, such as information technology and banking, rely on computers to input and analyze data in today's world. Malarvani et al. (2014) point out that workers cannot avoid using computer keyboards. Workers rarely get adequate rest, which causes pain in the shoulders, hands, and fingers. Meanwhile, individuals send messages, surf the web, and check social media via smartphones that have become indispensable everyday life activities thanks to low-cost mobile phone data plans and the availability and accessibility of free Wi-Fi. As a result, fingers, particularly thumbs, are used more frequently (Malarvani et al., 2014). Tenosynovitis of the Hand or Forearm was among the top three ailments in Hong Kong between 2002 and 2012, according to a data study from the Legislative Council Panel on Manpower (2013). This disease accounted for 24.6 percent of all illnesses in 2012, which is a substantial number.

According to the Labor Department's data (2019), the number of Tenosynovitis cases fluctuated in the period 2010 to 2019, and the condition was most common among salespeople, clerical support employees, and workers in elementary occupations. Regarding the Internet World Stats statistical report done by Miniwatts Marketing Group (2014), nearly three billion people worldwide used the internet in 2013, with Asia having the highest number of users and North America having the highest penetration percentage, with eight people using the internet for every ten people.

A study conducted by (PolyU, 2013) and the Hong Kong Physiotherapy Association (2013) has shown that 70% of adults and 30% of children and teenagers have experienced musculoskeletal symptoms in various parts of the body, with the symptoms being linked to the use of smart devices. Excessive texting with cellphones has been demonstrated in certain studies to promote tendon inflammation and articular degeneration in the thumb joint and index fingers. Malarvani et al. (2014) coined the name SMS syndrome – WhatsAppitis, which is also known as mother's wrist syndrome, De Quervain's syndrome, and other terms. The researchers conducted an experiment to assess wrist, index finger, and thumb muscle strength and a range of motion, and the results revealed substantial differences between the experimental and control groups. The pace at which people text is not a cause of creating muscular tiredness, according to the study.

Furthermore, according to Taneja (2014), people with a no-mobile phobia are terrified of not being able to use their phones for any reason. The dread of becoming socially isolated could be the reason. In recent years, posting images and updating status on social media has become commonplace. Those who do not check social media daily will most likely miss out on the most popular chatting subjects, will be unable to join in on their friends' leisure conversations, and will be tagged as old-fashioned. People check social media and submit comments more frequently in order to avoid feeling lonely, which causes the movement of thumbs to rise.

Rehabilitation refers to the extent to which body structure and functions, as well as activities, have returned to their pre-stroke form, whereas rehabilitation refers to the process of treatment (Bernhardt et al., 2017). Hart (2009) affirmed that rehabilitation can help patients overcome physical, psychological, and social-environmental issues. Both prevention and treatment are elements of rehabilitation, as the proverb goes, "prevention is better than cure."

Physical and occupational therapy help patients regain and repair muscle, bone, and nervous system function following amputations, burns, neurological difficulties, spinal cord injuries, stroke, and other ailments (Bernhardt et al., 2017). These two therapies are comparable and connected, however, they cannot be substituted for one another. Physical therapy focuses on functional aspects such as mobility, transfer, muscle and joint function, balance, neuromotor development, and so on, whereas occupational therapy focuses on the complete process from initial evaluation through ongoing assessment and subsequent assessment of an individual as a whole (Iconaru, 2014). Furthermore, physical therapy is typically used to treat physical illnesses, whereas occupational therapy is used to treat occupational diseases and a person's functional capacity (Creek & Bullock, 2008).

Motivation is critical in rehabilitation since only those patients who are willing to exercise have a higher recovery rate (De Mauro, 2011). In treatment, a serious game is used, which is more enticing and intriguing (Weiss et al., 2006). VR creates a "real-life" setting that allows users to forget they are in a testing environment. The actions and movements grow more natural. At the same time, patients' willingness to participate in training increases as they experience significantly less stress than they did during their initial recovery and find it more enjoyable (Levac & Galvin, 2013). VR has the potential to be an effective treatment for addictive behavior. The fight against smoking has always been a major issue. Teen smokers can reduce their nicotine cravings by using VR, which has appealing visuals (Wiederhold, 2006).

Numerous publications have been published that examine the usefulness of commercial VR games in rehabilitation for a variety of patients, including stroke, cerebral palsy, and Parkinson's disease. Chuang and Sung (2012) advocated conducting a randomized controlled experiment to see if using virtual reality in training for patients who had coronary artery bypass graft surgery was useful. The results demonstrated that there are significant perceived improvements in terms of physical capacity recovery. In a meta-analysis, Celinder and Peopies (2012) concluded that virtual reality applications are potential options for increasing therapy intensity and facilitating stroke patients' motor rehabilitation. Although there are numerous reviews, the spectrum of target patients is limited in these publications, there is no consistency in testing in terms of rating, and the sample size is typically small, making comparison difficult. Furthermore, there are just a few systematic reviews on the efficiency of virtual reality in rehabilitation, and there is no agreement on the effectiveness of improving physiological function, activities used, or participation levels. As a result, few studies support the usefulness in motor rehabilitation (Laver et al., 2017).

METHODOLOGY

There are six major steps to implement the methodology of this project (Figure 2). First, a SWOT analysis is undertaken to analyze the strengths, weaknesses, opportunities, and threats of VR in rehabilitation. Then, a questionnaire is conducted through the Internet to collect users' feedback towards the knowledge of tendonitis for the general public. Evaluation is designed to capture testers' opinions on game content, instruction, and feedbacks of the game at the end after the implementation and testing of the VR programme. The opinions collected are considered for analysis of the game as well as further developing and modifying the game in the future.

Figure 2. Flow of project implementation

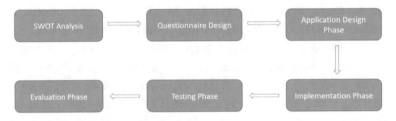

Strength, Weakness, Opportunities and Threats (SWOT) Analysis

In terms of rehabilitation, virtual reality offers a variety of advantages. It does, however, have its limitations. The four aspects of a SWOT analysis are strengths, weaknesses, opportunities, and threats. This analysis aids in a complete understanding of VR rehabilitation and also improves strategic planning or decision-making. A SWOT analysis for VR rehabilitation is shown in the table below (Rizzo & Kim, 2005).

VR allows patients to test and train in a safe setting, which is critical. This keeps patients safe during their recovery by preventing them from getting into an unwanted accident. VR improves stimulus control and consistency, and provides real-time feedback on performance, and helps students learn without making mistakes. It also

Figure 3. SWOT analysis for VR rehabilitation and therapy

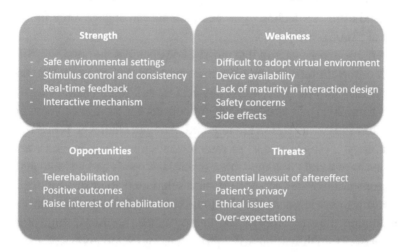

provides a secure environment for testing and training. Interaction mechanisms allow are a significant feature of using VR as it increases impressiveness. VR has been shown to help patients successfully and efficiently. However, there are still several weaknesses regarding VR usage in rehabilitation. Since therapists are typically forced to use existing technology to achieve the goal of therapy, patient engagement becomes considerably less natural, and learning to navigate the VE becomes a difficult task for patients with cognitive or physical limitations. Rapid changes in hardware capabilities and device availability, as well as a lack of maturity in interaction design, are some of the major roadblocks to establishing a useful VR rehabilitation system. Meanwhile, the required wires and connectors not only pose a safety risk, but also serve as a source of distraction for the patients (Rizzo & Kim, 2005). Despite the positive descriptions of VR as safe and useful, it does have certain negative side effects, which are classified as cybersickness and aftereffects. The images created by VR are not identical to the things, in reality, necessitating user recalibration. The possibility of experiencing cybersickness and post-exposure visual aftereffects increases when binocular vision is unstable (DiZio & Lackner, 1992).

McCue et al. (2010) recognized the possibility of VR rehabilitation. "The application of telecommunication, remote sensing and operation technologies, and computing technologies to aid with the provision of medical rehabilitation services at a distance" is how telerehabilitation is defined (Cooper et al., 2001). This strategy improves rural patient rehabilitation by reducing travel time to urban clinics, improving outcomes, and lowering expenses (Messinger et al., 2009). An experiment testing VR telerehabilitation games for teenagers who suffer from hemiplegic cerebral palsy gave a positive outcome in improvement in hand function and forearm bone health in patients (Golomb et al., 2010). Moreover, motivation for rehabilitation can be raised using VR technologies and patients can engage more in the training (Weiss et al., 2006).

One of the primary concerns that must be considered is the possibility of a lawsuit as a result of the aftereffects. As the parties who aid patients with VR technology, aftereffects may expose developers, physicians, and researchers to responsibility (Rizzo & Kim, 2005). In addition, patient consent for the use of virtual reality in rehabilitation and extra caution are required. Another challenge posed by evolving VR technology is ethical issues, as researchers, clinical applications, and patient populations have a right to know about potential hazards and advantages. In every ethical argument, there are almost no clear-cut solutions that can resolve all difficulties. Apart from the foregoing, because VR should be considered a professional instrument in rehabilitation, the credibility of VR therapy may be harmed if some practitioners lack the necessary qualifications to begin the therapy (Schulteis & Rothbaum, 2002). Once the new technology is used in routine therapy, users' expectations are raised and they become overly reliant on VR, posing a new threat. To address this issue, researchers must research the validity of virtual reality, and users must adapt their expectations.

Questionnaire Design

A survey was created to find out how much the general population knows about tendon problems. It was designed to understand the respondents' behaviors in using a smartphone or other device and was distributed online. The questionnaire consists of twelve questions divided into five sections that investigate respondents' computer accessory and smartphone activities, frequency of computer accessory and smartphone usage per week, frequency of hand and finger exercise per week, the severity of body discomfort, and awareness of tendonitis.

In the first part, questions were used to determine which types of activities respondents engage infrequently when using computer accessories and smartphones. In the second part, questions were designed posed to determine how much time the respondents spend using computer accessories and smartphones. In the third part, the amount of time spent on exercising hands and fingers every week was asked. In part four, questions were asked to determine the severity of the respondent's body discomfort, and if they have ever experienced continual fatigue as a result of extended usage of computer accessories or smartphones, as well as which regions of their body were affected. Part five contains questions aimed at determining the respondent's level of awareness of tendon problems. Respondents were asked if they are aware of the causes and implications of ten different types of tendonitis/ tendon condition, as well as other disease-related information such as linked syndromes and medical treatment options.

Application Design and Implementation

The hardware setup of the VR game-based training includes a private computer and a sensor to collect user hand motion data. In this project, we adopted the Leap Motion Controller (LMC) to collect the user's hand wrist, and fingers motions. LMC is a low-cost, contactless gesture sensor, and small device that does not requires a lot of space for training. LMC offers a high level of tracking precision, and there is an official online platform for developers to share their work and knowledge about LMC so that it can be used in rehabilitation. It also provides an official platform with resources and examples that makes the development of the virtual reality game much easier and faster. In the VR program development, the Unity3D game engine is selected for this project. Furthermore, Unity3D and 3DsMax are used in building game environments and assets.

This VR game-based training is designed to strengthen the user's finger and hand muscles. The upward movement may also help to lessen the risk of tendonitis in the arms and shoulders. We designed four tasks to complete in the application in which each part targets training different parts of the hand. Task one requires players to press the password. In order to press the number pad, "screen tap" movement is involved. "Screen tap" describes the motion using a finger to do a tapping action on a vertical computer screen. By doing so, fingers and wrist can be exercised. Task two requires players to push a door, involving push movement. When pushing the door, the biceps are extracted and relaxed. Hand, arm, and shoulder are trained in this task. Task three requires players to grab a cup from left to right and hold it to fill water. During this task, grabbing movement and holding movements are involved. The movement of the entire hand is involved in this task. For task four, players need to pick up objects and place them in designated spots. Pick-up movement is required for finger, wrist, hand, and arm to participate in the training process.

A timer is displayed in the top left corner of the screen, indicating how much time the player has left till the game is over. Players need to complete all tasks to obtain a training report with the amount of time indicating the effects and possible progress of VR training. Hence, players can trace the progress of training by saving the result reports.

RESULTS

Questionnaire Results

A survey of public awareness about tendon problems was undertaken via the Internet. There were 141 respondents, 78 women, and 63 men. Nearly two-thirds of those polled (63.8%) admitted to using a computer to check social media sites (Facebook, Instagram, Twitter). Over half of the respondents (58.9%) read and send an email on their computers. Two-fifths of respondents (44%) used computers to complete assignments or projects, while less than two-fifths of respondents (37.6%) used computers for office work. The majority of respondents (91.5%) used their cell phones to send and receive text messages (SMS, WhatsApp) and to monitor social media (Facebook, Instagram, and Twitter) (70.9%). More than half of the respondents (57.4% and 53.2%, respectively) used their smartphones to surf the Internet and make phone calls. Almost half of the respondents (47.5%) used their smartphones to read and send an email. Nearly a quarter of the respondents (28.4% and 21.3%, respectively) used their smartphones to perform calculations and other tasks.

Around 40% of those polled used computer accessories for more than 31 hours per week. The remaining respondents used for 21-30 hours, 11-20 hours, and fewer than 10 hours. A quarter of the respondents use their smartphones for 21 to 30 hours per week. Around 15% of respondents used it for 11-20 hours per week, while the rest use it for fewer than 10 hours per week.

Around half of the people polled (52.48% and 48.94%, respectively) said they only exercise their fingers and hands for less than 15 minutes every week. One-fifth of those surveyed (19.15% and 19.86%, respectively) exercise their fingers and hands for 15 to 30 minutes every week. Only around a tenth (9.22% and 7.8%, respectively) exercise their fingers and hands for 31 to 45 minutes per week. Around 20% of those polled spend more than 45 minutes exercising their fingers and hands. Moreover half of the respondents (56.03%) said they have never experienced continual exhaustion as a result of prolonged usage of computer peripherals or smartphones, implying that one out of every two people has experienced constant fatigue.

Figure 4 describes the distribution of body discomfort in the finger, wrist, upper arm, palm, forearm, shoulder, and others. 64 out of 141 people (45.4%) said they had shoulder pain. 26.2% and 20.5%, respectively, experienced soreness in their fingers and wrists. The upper arm, palm, and forearm discomfort were reported by 21, 11, and 5 of 141 respondents (15.9%, 7.8%, and 3.5%), respectively, and 16 of 141 respondents experienced discomfort in other body areas.

The average number of pain parts per respondent is shown in Figure 5. Due to lengthy use, 47 of 141 responders (33.3%) did not have any discomfort parts. Only one body area caused difficulty for 39 of the 94 respondents (41.5%). 34% and 16%

respondents experienced discomfort in two and three sections respectively, while less than a tenth of respondents (8 of 94) reported discomfort in four or more parts.

Figure 4. Parts that undergo discomfort

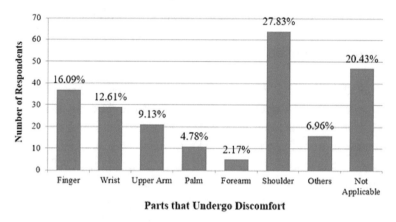

Figure 5. Numbers of parts that undergo discomfort

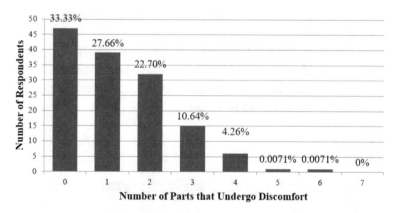

The causes and consequences of tendinitis are unknown to two-thirds of the respondents. The distribution of tendon disease phrases heard by the respondents. Shoulder Tendinitis was mentioned by 61 of 141 respondents (43.3%), Lateral Epicondylitis was mentioned by 57 of 141 respondents (40.4%), while De Quervain's Disease was mentioned by just 4 respondents (2.8%). Almost a third of the people polled had never heard of any of the labels for tendonitis. Another third of those polled had heard of at least one term. Only about a fifth of those polled had heard of two terms, and less than a fifth had heard of three or more. Table 4.5 shows respondents'

opinions on which hospitals patients with division tendon conditions should see. Almost a third of those polled (31.91%) have no idea where their patients should go. Patients should seek rehabilitation medicine, according to a fifth of respondents (19.86%), and orthopedics section, according to 16.31%. Pain management and neurosurgery come to mind for about a tenth of the responders. Patients should see general medicine, neurology, and general surgery, according to the rest.

VR Training Scenarios

This section illustrates the VR training scenarios developed in this project. We have developed four tasks under three scenes for different daily activities. Details of the VR training scenes and assessments can also be found from the authors previous publication in Fong et al. (2021). In scene one, as indicated in Figure 6, the first objective is to enter the password and then push the "OK" button. Above the password pad, a set of four-digit numbers is created at random and displayed. Players must enter the password that corresponds to the four-digit generated number, then hit "OK." When the password is entered incorrectly, the "CLEAR" button is pressed. In the meantime, a new four-digit password is generated. To complete the assignment, players must enter the newly generated password. Sound is released for each push of the password pad button as an indication to the players that the button is being pressed.

When the password is entered successfully, the word "DONE" appears in green above the password pad, and a sound is played as a symbol of success. Then it moves on to the next challenge, which involves shifting the screen and placing the door in the middle of the scene, as shown in Figure 6.

Figure 6. Scene 1 - password pad

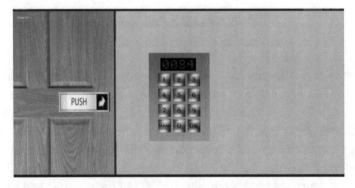

The second task in scene one is to push the door open. When the door is pushed, it opens as indicated in Figure 7, and a sound is made to indicate that the door has been opened. Then it moves on to the next scene. If you play this assignment for more than 30 seconds, the door will automatically open and you will be taken to the next scene.

Figure 7. Scene 1 – push door task

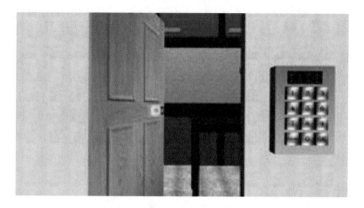

Scene two, seen in Figure 8, is where task three is designed. In this assignment, players must fill the cup with water and then return it to the left-hand table. The yellow cup on the left table must be picked up and moved to the pink cup location. The participants must then hold the cup in that position for 10 seconds in order to fill it with water. The cup is then returned to the pick cup location on the left table. Meanwhile, on the screen, there is an indicator bar that shows the time it takes to fill the water. The players must then return the cup to the left table in pink cup position after 10 seconds and the indication of completion.

Scene three, seen in Figure 9, is where task four is designed. Players must arrange nine objects in the scene's right-hand storage to complete this job. Three-ring folders, three markers, and three tapes are among the nine items on the table to the left of the scene. The locations for keeping the ring folder, marker, and tape are indicated by green, blue, and yellow lights, respectively. When the ring folder is placed under the green light, the light becomes red and the ring folder, as well as the marker and tape, are no longer touchable by players. In the meantime, the number next to the ring folder symbol in the top left corner of the screen changed from "3" to "2." The number of things that have not yet been assigned to their proper locations is displayed in the top left corner of the screen. When all of the objects are in position, all of the light indicators turn red, and the number in the upper left corner changes to "0" in green color. The game is then completed, and the game result is displayed. If the task is completed in more than 180 seconds, the unplaced objects are automatically stored, and the game is completed and the game result is displayed.

Figure 8. Scene 2 – cup detected

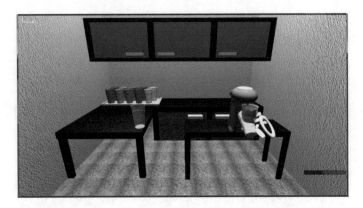

Figure 9. Scene 3 – storage room

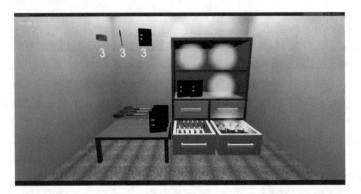

Figure 10 illustrates the game results after the player completed all tasks. The game result will be displayed for 30 seconds. The Status displays "completed" or "not completed" based on whether the player is able to accomplish the task within the time limitation. The number of objects successfully placed back by the players is displayed for task 4 in scene three. Finally, towards the bottom of the screen, the total playtime is displayed. Following the game result display, some information related to the cause of the usual tendon injury is provided. For instance, thumbs can be injured by excessive repeated movement, and other causes of tendon disorders are the excessive use of computers and smartphones.

Figure 10. Game result display

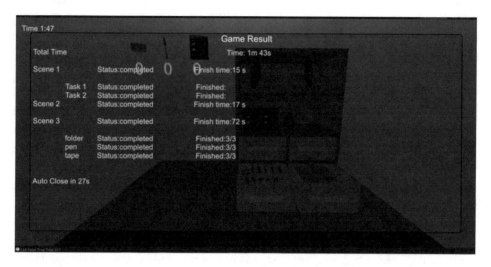

Evaluation and Users Feedbacks

According to the survey results, the majority of respondents spend more than 8 hours each day on computers and smartphones, while 70% exercise their hands and fingers for less than 15 minutes per week. In other words, people spend an average of 2.14 minutes each day exercising their hands and fingers, which is insufficient. Although the tendons and muscles of the thumb are quite strong, prolonged finger activity for eight hours a day combined with insufficient exercise or relaxation can result in tendinitis or tenosynovitis.

In terms of the level of physical discomfort, half of the respondents experienced pain in one to three body regions, the most common of which are the shoulder, finger, and wrist. Such fatigue can have catastrophic repercussions, and surgery to treat tenosynovitis may be required. Furthermore, those who do not currently experience any discomfort continue to engage in excessive activities with their hands and fingers, increasing their risk of developing tenosynovitis.

Tendon dysfunction has a low level of public awareness. Two-thirds of those polled were aware of the causes and consequences of tenosynovitis; half had heard of one to two terms, while one-third have not heard of any; and one-third had no idea where to go for tendon disease treatment. Excessive use of computers and cell phones can lead to major health problems if people are unaware of the causes and effects of tendon issues. As a result, in order to prevent treatment from being required, people must be encouraged to exercise their hands and fingers.

People rarely raise their hands to work out, so arm and shoulder muscles are rarely exercised. As a result, the designed application intended to focus on working body areas that aren't regularly worked. Players were expected to lift their arms during the entire game. Players' arms and shoulders are exercised as a result of this. The four exercises demand distinct portions of the body to participate, and all four tasks exercise the fingers, wrist, hand, arm, and shoulder. The player must enter the password, push the door, fill the cup, and insert the game accessories in order to complete the game. During the game, players concentrate on moving their fingers to complete the objective, and it appears that fingers are the sole element of the exercise. In fact, muscles in the hand and wrist are worked in order to move a finger. As a result, players are only required to concentrate on finger and hand movement and are not forced to decide which body component should be employed. As a result, players are simply required to enjoy the game and are not under any obligation or pressure to exercise, which is a good way to consider exercise. After the player has completed all of the tasks, a game result is presented, which includes the total time spent in all scenes and individual scenes, as well as the status of whether or not the tasks have been accomplished. This creates a record for the player, allowing them to compare prior and new plays over time. The goal for the players is to outperform the previous play. As a result, progressive exercise training is provided.

Finally, because public awareness of tendon disorders is insufficient, at the end of the VR game, brief information about tendon disorders is displayed. As a result, players can gain some background information on their tendon condition and reveal activities they did during the game after exercising in the game. Furthermore, gamers are taught the consequences of excessive computer and smartphone use. As a result, more people will be aware of tendon disorders.

Following the game test, testers are required to complete an evaluation form. The testers' thoughts are solicited in four sections of the assessment form: game content, instruction and feedback, bodily comfort, and general comments. The techniques of playing are fairly decent, according to testers, and the game premise is really good. It is, nevertheless, rather difficult to play. Visual and auditory feedback is sufficient. However, users said they were exhausted after playing the game. They also believe that the game will aid in the prevention of weariness caused by prolonged use of computers and cellphones. Positively, users noted that even though some of the exercises are tough to complete, the act of striving to complete the assignment still works the muscles, which is a good outcome. On the downside, the detecting area in job four is very narrow, making it impossible to return all of the game accessories. Furthermore, the LMC is not user-friendly and difficult to operate. In addition to the foregoing, one of the users suggested that the game be adjusted to allow the elderly to exercise their muscles.

CONCLUSION

Smartphones and computers are indispensable in our daily lives. Yet, if people do not keep up with current events or issues, they may be disregarded or discriminated against. As a result, it is unavoidable to abandon the use of smartphones and laptops. Meanwhile, excessive use of cellphones and computers causes a great deal of strain on the fingers and hands, increasing the risk of cumulative trauma illnesses and tendonitis. With documented cases of Tenosynovitis of the hand or forearm, and a survey finding that public knowledge of tendonitis is extremely low, the issue is significant. Thus, it is a prerequisite to act to arouse public awareness on this issue and to prevent tendonitis. As a consequence, it is essential to take steps to raise public awareness about this issue and to prevent tendon disorders. Therefore, this project develops a preventive VR rehabilitation game to raise public awareness and avoid tendon conditions. The game consists of four tasks that target muscles in the upper limbs, such as the shoulder, arm, hand, wrist, and finger, with the planned workout focusing on those muscles that aren't generally exercised. The game was tested by five volunteers who work in the computer industry. The findings demonstrate that this game can help avoid weariness caused by prolonged computer and smartphone use, and that it is ideal for rehabilitation treatment, although certain changes can be made to the game.

There are some limitations upon completion of this project and future work can be done to improve several obstacles. Some of the exercises were created to be included in the game. Because LMC does not supply that exact gesture script and time is restricted, a C# library for the precise motions cannot be built. As a result, several of the workouts have been deleted. Furthermore, there is a lot of rehabilitation exercise for different conditions, but there isn't a clear definition or agreement on which types of exercises can reduce the risk of specific disorders. Attempting to train linked muscles and tendons is a common rehabilitation practice for tendonitis. Therefore, the exercises devised for this project primarily target those muscles that aren't typically exercised in order to improve their strength and endurance. This is an attempt to reduce the risk of tendon problems. According to the testers, the item detection region is rather limited, and placing the game accessories into the storage in job four is quite challenging. The difficulty of this assignment is exacerbated by the narrow detecting area.

This project aims to raise public knowledge about tendonitis and to aid in their prevention. It is difficult to quantify and evaluate whether the game achieved the goal of raising public awareness. At this time, the only thing that can be said is that the game is appealing and people want to play it. People will become more aware of when they apply too much pressure and movement on their hands and fingers. This project is regarded as a pilot study. A group of samples to test the game's ability to prevent tendonitis is required for at least a half year to test the game's ability to prevent tendonitis. Because of the amount of time required to design the game, there isn't enough time to conduct thorough testing on the possibilities of preventing tendon conditions in this game. Furthermore, because rehabilitation is professional employment, only rehabilitation experts can conduct a more thorough investigation of the game. Furthermore, the activities that were designed in this game can be substantiated with stronger proof thanks to their knowledge.

While the level of difficulty can be added to the training in order to enhance the game element of the program. Challenges can be created by increasing the level of difficulty, to enhance the initiative of users participates in the game-based training. It is because increasing the amount of time spent exercising is believed to directly improve muscles and allows players to engage in progressive muscle training. Tasks one, three, and four can increase the difficulty level. For instance, players may be required to enter more than one password in task one. In task three, as the level rises, the holding time for filling the cup with water can be increased. In the next level, the number of gaming accessories that must be placed in the storage can also be increased.

This training game was created to prevent tendonitis. The exercises are designed to be generic and do not require any special techniques to complete, so they can benefit not just persons who are preventing tendonitis, but also stroke patients and other sorts of patients. Furthermore, only rehabilitation experts are knowledgeable about which exercises are appropriate for different sorts of patients. As a result, it is suggested that more study can be undertaken by rehabilitation professionals to adjust the game's workout so that it is more specialized for different sorts of patients, as well as to assess whether the game is beneficial to a particular group of patients.

REFERENCES

Bernhardt, J., Hayward, K., Kwakkel, G., Ward, N., Wolf, S., Borschmann, K., Krakauer, J. W., Boyd, L. A., Carmichael, S. T., Corbett, D., & Cramer, S. (2017). Agreed definitions and a shared vision for new standards in stroke recovery research: The Stroke Recovery and Rehabilitation Roundtable taskforce. *International Journal of Stroke*, *12*(5), 444–450. doi:10.1177/1747493017711816 PMID:28697708

Celinder, D., & Peoples, H. (2012). Stroke patients' experiences with Wii Sports® during inpatient rehabilitation. *Scandinavian Journal of Occupational Therapy*, *19*(5), 457–463. doi:10.3109/11038128.2012.655307 PMID:22339207

Cho, S., Ku, J., Cho, Y. K., Kim, I. Y., Kang, Y. J., Jang, D. P., & Kim, S. I. (2014). Development of virtual reality proprioceptive rehabilitation system for stroke patients. *Computer Methods and Programs in Biomedicine, 113*(1), 258–265. doi:10.1016/j. cmpb.2013.09.006 PMID:24183070

Cooper, R. A., Fitzgerald, S. G., Boninger, M. L., Brienza, D. M., Shapcott, N., Cooper, R., & Flood, K. (2001). Telerehabilitation: Expanding access to rehabilitation expertise. *Proceedings of the IEEE, 89*(8), 1174–1193. doi:10.1109/5.940286

Creek, J., & Bullock, A. (2008). Assessment and outcome measurement. *Occupational Therapy in Mental Health*, 83–114.

De Mauro, A. (2011). Virtual reality based rehabilitation and game technology. *CEUR Workshop Proceedings, 727*, 48–52.

Djukic, T., Mandic, V., & Filipovic, N. (2013). Virtual reality aided visualization of fluid flow simulations with application in medical education and diagnostics. *Computers in Biology and Medicine, 43*(12), 2046–2052. doi:10.1016/j. compbiomed.2013.10.004 PMID:24290920

Ebert, L., Flach, P., Thali, M., & Ross, S. (2014). Out of touch – A plugin for controlling OsiriX with gestures using the leap controller. *Journal of Forensic Radiology and Imaging, 2*(3), 126–128. doi:10.1016/j.jofri.2014.05.006

Fidopiastis, C., Stapleton, C., Whiteside, J., Hughes, C., Fiore, S., Martin, G., Rolland, J. P., & Smith, E. (2006). Human Experience Modeler: Context-Driven Cognitive Retraining to Facilitate Transfer of Learning. *Cyberpsychology & Behavior, 9*(2), 183–187. doi:10.1089/cpb.2006.9.183 PMID:16640476

Fong, N. K. N., Tang, Y. M., Sie, K., Yu, A. K. H., Lo, C. C. W., & Ma, Y. W. T. (2021). Task-specific virtual reality training on hemiparetic upper extremity in patients with stroke. *Virtual Reality (Waltham Cross)*. Advance online publication. doi:10.100710055-021-00583-6

Freitas, V., Carlos de Abreu Mol, A., & Shirru, R. (2014). Virtual reality for operational procedures in radioactive waste deposits. *Progress in Nuclear Energy, 71*, 225–231. doi:10.1016/j.pnucene.2013.11.003

Gershon, J., Zimand, E., Pickering, M., Rothbaum, B. O., & Hodges, L. (2004). A pilot and feasibility study of virtual reality as a distraction for children with cancer. *Journal of the American Academy of Child and Adolescent Psychiatry, 43*(10), 1243–1249. doi:10.1097/01.chi.0000135621.23145.05 PMID:15381891

Golomb, M. R., McDonald, B. C., Warden, S. J., Yonkman, J., Saykin, A. J., Shirley, B., Huber, M., Rabin, B., AbdelBaky, M., Nwosu, M. E., Barkat-Masih, M., & Burdea, G. C. (2010). In-home virtual reality videogame telerehabilitation in adolescents with hemiplegic cerebral palsy. *Archives of Physical Medicine and Rehabilitation*, *91*(1), 1–8. doi:10.1016/j.apmr.2009.08.153 PMID:20103390

Grajewski, D., Górski, F., Zawadzki, P., & Hamrol, A. (2013). Application of Virtual Reality Techniques in Design of Ergonomic Manufacturing Workplaces. *Procedia Computer Science*, *25*, 289–301. doi:10.1016/j.procs.2013.11.035

Guzsvinecz, T., Szucs, V., & Sik-Lanyi, C. (2019). Suitability of the kinect sensor and leap motion controller-A literature review. *Sensors (Basel)*, *19*(5), 1072. doi:10.339019051072 PMID:30832385

Hart, T. (2009). Treatment definition in complex rehabilitation interventions. *Neuropsychological Rehabilitation*, *19*(6), 824–840. doi:10.1080/09602010902995945 PMID:19544183

Iconaru, E. (2014). Similarities and Differences between Evaluation Protocols in Physical Therapy and Occupational Therapy – A Case Study. *Procedia: Social and Behavioral Sciences*, *116*, 3142–3146. doi:10.1016/j.sbspro.2014.01.723

Lan, C., Chen, S. Y., & Lai, J. S. (2012). *Exercise training for patients after coronary artery bypass grafting surgery*. In M. Brizzio (Ed.), *Acute Coronary Syndromes* (pp. 117–128). IntechOpen.

Lau, Y. Y., Tang, Y. M., Chan, I., Ng, A. K., & Leung, A. (2020). The deployment of virtual reality (VR) to promote green burial. *Asia Pacific Journal of Health Management*, *15*(2), 53–60. doi:10.24083/apjhm.v15i2.403

Lau, Y. Y., Tang, Y. M., Chau, K. Y., & Hui, H. Y. (2021). Pilot Study of Heartbeat Sensors for Data Streaming in Virtual Reality (VR) Training. *International Journal of Innovation. Creativity and Change*, *15*(3), 30–41.

Laver, K., George, S., Thomas, S., Deutsch, J., & Crotty, M. (2015). Virtual reality for stroke rehabilitation. *Cochrane Database of Systematic Reviews*, *2015*(2), CD008349. PMID:25927099

Laver, K. E., Lange, B., George, S., Deutsch, J. E., Saposnik, G., & Crotty, M. (2017). Virtual reality for stroke rehabilitation. *Cochrane Database of Systematic Reviews*, *11*. PMID:29156493

Legislative Council Panel on Manpower. (2013, Dec.). *Occupational Diseases in Hong Kong*. Government of the Hong Kong Special Administrative Region. https://www.legco.gov.hk/yr13-14/english/panels/mp/papers/mp1217cb2-491-12-e.pdf

Levac, D. E., & Galvin, J. (2013). When is virtual reality "therapy"? *Archives of Physical Medicine and Rehabilitation*, *94*(4), 795–798. doi:10.1016/j.apmr.2012.10.021 PMID:23124132

Liu, C., Yip, K., & Chiang, H. (2020). Investigating the optimal handle diameters and thumb orthoses for individuals with chronic de Quervain's tenosynovitis - a pilot study. *Disability and Rehabilitation*, *42*(9), 1247–1253. doi:10.1080/09638288.2018.1522548 PMID:30689463

Malarvani, T., Ganesh, E., Nirmala, P., Kumar, A., & Singh, M. K. (2014). WhatsAppitis: Recent Study on SMS Syndrome. *Scholars Journal of Applied Medical Sciences*, *2*(6B), 2026–2033.

Malloy, K. M., & Milling, L. S. (2010). The effectiveness of virtual reality distraction for pain reduction: A systematic review. *Clinical Psychology Review*, *30*(8), 1011–1018. doi:10.1016/j.cpr.2010.07.001 PMID:20691523

McCue, M., Fairman, A., & Pramuka, M. (2010). Enhancing quality of life through telerehabilitation. *Physical Medicine and Rehabilitation Clinics of North America*, *21*(1), 195–205. doi:10.1016/j.pmr.2009.07.005 PMID:19951786

Messinger, P. R., Stroulia, E., Lyons, K., Bone, M., Niu, R. H., Smirnov, K., & Perelgut, S. (2009). Virtual worlds—past, present, and future: New directions in social computing. *Decision Support Systems*, *47*(3), 204–228. doi:10.1016/j.dss.2009.02.014

Miniwatts Marketing Group. (2014). *Internet Usage Statistic*. The Internet Big Picture. https://www.internetworldstats.com/stats.htm

Mujber, T., Szecsi, T., & Hashmi, M. (2004). Virtual reality applications in manufacturing process simulation. *Journal of Materials Processing Technology*, *155-156*(1-3), 1834–1838. doi:10.1016/j.jmatprotec.2004.04.401

Occupational Safety and Health Branch. Labour Department. (2020, September). *Occupational Safety and Health Statistics 2019*. https://www.labour.gov.hk/eng/osh/pdf/archive/statistics/OSH_Statistics_2019_eng.pdf

Olasky, J., Sankaranarayanan, G., Seymour, N., Magee, J., Enquobahrie, A., Lin, M., Aggarwal, R., Brunt, L. M., Schwaitzberg, S. D., Cao, C. G. L., De, S., & Jones, D. (2015). Identifying Opportunities for Virtual Reality Simulation in Surgical Education. *Surgical Innovation, 22*(5), 514–521. doi:10.1177/1553350615583559 PMID:25925424

Rachel, T. (2010). *How I Do Treat My De Quervain's Tenosynovitis?* https://ecfamilyclinic.wordpress.com/2010/10/13/how-i-do-treat-my-de-quervains-tenosynovitis/

Reid, D. (2004). The influence of virtual reality on playfulness in children with cerebral palsy: A pilot study. *Occupational Therapy International, 11*(3), 131–144. doi:10.1002/oti.202 PMID:15297894

Rizzo, A., & Kim, G. (2005). A SWOT Analysis of the Field of Virtual Reality Rehabilitation and Therapy. *Presence (Cambridge, Mass.), 14*(2), 119–146. doi:10.1162/1054746053967094

Ruthenbeck, G. S., Hobson, J., Carney, A. S., Sloan, S., Sacks, R., & Reynolds, K. J. (2013). Toward photorealism in endoscopic sinus surgery simulation. *American Journal of Rhinology & Allergy, 27*(2), 138–143. doi:10.2500/ajra.2013.27.3861 PMID:23562204

Schulteis, M. T., & Rothbaum, B. O. (2002). *Ethical issues for the use of virtual reality in the psychological sciences. Ethical issues in clinical neuropsychology.* Swets & Zeitlinger.

Schultheis, M., & Rizzo, A. (2001). The Application of Virtual Reality Technology in Rehabilitation. *Rehabilitation Psychology, 46*(3), 296–311. doi:10.1037/0090-5550.46.3.296

Sherman, W., & Craig, A. (2019). Understanding virtual reality: Interface, application, and design (2nd ed.). Morgan Kaufmann.

Steinicke, F., Ropinski, T., & Hinrichs, K. (2005). A generic virtual reality software system's architecture and application. *Proceedings of the 2005 International Conference on Augmented Tele-Existence, 157,* 220-227. 10.1145/1152399.1152440

Taneja, C. (2014). The psychology of excessive cellular phone use. *Delhi Psychiatry Journal, 17*(2), 448–451.

Tang, Y. M., Ng, G. W. Y., Chia, N. H., So, E. H. K., Wu, C. H., & Ip, W. H. (2021). Application of virtual reality (VR) technology for medical practitioners in type and screen (T&S) training. *Journal of Computer Assisted Learning*, *37*(2), 359–369. doi:10.1111/jcal.12494

The Hong Kong Polytechnic University. (2013). Health effects of using portable electronic devices studied. *ScienceDaily*. www.sciencedaily.com/releases/2013/09/130905160452.htm

Wang, C., Li, H., & Kho, S. (2018). VR-embedded BIM immersive system for QS engineering education. *Computer Applications in Engineering Education*, *26*(3), 626–641. doi:10.1002/cae.21915

Weichert, F., Bachmann, D., Rudak, B., & Fisseler, D. (2013). Analysis of the accuracy and robustness of the Leap Motion Controller. *Sensors (Basel)*, *13*(5), 6380–6393. doi:10.3390130506380 PMID:23673678

Weiss, P., Kizony, R., Feintuch, U., & Katz, N. (2006). Virtual reality in neurorehabilitation. In *Textbook of Neural Repair and Rehabilitation* (pp. 182–197). Cambridge University Press. doi:10.1017/CBO9780511545078.015

Wilson, G. (1992). The Rise and Rise of the Computer -- The Dream Machine: Exploring the Computer Age by John Palfreman and Doron Swade. *New Scientist, 133*(1812).

Chapter 6
Designing a Conceptual Virtual Medical Research Initiative in the Virtual Reality Environment

N. Raghavendra Rao
FINAIT Consultancy Services, India

EXECUTIVE SUMMARY

Many technologies tend to be applicable only in a specific industry or defined area of operation in business. The case of information and communication technology is different. The potential of information and communication technology in any sphere of activity in any discipline is more useful. Information and communication technology is a driving force in providing a good scope in making use of the various concepts in this discipline for designing models as per the requirements of a particular application. The concepts of cloud computing and virtual reality have proved to be significant particularly in the healthcare sector. This chapter gives an overview of the above concepts and related technology. Further, this chapter explains the case illustrations by adopting the above concepts for designing a virtual medical research initiative in the virtual reality environment.

INTRODUCTION

Hospitals are the most important entity in the healthcare system. Health issues and the needs of patients are increasing. Healthcare issues are also becoming more complex. While providing service to the patients, a lot of data is generated. Data in the healthcare systems are available as disperse elements. Once it is compiled into the meaning pattern, then it becomes information. When the information is

DOI: 10.4018/978-1-7998-8790-4.ch006

converted into a valid basis for action, then it becomes knowledge. This knowledge will facilitate in creating knowledge for medical research initiatives in the healthcare sector (Nagafeeson Madison, 2014).

The data in the systems of the hospitals are based on the diagnosis of the patients. Then the treatment is suggested to the patients with the prescription of medicines. Their diagnosis and treatment are stored in the system in respect of each patient consulted them (Vijayrani S, 2013). Doctors may not have time to analyse the data of various patients from the perspective of research. Over a period, their computer systems become slow due to huge data is stored in their systems. It is the practice of many hospitals, they take back up of the data from their systems in the external devices (Charles R McConnell, 2020). Then the data is deleted from their existing computer systems. Most of the hospitals do not make use of the historical data stored in external devices for analysis and research purposes. It would be a good approach if the historical data stored in the external devices by the various hospitals are integrated for research purposes. This integration will provide a good scope for designing models in the healthcare sector. These models will benefit the medical fraternity who have a bent of mind for research. It will be also useful for medical students making use of them for evidence-based learning (Sunitha C, Vasanthakokilam K, & Meena Preethi B, 2013).

BACKGROUND

For years research in medicine was related closely to natural sciences. This research was mainly related to developing new drugs. Rapid advancements in telecommunication technology enabled the healthcare sector to develop Telemedicine for the benefit of patients across the globe. It will be interesting to recall the approach followed by Middlesex University in the UK when telecommunication was becoming popular. Middle Sex University has created a central disease management system. Asthma patients and those with the chronic obstructive pulmonary disease would use a portable monitoring device to record their breathing patterns up to four times a day in the comfort of their homes. The data was sent via modem and telephone lines to the central disease management system. It was processed and results were sent to the patient's doctor using the cable and wireless secure internet way. This system would record the date and time, temperature, and humidity measures critical for analysing the health of asthma patients surrounding such as air pollution and quality of the air. This information would assist in providing the correct treatment and diagnosis for individual patients. The patients' symptoms and use of medication as well as their lung functions data were recorded in the central disease management. This disease management system would contain two parts of data in respect of asthma patients. One part of data would be in respect of patient's data about date and time, temperature, and humidity measurements. The second part of the data would relate to environmental conditions, air pollution, and quality. This approach facilitated the doctors to treat their patients (Sharon Wulfovich, 2019 & Krishna Kumar L Jimmy Joy, 2013).

Need for Knowledge-Based System

Integrating the knowledge and experience of the medical experts is very important for the benefit of patients. Collective intelligence is required to address the healthcare issues and requirements of the patients. Some of the concepts in information and communication technology will facilitate a proactive approach in healthcare systems. Great accomplishments are most likely to occur in the collaboration environment. There are two types of approaches prevalent in the health sector. They are the "Conservative Approach" and "Adaptive Change Approach". The first approach can be said to follow a beaten path and there will be no deviation in thinking. The elements in the second approach are reasoning, knowledge-based understanding and enlightened creative wisdom blended with professional values (Christensen C M, Grossman J H & Hwang J, 2008).

Approach Followed in This Chapter

Many concepts have been emerging in the discipline of information and communication technology. Every concept has some special features. These features are to be understood clearly before applying them in a particular application. The concepts such as virtual reality, virtual environment, and cloud computing are identified for designing this medical research initiative model. Collaborative concepts such as data warehouse, and data mining are also part of this design. This chapter is dived into five sections. Section-1 gives an overview of the above three concepts. Section-2 highlights the important aspects of the collaborative concepts such as Data ware house and data mining. Section-3 talks about medical databases Section-4 presents the scenario of healthcare services in India Section-5 deals with the case illustrations. Section-6 consists of future trends and conclusion paragraph.

MAIN CONCEPTS OF THE MODELS IN THIS CHAPTER

The following concepts provide insight into creating a virtual medical research centre.

Concept of Virtual Reality

The concept of virtual reality facilitates in visualizing new ideas for business purposes. The element constituting virtual reality are audio voice, graphics, images, sound, and motion sensing. These elements along with numerical and textual data facilitate the creation of real-time simulation. Business enterprises have choices to evaluate their new ideas by making use of the concept of virtual reality. Simulated outputs resulted from virtual reality application programs help to visualize and visibilize the proposed ideas of business enterprises. These outputs help to visualize hypothetical cases in business and interact with the applications developed under the virtual reality concept. It may be noted that the concept of multimedia is required in virtual reality applications. The concept of virtual reality is the seed of innovation for developing business models (Chorafas Dimitri's N & Steinmann, 1995).

Visualization

Information and communication technology has made the visualization process an important component in the development of advanced business applications. Presentation of output through simulated data helps to analyse and make decisions.

Visibilization

Visibilization makes mapping of physical reality with virtual reality for end-users to understand the output generated through simulated data.

Visitraction

Visitraction is the process of visualization of concepts, characteristics, or phenomena lacking a direct physical interpretation. This results in establishing the link between the concepts and ideas.

Advantages of the Concept of Virtual Reality

Virtual reality refers to the presentation of system-generated data. This data is made available in such a way that those who use it perceive the information at their disposal as having similar or enhanced characteristics in business models. The line dividing simulated tasks and their real-world counterparts are very thin. The ability to get real-world perceptions interactively through computer systems explains the interest associated with three-dimensional graphics in virtual reality. The synergy between real and simulated facts yields real effectiveness. It will be more effective if the system and its artefacts are to be active rather than a passive display. The essential element of virtual reality is that interactive simulation with navigation among widely scattered heterogeneous databases. This results in logical, numerical processing and a wide range of visualization functions. The virtual reality concept helps to unlock innovative thinking in enterprises for carrying out incremental and radical innovation in their organization. The virtual reality concept helps enterprises to accomplish their ambitious goals with innovation improvements initiatives. The new initiatives help to generate alternative ideas by taking inputs from different sources and structuring them through virtual reality applications. The virtual reality concept will increase the chances of successfully diffusing knowledge, technology, and process. It will provide scope for innovation to emerge (Raghavendra Rao N, 2011).

History of Virtual Reality

Digital simulation has emerged after the advent of computer systems. Contribution to the concept of the simulation was a video presentation combined with the mechanical flight simulator in 1952. It was considered the birth of virtual reality in that year. The US Air Force, US Navy, and NASA have provided the funds to the university laboratories for the activities related to virtual reality. The US Air Force had planned to immerse pilots into training simulators at Wright Patterson Air Force base in Dayton, Ohio. The pilots got the simulated experience of being inside an Air Craft by being able to test specific flight situations at any point in time. This and projects similar to this, have indicated that computer simulation and the associated visualization could be applied to create a valuable scenario for training.

Another application related to virtual reality has taken place by the development of fuel-flow simulators for the space shuttle. This helped the technicians to monitor fuel storage and usage. This was known as the virtual environment workstation project. The main focus of this project was to combine sources as process monitoring, live video, and workstation input. As the technology got integrated it has provided a single environment in which the user world has control over various information sources through the use of dynamic interactive windows. Consequent to this the new uses of virtual reality have started gaining importance, funding for the project related to virtual reality has also increased.

Role of Virtual Reality

The practical applications of virtual reality are made use of in the areas such as architecture and engineering. Both architecture and engineering are handling big complex data sets. The Healthcare sector also has big complex data sets. This concept is particularly more useful in the healthcare sector for teaching, demonstrating surgical operations on the simulated human body. It is useful for designing a drug.

Real-Time Simulation Approach

Real-time thinking is possible through modelling and feature-based simulation. Real-time simulation and visualization provide competitive benefits to the end-user. The components required for this type of venture are software and hardware that integrate modelling and interpretation by the medical fraternity who are ready to learn and adapt the real-time simulation approach in a human body. This will facilitate them to achieve their research initiative in their area of specialization.

Virtual Environment

One of the big changes that are emerging in the present globalization scenario in the virtual environment. This has given scope for virtual medical conferences, virtual consultations, and even virtual hospitals. The professional isolation that is experienced by so many professionals working away from distant places has become largely a thing of the past. Now they can take part in interactive exchanges and have access to online knowledge bases and expertise as anyone and anywhere in the World. The idea behind suggesting private cloud is to provide health care services under a virtual environment.

Virtual Reality in Virtual Environment

Virtual reality is a way of creating a three-dimensional image of an object or scene. The user can move through or around the image. Virtual reality imitates the way the real object or scene looks and changes. Information system helps to use information in databases to stimulate. The line dividing simulated tasks and their real-world counterparts are very thin. Virtual reality systems are designed to produce in the participant the cognitive effects of feeling immersed in the environment created by a computer system. The computer system uses sensory inputs such as vision, hearing, feeling, and sensation of motion. The concept of multimedia is required in the virtual reality process. The components of multimedia are tactile (Touch), Visual (Image), and auditory (Sound).

The concept of virtual reality is more useful for showing the advancements taking place in the health care sector especially in the area of surgery. Medical students will be benefited by upgrading their knowledge. Simulated tasks replicate the real medical tasks.

Features in Cloud Computing Infrastructure

Cloud computing is a generic term that involves delivering a host of services over the internet. The name cloud computing is said to have been derived from the cloud symbol that is often used to represent the internet. Another interpretation can also be given that the cloud is visible in the sky from any part of the universe. Similarly, the services through the concept of cloud are also available to an end-user from any part of the world (Raj Kumar Buyya, Christian Vecchiola, & Thamaraiselvi S, 2013).

Concept of Cloud Computing

Cloud computing is a concept generally defined as a group of scalable and virtualized resources which make use of the internet to provide on-demand services to end-users (Thomas ERL, 2014). The national institute of standards and technology (NIST) describes it as "a model for enabling convenient on-demand network access to a shared pool of configurable computing resources that can be rapidly provisioned and released with minimum management effort or service provider interaction. This cloud model promotes availability and is composed of five essential characteristics such as on-demand self-service, broad network access, resource pooling, rapid elasticity, and measured service ".

The following characteristics can be considered as advantages for enterprises.

1. On-demand service
2. Ubiquitous network access
3. Location-independent pooling of resources
4. Elasticity and scalability
5. Pay- as - you use to approach

Cloud Computing Environment

Cloud computing provides four types of environments to end-users. An enterprise can choose any of the following environments for its requirements.

1. Private Cloud
   This type of infrastructure is owned or leased by a single enterprise and is operated solely for that enterprise.

2. Community Cloud
   This type of cloud infrastructure is shared by several enterprises and supports a specific community.

3.   Public Cloud

This type of cloud infrastructure is owned by an enterprise providing cloud services to the general public or a large industrial or business group.

4.   Hybrid Cloud

This type of cloud infrastructure is a composition of two or more cloud environments such as internal community or public that remains unique entities. They are bound together by standardized or proprietary technology that enables data and application portability.

Advantages in Cloud Computing Environment

Cloud computing offers various components from deployment models. These models provide mix and match solutions that are sought. An enterprise can make use of a component such as storage-as-a-service from one service provider, database-as-a-service from another, and even complete application development and deployment of a platform from a third service provider. Enterprises need to remember that cloud computing facilitates the use of cloud computing deployment models over the internet

Data-Intensive Applications

Cloud computing is more useful for data Intensive applications in the sectors such as manufacturing, financial institutions, hospitality, and healthcare. Research scholars particularly require mechanisms to transfer, publish, replicate, discover, share and analyse data across the Globe. Similarly, the above sectors need to maintain a database consisting at the country level, or worldwide level. Every sector has different characteristics both in the use of data and volumes of data. The applications in the cloud computing environment are required to be designed for managing data replication, data recovery, and responding dynamically to changes in the volume of data in databases.

Storage of Data in Cloud Computing Environment

The main use of cloud computing is for the storage of data. Data is stored in multiple servers rather than in the dedicated servers used in the traditional network data storage system. An end-user sees it as a virtual space carved out of the cloud. In reality, the user's data can be stored in any or more servers used to create a cloud computing environment (Chaka C, 2013)

Virtualization

There are many advantages in virtualization some of the advantages of virtualization are given below

Virtualization facilitates to consideration of infrastructure, thereby reducing the space and requirement of power (Schulz G, 2012).

1. Utilization
   Virtualization helps in increasing the utilization of hardware and software and decreasing capital investments.

2. Cost containment
   Virtualization is beneficial for the reduction in maintenance costs in respect of hardware and software, and operational costs also.

3. Business Continuity
   Virtualization allows the business process to run independently of the hardware thereby enabling it to move the process to the other system at runtime.

4. Data Recovery
   The data may be replicated in multiple storage servers thereby enabling data to be recovered rapidly with a minimum loss of time

5. Management
   Virtualization helps the system group to use the system with fewer problems.

COLLABORATIVE CONCEPTS

The following concepts play an important role in storing and analysing healthcare data for medical research purposes.

Dataware House

The data warehouse concept facilitates hospitals to store huge volume of data for analysis and research. The Data warehouse is a central store of data that is extracted either from the operational database or from a historical database. The data in data warehouses are subject-oriented, non-volatile, and of a historical nature. So data warehouse tends to contain extremely large data sets. It can be inferred that the purpose of a data warehouse is 1) To slice and dice through data 2) To ensure that past data is stored accurately 3) To provide one version of data 4) To operate for analytical process and 5) To support the decision process (Joe Kraynak, 2017 & Paul raj Ponniah, 2012).

Data Mining

Data Mining is a concept used in Data warehouses. Data Mining deals with discovering hidden data and unexpected patterns and rules in a large database. A good foundation in terms of a data warehouse is a necessary condition for effective implementation. Four types of knowledge can be identified in Data Mining. They are 1) Shallow Knowledge 2) Multidimensional Knowledge 3) Hidden Knowledge 4) Deep Knowledge (Arun K Pujari, 2003 & Pieter Adriaans and Dolf Zantinge, 1999).

Shallow Knowledge

Information can be easily retrieved from databases using a query tool such as structured query language (SQL)

Multi-Dimensional Knowledge

Information can be analysed using online analytical processing tools.

Hidden Knowledge

Data can be found relatively easily by using pattern recognition or machine learning algorithms.

Deep Knowledge

Information that is stored in the database can be located if one has a clue that tells the user where to look.

MEDICAL DATABASES

The following information will be useful for the medical research initiative.

International Code of Diseases (ICD)

International Code of Diseases is a specific standard for all general epitomical and many health management purposes. ICD11 contains the classification of diseases.

DICOM

Medical images have codes. These codes are classified in DICOM (Digital Imaging and Communication in Medicines.

Biological Data

The properties that characterize a living organism (Species) are based on its fundamental set of genetic information. It is important to understand the fundamental terms of aspects such as DNA, RNA, Protein, and their information concerning the Genome (Jean Michael Claverie & Cedric Notre dame, 2011).

Different sequences of bases in DNA specify different sequences of bases in RNA. The sequence of bases in RNA specifies the sequences of amino acids in proteins. The central dogma states that DNA is transcribed into RNA, which is then translated later into protein. The main advantage of the Bioinformatics discipline is biological data are available on various websites. The databases on these websites can be classified into two types such as generalized and specialized databases. The generalized databases contain information related to DNA, Protein, or similar types. The generalized databases can again be further split into sequence databases and structured databases. Sequence databases hold the individual sequence records of either nucleotides or amino acids or proteins. Structured databases contain the individual sequence records of bio-chemically solved structures of macromolecules.

Specialized databases are 1) EST (Expressed Sequence Tags) 2) GSS (Genome Survey Sequences) 3) SNP (Single Nucleotide Polymorphism) 4) STS (Sequence Tag Sites) 5) KABAT for Immunology Proteins and LIGAND for enzymes reaction legends. These databases can be further split into three types based on the complexity of the data stored.

1. Primary Databases
   These databases contain data in their original form from the sequences.

2. Secondary Databases
   These databases have value-added data and derived information from the primary databases.

3.   Composite Databases
      Composite databases amalgamate a variety of different primary databases, structured into one. There are various software tools available to facilitate searching the above databases.

Developing or designing a drug is possible by making use of the information in the diverse chemical libraries along with the information about biological functions stored in the above databases before starting laboratory-based experiments. It is always possible to generate as much information as possible about potential drug and target interaction from the above databases and chemical libraries.

SCENARIO OF HEALTHCARE SECTOR IN INDIA

This section explains the healthcare sector in India and the initiatives are taken by some doctors for the creation of a virtual medical research center.

Overview of Healthcare Services Provided to Patients

Mainly four types of hospital enterprises are providing healthcare services to the patients in India. They are 1-Hospitals managed by the corporate sector, 2-Hospitals managed by the government agencies, 3-Hospitals managed by a group of trustees, and 4-Nursing homes managed by a doctor or a group of doctors. In addition to these services, there are clinical testing laboratories and diagnostic centres. They are also playing an important role in the health care sector.

It is the practice in India doctors who do not have their own clinics and specialists are associated with some of the hospitals mentioned under the four categories (Govil D & Purohit N, 2011). These doctors provide either consultancy services or perform surgeries. Some of the doctors provide both types of services mentioned above. Doctors who have flair for teaching, take up teaching assignments also as visiting professors in the medical colleges. A few doctors have made it a point to meet at regular intervals in a month and share their professional experience in providing medical services and the medical conferences attended by them. Some of them highlighted the advancements in information and communication technology who attended the medical informatics conferences. They have also explained about the doctors who made use of the discipline of information and technology in their areas of medical services. This information has motivated some of the doctors who were participants in the meetings to start a virtual medical research institute. Any research needs data, medical research is no exception. Six doctors have taken the initiative to request the management of the hospitals associated with them about their medical research institute venture (Sandro Galea, 2019).

The management of the hospitals has agreed to provide the required infrastructure for the virtual medical research centre (Reur J Arino J & Olk P, 2011). It has been agreed by the management of the hospitals to transfer the historical data of their patients to the Centralized Data ware for research, designing a drug and evidence-based learning purpose only. The transferred data will contain the information about 1-History of the patients covering their habits and health issues, 2- Procedures followed, tests conducted and the results of the tests, 3-Treatment suggested and medicines prescribed,4- Reaction of the medicines experienced by the patients, and 5- Reports of the surgeries conducted by the surgeons. The clinical testing laboratories and the diagnostic centres have agreed to transfer the data of the results of the tests conducted for the patients referred by the hospitals and the doctors to the Centralized Data ware house. Figure-1 Medical data from the above sources in the healthcare sector and Figure-2 Basic data segregated and categorized in the Data ware house give an idea of the data stored in the centralized Data ware house.

Figure 1.

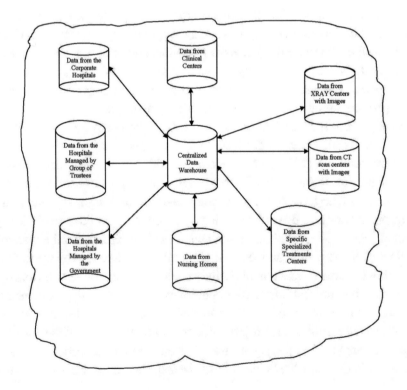

Figure 2.

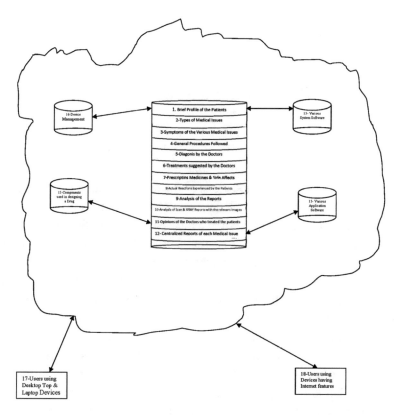

Creation of Virtual Medical Research Centre

The infrastructure consists of the centralized data warehouse uploaded in the private cloud computing environment (Semolic & Baisya, 2013). This centre is located at one of the corporate hospitals in Chennai. The investment cost of the hardware infrastructure, software, software professionals' salaries, and maintenance of the research centre is shared by the four types of hospitals mentioned in the above case illustration. The doctors who have evinced interest to be associated with this research centre are given formal training in making use of the infrastructure by the software professionals. A core team has been formed consisting the doctors who have a research bent of mind and software professionals. The core team has assumed the responsibility of managing the virtual medical research centre. Software professionals have also taken interest in updating their knowledge related to the healthcare sector. Based on guidance provided by the doctors the data in the centralized data ware house is codified by making use of ICD 11a and DICOM. The centralized data ware house is termed as the patient data ware house.

CASE ILLUSTRATIONS

This section discusses the case illustrations related to the medical research initiatives taken by the medical fraternity in India.

Case Illustration Relating to Analysis and Teaching

The doctors who have bent of mind in research activities have taken part by making use of the data in the centralized data warehouse. The patient data ware house is in the private cloud computing environment (Anahory S & Hurray D, 2011). The doctors who are working at the different locations of the hospitals can make use of the data for their research purposes. A simulated version of the human body can be created for demonstrating the surgeries in the virtual reality environment (Ilkakunna Mo, 2015). Doctors can get an opportunity to update their knowledge in surgery by observing the virtual surgery conducted on the simulated human body. The three elements of the virtual reality concept 1-visualization, 2-visibilization, and 3-visitraction have helped the surgeons to demonstrate their surgery in the simulated version of the human body. The doctors who have taken up the teaching assignments in the medical colleges helped them to teach the procedures in the surgery on the simulated version of the human body.

In this case illustration, it may be noted that the doctor who is involved in research activities has used the features in the data mining tool such as multidimensional knowledge, hidden knowledge, and deep knowledge in the context of a particular disease of their research topic. The results after their analysis are tested on the simulated human body. They form their conclusions based on their analysis and results. Their research findings can be explained in the virtual medical conference

Case Illustration Relating to Designing a Drug

The doctors have been highlighting some of the side effects of the drugs prescribed by them to their patients at various medical conferences. The doctors who are already associated with virtual medical research centres can make use of the data in the patient data warehouse for designing a drug. Primary databases, secondary databases, and composite databases in biological data environment can be made use of designing a drug under a rational approach. A data mining tool is used for the analysis of the research. The method of designing a drug followed by medical doctors in the core team is explained in the following paragraph. The proposed design of the drug is to be tested by the doctors on the simulated version of the human body. Later it can be given to a pharmaceutical company for testing by their R & D department before actual production is scheduled to plan (Linwoes, 2015 & Khon M S and Skarulis, 2012).

Figure 3. Rational base approach

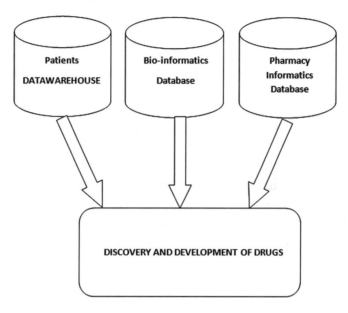

Role of Bioinformatics in Drug Discovery

Bio Informatics is the storage, manipulation, and analysis of biological information by making use of information technology. Bio Informatics is an essential infrastructure underpinning biological research. The adoption of a Bioinformatics based approach to drug discovery provides an important advantage in a rational approach (Ignacimuthu, 2005).

Role of Virtual Reality in Drug Design

The software professionals who are part of a drug discovery research project have created a simulated version of a human body with all the internal parts in the human body visible under a virtual reality environment. They can take the data from the patient data warehouse in respect of the reactions to the drugs for highlighting them in the simulated human body system. Various reactions such as feeling restless, screaming with pain, drowsy, not getting a sound sleep and digestive problems can be viewed in the simulated version of the human body. This will facilitate the research team members to visualize the reactions of a drug in the simulated version of a human body. Each member of the research team can analyse the visual reactions in the simulated human body system (Jain Vivek, 2020). Each member of the research team can suggest the various components are to be used in designing a new drug.

The entire research team can analyse and discuss among themselves each member's suggestion of composition for a drug (Damayanti Bandopadhyay, 2013). After the discussions among themselves, they can mutually ages to a particular composition for a new drug. The advantage of creating a simulated human body system under the virtual reality environment can facilitate the research team members to visualize the pain and suffering due to the side effects of a drug. The drug designed under this environment can be given to a laboratory at a pharmaceutical company to produce a drug and test it before the actual manufacturing of a drug takes place (Sean Masaki Flynn, 2019).

Case Illustration Relating to Evidence Based Learning

Learning any subject in-depth understanding requires that learners construct their meanings of the topics they learn and integrate with their prior knowledge and skills. Medical students can apply their knowledge to a simulated version human body under a virtual reality environment by using the patient data warehouse. This approach facilitates medical students to enhance themselves with knowledge and improving both competence and confidence. Patient Data ware house is useful for evidence-based learning by medical students.

A group of medical students has decided to form a "Knowledge Sharing Team" for discussion on medical-related subjects and topics. They have requested Virtual Medical Research Centre to make use of their patient data warehouse for knowledge-sharing purposes. They have agreed to their request and stipulated that it should be exclusively used for their academic discussion only.

A few members among the "Knowledge Sharing Team" have been identified to prepare a case study based on the data related to diseases/disorders treated stored in the patient data warehouse and the actual treatment given to the patients is not mentioned in the case study. Each member of the group is expected to go through each case study. After studying the case study each member suggests a treatment based on the member's knowledge. Two or three medical students can together suggest a treatment. Later all their suggested treatments are stored in the patient data warehouse. A data mining tool is used for learning and analysing the data in the patient data warehouse. Then the discussion takes place on the suggested treatments. After their discussion, they will compare with the actual treatment given to the patient. They have also made use of the simulated human body for the medical procedure. Under the guidance of they have attempted medical surgery in the simulated human body in the virtual reality environment. This method facilitates them to update their knowledge. Further, it sharpens their professional thinking.

Figure 4. Evidence-based learning

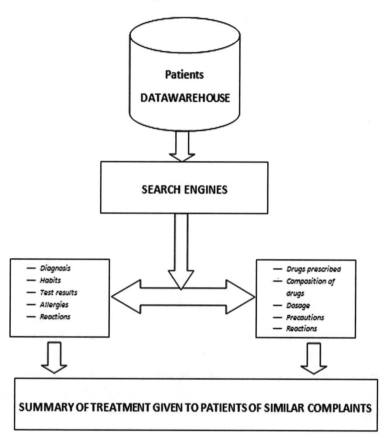

Case Illustration Relating to General Health Information

A group of social workers in South India visits the various rural parts of their social work. During their visits, they make it a point to explain to the rural people the importance of hygiene and the good health habits to be followed by them. During their talk, they use various charts and diagrams related to basic health education. They use to interact with them after their talk. During their interaction, they felt that there is not a good impact of their health-related tips mentioned in their talk of the rural people. They felt there was a need to change the method of presenting their health-related tips to rural people. They have met the management of the virtual medical research centre for getting their guidance in conducting the basic health-related talk (Lals, 2018).

The management of the centre has agreed to help them and considered it as a corporate responsibility to society. They have decided to create a "General Health

Data Warehouse" in their infrastructure. This database mainly talks about the salient features in health care information to be explained to the rural people. A simulated version of the human body has been created. Medical students are involved in this venture. The internet facility is available in the rural parts of South India. Medical students have made use of the simulated version of the human body under a virtual reality environment for explaining basic health education. The medical students are happy that they can make an impact on the rural people with the new approach (Sarah E Boslaugh, 2013).

FUTURE TRENDS AND CONCLUSION

Future Trends

Many more requirements in the area of medical informatics will be needed. There is a good scope for research scholars to develop innovative models in the health care sector. The interdisciplinary development process is becoming important because no science in itself answers all the prerequisites that exist in an expanding implementation field. This is true of the sciences at large as well as the perspectives of the particular application. The concept of virtual reality helps to design in addressing the needs of scientific and in any domain which is now being cross-fertilized. There is a good scope for designing and developing models for the health care sector in the artificial intelligence environment with the concept of virtual reality.

Conclusion

In today's knowledge-rich environment, information and communication technology has increased particularly virtualization in the activities of the health care sector and ways of working. The term "Virtual" is now appearing in many forms. Knowledge-based health care system at the virtual medical research centre explains the need for adopting an innovative approach in involving the medical fraternity by applying the concept of "Mind invoking".

It may be observed that the virtual medical research center has made use of the services of the core team in designing and developing a system for the health care sector. Hospitals will find that private cloud is a better solution for them in leveraging the benefits of cloud computing within their firewall. The medical research centre has proved the usefulness of the concept of virtual reality in the cloud computing environment. It will be beneficial for virtual hospitals to share the common resources for computing power and accessing data across the globe (Walshe, 2014).

REFERENCES

Adriaans & Zantinge. (1999). *Data Mining*. Addison Wesley Longman.

Anahory, S., & Hurray, D. (2011). *Data Ware Housing in the Real World*. New Delhi: Pearson.

Arun, K. P. (2003). Data Mining Techniques. Universities Press (India) Private Limited.

Attwood, T. K., & Parry-Smith, D. J. (2005). *Introduction to Bioinformatics; New Delhi: Pearson Education*. Private Limited.

Bandopadhyay. (2013). A Technology Lead Business Model for Pharma – Collaborative Patient Care. *CSI Communications Journal, 37*(9), 12-13, 26.

Boslaugh, S. E. (2013). *Healthcare Systems around the world A Comparative Guide*. Sage Publishing. doi:10.4135/9781452276212

Buyya, Vecchiola, & Selvi. (2013). *Mastering Cloud Computing*. McGraw Hill Education (India) Private Limited.

Chaka, C. (2013). *Virtualization and Cloud Computing Business Models in the Virtual Cloud*. IGI Global.

Chorafas & Steinmann. (1995). *Virtual Reality Practical Applications in Business and Industry*. Prentice Hall.

Christensen, C. M., Grossman, J. H., & Hwang, J. (2008). *The Innovator's Prescription: A Disruptive Solution for Healthcare*. McGraw Hill.

Claverie & Notredame. (2011). *Bioinformatics for Dummies*. John Wiley & Sons.

Flynn. (2019). *The Cure That Works: How to have the World Best Healthcare*. Regnery Publishing.

Galea. (2019). *Well What We Need to Talk about When We talk about Health*. Oxford University Press.

Govil, D., & Purohit, N. (2011). Healthcare Systems in India. In H. S. Rout (Ed.), *Healthcare Systems –A Global Survey*. New Century Publications.

Ignacimuthu, S. (2005). *Basic Informatics*. New Delhi: Narosa Publishing House.

Khon & Skarulis. (2012). IBM Watson Delivers New Insights for Treatment and Diagnosis. *Digital Health Conference*.

Kraynak. (2017). *Cloud Data Warehousing Dummies*. John Willey & Sons.

Kumar & Joy. (2013). Application of Zigbee Wireless Frequency for Patient Monitoring System. *CSI Communications Journal, 37*(9), 17–18.

Lals. (2018). *Public Health Management Principles.* CBS Publishers & Distributors.

Linowes. (2015). *Virtual Reality Projects.* Pack7.

Madison, N. (2014). *Health Information Systems, Opportunities, and Challenges.* Http//commons.nmu.edu/facwork book chapters/14

McConnell, C. R. (2020). *Hospitals and Healthcare Systems: What they are and how they work.* Jones & Bartlett Learning.

Mo. (2015). How to Build an Ideal Health Care Information System. In *The World Book of Family Medicine.* Academic Press.

Rao. (Ed.). (2011). *Virtual Technologies for Business and Industrial Applications: Innovative and Synergistic Approaches.* IGI Global.

Reur, J., Arino, J., & Olk, P. (2011). *Entrepreneurial Alliances* (Vol. 1). Boston: Pearson Higher Education.

Schulz, G. (2012). *Cloud and Virtual Data Storage, Networking.* Taylor & Francis Group.

Semolic & Baisya. (2013). *Globalization and Innovative Business Models.* New Delhi: Ane Books Private Limited.

Sunitha, Kokilam, & Preethi. (2013). Medical Informatics-Perk up Health Care through Information. *CSI Communications Journal, 37*(9), 7-8.

Thomas, E. R. L. (2014). *Cloud computing Concepts, Technology, and Architecture.* Pearson.

Vijayrani, S. (2013). Economic Health Records- An Overview. *CSI Communications Journal, 37*(9), 9-11.

Vivek, J. (2020). *Review of Preventive & Social Medicine (Including Bio-Statistics).* Jaypee Brothers Medical Publisher.

Walshe. (2014). *Healthcare Management.* McGraw-Hill.

Wulfovich. (2019). Digital Health Entrepreneurship. Springer.

Chapter 7
Anatomy–Based Human Modeling for Virtual Reality (VR)

Yuk Ming Tang

(iD) https://orcid.org/0000-0001-8215-4190
Hong Kong Polytechnic University, China

Hoi Sze Chan
Hong Kong Polytechnic University, China

Wei Ting Kuo
Hong Kong Polytechnic University, China

EXECUTIVE SUMMARY

The authors proposed an anatomy-based methodology for human modeling to enhance the visual realism of human modeling by using the boundary element method (BEM) and axial deformation approach. To model muscle deformation, a BEM with linear boundary elements was used. The significance of tendons in determining skin layer deformation is also discussed. The axial deformation technique is used to allow for quick deformation. To control tendon deformation, the curve of the axial curve is changed. Each vertex of the skin layer is linked to the muscles, tendons, and skeletons beneath it. The skin layer deforms in response to changes in the underlying muscle, tendon, and skeleton layers. This chapter made use of human foot modeling as the case study. Results have illustrated that the visual realism of human models can be enhanced by considering the changes of tendons in the deformation of the skin layer. The lower computational complexity and enhanced visual realism of the proposed approaches can be applied in human modelling for virtual reality (VR) applications.

DOI: 10.4018/978-1-7998-8790-4.ch007

INTRODUCTION

Human model modeling and animation have long been a research goal in the aspect of computer graphics. Computer human modeling can be widely used in many areas including virtual reality (VR), surgery simulation, footwear design, gait analysis, etc. For instance, applications of human foot simulation are used in surgery simulation (Bro-Nielsen & Cotin, 1996; Cotin, 1999; Charles et al., 2021), footwear design, gait physical therapy (Yano, 2003), etc. Nevertheless, due to the complexity in the modeling of a human character, not much physics-based approach in the modeling and simulating of human foot model has been reported for VR applications. Although different approaches have been developed for interactive deformation, the performance of the simulation is still far from satisfactory.

Nowadays, there are various approaches for modeling in VR and related computer graphics applications. First of all, is the geometry-based approach to design based on the manual processes by graphical designers. This approach involves the design using a generic three-dimensional (3D) model or a statistical human model. In a generic 3D model, designers can design the human model freely based on their senses and experience. In a statistical human model, the model postures can be learned from statistical databases. The statistical databases have developed valuable tools for solving a variety of visual and graphic problems for 3D modeling. Blender, SketchUp, ZBrush, AutoCAD, SolidWorks, Rhino3D, 3Ds Max, Maya, CATIA, and other commercially accessible 3D modeling programs are currently available to help with design work. Autodesk 3Ds Max is a 3D computer graphics software that has gained popularity among both professional and amateur animators due to its versatility. It provides effective, rapid, and efficient performance and workflows to help increase the processing complex's overall efficiency. Autodesk Maya is another popular 3D animation program. Maya also comes with a simple simulation tool. Cinema 4D, unlike Autodesk 3Ds Max and Autodesk Maya, is not only popular among animators, but is also recommended for beginners because it is less complex than 3D Studio Max and Maya.(Hendriyani, & Amrizal, 2019). Professional and industrial applications are among the most often utilized modeling tools. These tools are used not only for computer-aided design (CAD), but also for computer-aided engineering (CAE) analysis, additive manufacturing (AM), and 3D printing. (Tang, & Ho, 2020).

Another approach is based on computer simulation methods. The methods including physics-based and anatomy-based approaches. Simulating human walking is a difficult topic from the standpoint of computational analysis. In the research, inverted pendulum models, passive dynamic walking, and approaches based on zero moment points have all been used to generate realism and natural human walking using mechanical models (ZMP). Simulation science has advanced significantly in recent years. The literature on human walking simulation is mostly divided into two categories: biped robot research and physical mechanics study. Real-time biped walking control is a major topic in robotics, and simpler walking models such as inverted pendulum models and passive power walking are commonly used for this. Furthermore, the ZMP-based trajectory planning approach seeks to follow the pre-planned ZMP trajectory. (Refai et al., 2019). Although biped robots have made significant progress in walking synthesis, many aspects of human walking cannot be replicated by biped robots. Gait analysis based on biomechanics and musculoskeletal models can provide more physiological information about human walking. Muscles, weariness, and injuries are all hot topics in science right now. (Xiang, Arora & Abdel-Malek, 2010).

In the field of computer graphics and simulation, anatomy-based modeling is critical. Medical imaging using multiple modalities allows us to visualize and comprehend the changes of the full living human body in 3D space throughout time. A clearer picture of anatomical dynamics could aid in the resolution of contemporary medical issues. In surgical data science, the most significant component is the modeling of individualized digital patients. (Maier-Hein et al., 2017). The origins of computational anatomy may be traced back to 1917, when D'Arey Wentworth Thompson wrote his classic book "Shape and Growth". (Xiang, Arora & Abdel-Malek, 2010). It emphasizes the importance of physics and mechanics in determining the morphology and structure of organisms, as well as the fact that morphological differences between related animals can be explained using simple mathematical procedures. Modern computational anatomy is evolving into a science devoted to the quantitative analysis of organ shape variability and its application to computer-aided diagnosis (CAD) and computer-assisted surgery (CAS). Modern computational anatomy provides a technical framework for a better understanding of anatomical diversity, simplifies illness detection, and allows for the simulation of surgical intervention in light of these improvements.

For novel advanced technologies based on mathematics, engineering, and medical research, a new model of Multidisciplinary Computational Anatomy (MCA) must be constructed (Kobatake & Masutani, 2017). Its objectives are to discover the significant meaning and statistical relationship between various modalities of medical images, integrate a large amount of information about human body structure and life phenomena, envision various types of information, and develop mathematical statistics principles and models. A method for more readily accessing or searching for information. Comprehensive interdisciplinary knowledge is implemented to medical judgment or decision-making by thoroughly comprehending the anatomy and the real strategy before the activity (Hashizume, 2021).

The anatomy-based approach not only enhances the visual realism but is also able to simulate the anatomical structure, as well as simulate the models based on physics. With the recent advancement of the graphics card and computational power of the personal computer, real-time interactions can also be achieved. The goal of this chapter is to discuss an anatomy-based approach for interactive simulation of the human foot. Muscle, skeleton, tendon, and skin are among the components that make up the foot model. To achieve accurate and interactive deformation, various physics-based approaches are adopted. The Boundary element method (BEM) with linear boundary elements is adopted to model the deformation of foot muscles. The axial deformation technique is used to deform foot tendons. This approach has potential application in animated movies, computer games, shoes design and manufacturing, and other activities in VR, augmented reality (AR), and mixed reality (MR). Based on the deformation of the underlying skeleton, muscle, and tendon layers, the deformation of the skin layer is calculated in real-time on a personal computer.

This chapter is organized as follows. The human anatomy including human biomechanics, the human skeleton and joint, musculotendon unit are firstly reviewed. The methodology including physics-based, tendon deformation, and skin deformation is illustrated in the next section. We present the results of muscle deformation, modeling toses raising, and human gait modeling, followed by the conclusion section.

REVIEW ON HUMAN ANATOMY

Human Biomechanics

It is a prerequisite for the description of human biomechanics in the following sections of this thesis. Fundamental biomechanics of human anatomy can be found in many references (Tang et al., 2010, Charles et al., 2021). Anatomists have introduced terms to identify specific planes and the corresponding axis perpendicular to these planes to describe relative movements of different body parts. Figure 1 illustrates the three perpendicular planes: frontal, sagittal, and transverse planes, and the corresponding axes that pass perpendicularly through the planes: anteroposterior, mediolateral, and longitudinal axes.

After the plane or the axis of motion is identified, the joint movement of different parts of the body can be easily identified. Movements of joints around the transverse axis include flexion, extension, and hyperextension, which occur at the wrist, elbow, shoulder, hip, knee, and intervertebral joints. In the sagittal plane, flexion and extension relate to a decrease and increase in joint angle respectively. Hyperextension is the movement to the extremities of the range of motion. Dorsiflexion and plantar flexion are joint actions that occur at the ankle (Medeiros & Martini,

2018). Dorsiflexion and plantar flexion occur around the transverse axis through the ankle joint and cause the foot to move in the sagittal plane. The upward motion of the foot in dorsiflexion and the downward motion of the foot are known as plantar flexion. Figure 2 illustrates the joint actions in the sagittal plane.

A body standing flat and erect, and facing forward is called anatomical position. Motion at the shoulder and hip joints starting from the anatomical position around the anteroposterior axis is the abduction, while moving back to the anatomical position is called adduction. Inversion and eversion are the frontal plane movement along the anteroposterior axis at the ankle joint. Starting from the anatomical position, an inversion occurs when the foot is lifted to the medial side. The return movement of the foot is eversion. Figure 3 shows some examples of frontal plane joint actions.

Figure 1. Anatomical planes and axes of human body
(Knudson, 2003)

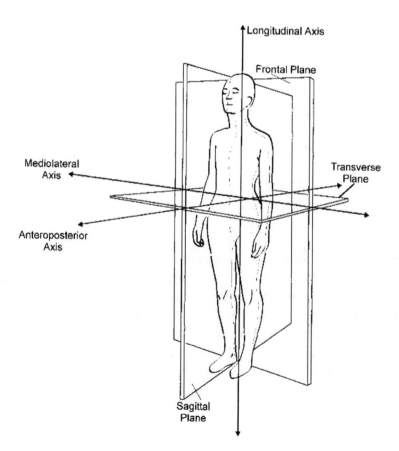

Figure 2. Joint actions in the sagittal plane
(McGinnis, 1999)

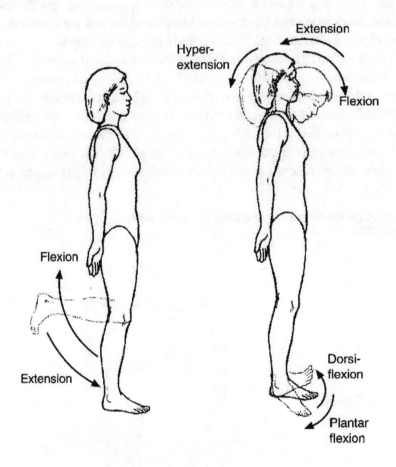

Pronation and supination, which refer to the complicated motions of the subtalar joint (a joint at the foot ankle), are two other examples of special joint motion terms. Pronation combines the anatomical actions of eversion, plantar flexion, and abduction while the opposite motion is called supination. Figure 4 illustrates the pronation and supination of the foot. These arches are supported by the foot's muscles, tendons, ligaments, and fasciae. A detailed discussion of the anatomy of the human foot may be found in (Barcsay,1973; Goldfinger,1991; Sheppard,1992; Holowka & Lieberman, 2018; McNutt, Zipfel & DeSilva, 2018).

Figure 3. Joint actions in frontal plane
(McGinnis, 1999)

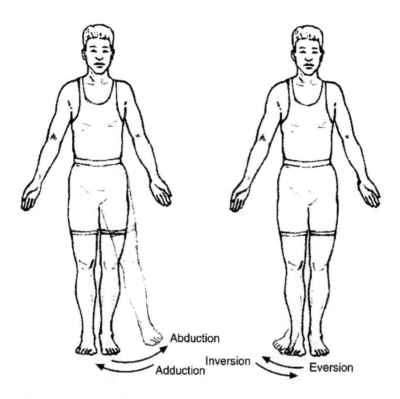

Figure 4. Pronation and supination of the foot
(Knudson,2003)

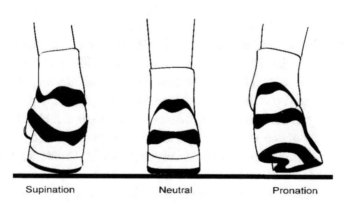

Human Skeleton and Joint

The human body is made up of 206 bones that are separated into three sections: the head, trunk, and limbs. They are distributed in different parts of the body, supporting the body, protecting the internal organs, and at the same time being assisted by muscles to perform various activities. All the bones of the human body are different in shape and size. Some are larger, such as tibia and humerus, and some are very small, such as phalanges. Long bones, short bones, flat bones, irregular bones, and air-bearing bones are the five types based on shape. The flat bones cover the interior organs, such as the skull, which protects the brain, while the rod-shaped bones, such as the limb bones, are important for human mobility. The vertebrae are bones that run through the center of the body from the neck to the buttocks. From top to bottom, they are cervical vertebrae (7), thoracic vertebrae (12), lumbar vertebrae (5), sacrum, and tailbone. There are convex bones on the spine that can be touched from the outside, which is an important basis for finding acupuncture points.

If human bones are as rigid as a pillar, people will not be able to move. The key to people's freedom of movement is that they have joints. A joint is the portion of the body that connects two or more bones. Some of these joints are huge enough to support the entire human body's weight, while others are so little that they are invisible to the naked eye. It is with joints that our body can make a variety of movements. Joints can be divided into fixed joints, semi-moving joints, and movable joints. The bones in the human body can barely move after some joints are joined. Fixed joints are the name for these types of joints. The freedom of mobility of neighboring bones is greatly reduced when the joints in the human body are joined. This kind of joint is called a semi-moving joint. In fact, most joints in the human body are movable joints. The types of movable joints are axle joints, saddle joints, elliptical joints, club and socket joints, flexor joints, and flat joints.

A typical joint is generally composed of three parts: articular surface, joint capsule, and joint cavity. The articular surface can be divided into the joint head and the joint socket; the joint capsule is the connective tissue attached around the joint surface; the joint cavity is the space between the joint surfaces in the joint capsule. The human body in medicine generally includes rotation and circulation, flexion and extension, abduction and adduction, and plantar flexion and dorsiflexion.

The foot's skeleton is made up of twenty-eight skeletal bones kept together by, ligaments, muscles, and tendons. There are three types of phalanges: phalanges, metatarsus, and tarsus. In the toes, there are 14 bones called phalanges. A phalanx is a long bone that can be proximal, middle, or distal, with the exception of the big toe, which has only proximal and distal phalanxes. Between the tarsus and the phalanx is the metatarsus, which is a lengthy bone. The tarsus is made up of seven bones: the talus, calcaneus, cuboid, navicular, and three cuneiforms. The foot articulates with the long bones of the lower leg, tibia, and fibula. There are 28 bones and over 30 joints in the foot. Ligaments hold the bones and joints in place. The ankle, subtalar joint, metatarsophalangeal (MTP), and interdigital (IP) joints are the primary joints of the foot.

Musculotendon Unit

In order to facilitate the simulation of the musculotendon unit (Yamamoto et al., 2020), it is important to identify the structure of the foot muscles and tendons and the types of muscle movements. Next, we will introduce the structure of muscles and tendons, and classify the types of muscle movements. On this basis, the muscle model of Hill and Zajac is introduced. Finally, the foot kinematics related to tendon length, tendon strength, and moment arm is introduced.

Three types of muscles including skeletal, cardiac, and smooth. Skeletal muscle takes up a significant portion of an animal's body (Sarver et al., 2017). It is the primary mover in animals' locomotion and is controlled by nerves. The movement of the bones that they link is caused by alternating between contractions and relaxations. Skeletal muscles are the muscles on the bottom of the foot. Muscle belly and two end tendons make up the general anatomy of skeletal muscles (Tieland, Trouwborst & Clark, 2018). When an active muscle lengthens, the muscle torque is smaller than the resistance torque, resulting in an eccentric movement (Schoenfeld et al., 2017). At the MTP joint, the foot tendons are frequently visible on the skin surface (Van Royen et al., 2020). The active force is created by the contractile elements of the muscle. Stored chemical energy is consumed during the motions. The elongation of the musculotendon unit's connective tissues produces passive force. We assume that all created forces are active forces, and that only the muscle's concentric activities are taken into account.

The muscle models are usually adopted by Hill's muscle model (Hill,1938; McMahon,1984; Bujalski, Martins & Stirling, 2018). Hill's approach considers both the active and passive aspects of the muscle. The active tension of the muscle is represented by the contractile element, while the passive tension is represented by the elastic element (spring), which is connected in series and parallel to the contractile element. Similar to Hill's muscle model, Zajac developed a "dimensionless" model of a musculotendon unit (Zajac, 1986; Zajac, 1989; Laclé & Pronost, 2017). By adjusted a few parameters, a generic muscle model based on these parameters can be obtained.

Although a muscle generates a force F^M along the line of action, motions at joints are rotary. The geometry of the line of action of the muscles can be found in (Allard, 1995). The rotary torque T can be computed by (Rassier, 1999, Salathea, 2002)

$$T = F^M r, \tag{1}$$

The moment arm about the joint is denoted by r. The moment arm is the perpendicular distance between the joint and the muscle's path of action (Hoy et al., 1990; Maganaris,2001; Desmyttere et al.,2020)

During joint motions, muscles and tendons change their length due to the active and passive forces. The change in musculotendon length, Δl^{MT} and the change in joint angle $\Delta\theta$ is related by (Hoy et al., 1990)

$$\Delta l^{MT} = r\Delta\theta. \tag{2}$$

This relationship is widely used for computer simulation (Delp, 1990, Delp, 1995; Zhang et al., 2019). Blemker et al. (2005) computed the individual fiber moment arm from the muscle fiber lengths using Equation (2).

METHODOLOGY

In anatomical-based modeling, several methodologies are adopted to simulate the deformation of different layers of a human model. In this chapter, a boundary element method (BEM) was used to perform a physics-based simulation of the muscles. The tendons are simulated using the deformable axial curves. The human bone movement was driven by the deformation of muscles and the tendons. Finally, the underlying muscles, tendons, and bones determine the appearance of the skin layer. The purpose of this chapter is to explain how to represent muscle, tendon, and skin deformation. Our goal is to simulate a human anatomical model for animation purposes. The deformation of each layer should be realized at the interactive frame rate. An anatomical foot model including skin, muscle, tendon, and bone layers is proposed as the case study in this chapter.

Anatomical Model

To perform the anatomy-based modeling, an anatomical model needs to be obtained at the beginning. In this chapter, a commercially available foot skeleton and tissue model is used as the case study. The 3-D foot skin data is provided by the Department of Sports Science and Physical Education. The foot skin data is obtained by scanning a real human foot using a 3-D foot scanner. The anatomical foot model is composed of three rigid segments that allow for two joint motions. Five Phalanges make up the initial segment. The tarsus and five metatarsals make up the second segment. The third segment is formed by the lower leg's end. The MTP joint joins the first and second segments, and the ankle joint articulates the second and third segments. We designed the ankle and MTP joints with fixed instantaneous centers of revolution, only dorsiflexion and plantar flexion are allowed at the ankle joint, and only flexion and extension of the toes are allowed at the MTP joint.

Physics-Based Deformation

Two basic physics-based deformation techniques, finite element method (FEM) and boundary element method (BEM), have been widely used in interactive object simulation issues (Tang, 2010). However, due to the conflicting requirements for accuracy and speed, this is still a huge challenge in computer graphics. Surgery simulation done by Bro-Nielsen (1996) and Cotin (1999) is an example of this, because it demands accurate deformation as well as real-time interaction. Nevertheless, due to the complexity of human organs and tissues, real-time deformation can only be performed using a relatively simplified model.

The use of FEM (Hui et al., 2002b) provides more accurate physical simulation and analysis (Tang et al, 2014). However, the method's main shortcomings are the complexity of using FEM and the high computational cost of calculating deformation. Additionally, from the geometric model, the finite element method must generate solid elements., which is a time-consuming and tedious procedure. In engineering analysis and application, the boundary element method is a prominent technique (Katsikadelis, 2002). Yet, it is not widely used to simulate deformable objects in computer graphics (Hui et al., 2002a). The same boundary mesh can be utilized for deformation and rendering owing to boundary elements. Furthermore, the boundary grid makes it simple to create popular graphical packages. This saves time and effort while creating solid volume finite element elements. James et al. (1999) proved that the use of the boundary element method can simulate deformable objects in real-time. A detailed comparison between the FEM and BME was performed by Tang et al. (2005 and 2006).

The idea behind BEM is to discretize the model's border into a sequence of elements using a numerical approach. Previous research was conducted to investigate the muscle deformation based on the BEM (Zhou et al., 2006 and Tang & Hui, 2011). In the m-th element, the displacements u_m and tractions t_m at a point of the element are approximated by interpolating the nodal displacements u_m^n and tractions t_m^n using the shape function Φ such that

$$u_m = \sum_{n=1}^{N} \Phi^n u_m^n \qquad (3)$$

and

$$t_m = \sum_{n=1}^{N} \Phi^n t_m^n, \tag{4}$$

where N is the number of nodal points in each element which is equal to one for constant element and three for linear element.

Suppose the boundary of the object is discretized into a set of M triangular elements, and using Equations (3) and (4), by turning the surface integrals into the sums of integrals, the expression across each boundary element can be recast. This gives

$$c_k u_k + \sum_{m=1}^{M} \sum_{n=1}^{N} \left(\int_{\Gamma_m} t_k^* \Phi^n d\Gamma \right) u_m^n = \sum_{m=1}^{M} \sum_{n=1}^{N} \left(\int_{\Gamma_m} u_k^* \Phi^n d\Gamma \right) t_m^n, \tag{5}$$

where Γ_m is the surface of the mth element.

Grouping all the integrals of the same node together, we have

$$c_k u_k + \sum_{l=1}^{L} \hat{h}_{kl} u_l = \sum_{l=1}^{L} g_{kl} t_l, \tag{6}$$

where L is the total number of nodal elements which is equal to the number of nodes of the linear element, $\hat{h}_{kl}$ and g_{kl} are the integrals of the fundamental solution for the displacements and tractions respectively.

Define elements h_{kl}, $k \neq l$, as $\hat{h}_{kl}$, and letting $h_{kk} = c_k + \hat{h}_{kk}$. Equation (6) yields

$$\sum_{l=1}^{L} h_{kl} u_l = \sum_{l=1}^{L} g_{kl} t_l. \tag{7}$$

Assembling all the elements together and using matrix notation, Equation (7) can be written as

$$HU = GT, \tag{8}$$

where

$$U = \begin{bmatrix} u_{1x} & u_{1y} & u_{1z} & u_{2x} & u_{2y} & u_{2z} & \cdots & u_{Lx} & u_{Ly} & u_{Lz} \end{bmatrix}^t,$$

$$T = \begin{bmatrix} t_{1x} & t_{1y} & t_{1z} & t_{2x} & t_{2y} & t_{2z} & \cdots & t_{Lx} & t_{Ly} & t_{Lz} \end{bmatrix}^t,$$

H is a $3L{\times}3L$ matrix with elements that are functions of h_{kl} and
G is a $3L{\times}3L$ matrix with elements that are functions of g_{kl}.

Modeling Tendon Deformation

Recently, there has not been a lot of research done recently on the distortion of the skin's surface caused by underlying tendons. Tendons, in particular on the foot and hand, play a vital role in influencing skin surface deformation. Tendon deformation procedures are utilized to determine the skin layer's distortion, which improves the visual realism of foot modeling. We propose that the axial deformation technique may be utilized to regulate the deformation of foot tendons based on the axial curves in order to achieve interactive deformation of tendon models (Tang & Hui, 2009). To estimate the shape of the axial curves that prescribe tendons deformation, both geometry-based and physics-based techniques are proposed. Using the basic functions to determine the degree of deformation of the tendons, this chapter demonstrated a simple way to improve the realism of the foot simulation in the geometry-based approach. A method for calculating the basis function from photos is provided, which collects images with a low-cost camera. The updated position of the "via points" that define the axial curves was computed using the mass-spring system in the physics-based technique. (Choi et al., 2007). Tendon deformation is determined by the stiffness of the foot tendon. The stiffness of the angular springs can be adjusted to affect how visible the tendons are on the skin near the joints. Finally, the skin layer is distorted in accordance with the distortion of the underlying layers.

Skin Deformation

This section discusses the method for deforming the skin layer. After determining the distortion of the underlying layers, the skin layer is deformed correspondingly. To attain fast deformation, a simple method by translating the vertices of the skin layer according to the summation of the displacement of the weighted correspondences based on Tang & Hui (2007) was adopted. The technique connects the skin vertices with the vertices of the underlying layers in a one-to-N relationship. Each vertex of the skin layer is associated with N vertices of the underlying muscle, tendon, or skeleton layers. The distortion of the underlying layers affects the vertices of the skin layer.

We compute the shortest distances between the skin vertices and the underlying layers to find the correspondences. Denote U_s be the set of vertices of the skin layer and U_u be the set that contains the number of vertices of the muscle, tendon, and skeleton layers. A total of I_s skin vertices, $v_i^s, i \in U_s$ are defined to represent the 3-D coordinate of the ith vertex of the skin layer, and a total of I_u vertices of the underlying muscle, tendon, and skeleton layers, $v_i^u, i \in U_u$ are defined to represent the 3-D coordinate of the ith vertex of the underlying muscle, tendon and skeleton layers.

Assume $d_{n,i}^c, i \in U_s$ to be the 3-D displacement vector of the nth correspondence associated with the ith skin vertex. The ith 3-D displacement vector that transforms v_i^s, $d_i^v, i \in U_s$ is determined by

$$d_i^v = \sum_{n=1}^{N} w_n d_{n,i}^c ,$$ (9)

where w_n is the weighting of the nth correspondence which satisfies $\sum_{n=1}^{N} w_n = 1$.

Then, the skin vertex is simply updated by

$$v_i'^s = v_i^s + d_i^v .$$ (10)

RESULTS

The modeling of the human foot based on anatomy is visualized using experimental software. The simulation program was developed using graphics engine Microsoft Visual C++ and adopted OpenGL. It accepts 3-D models with various file formats such as "ASE", "DXF" and "OBJ" and exports the simulated model in "OBJ" format. The simulations were run on a computer with a 3.2GHz processor and 2GB of RAM. In each of the following experiments, the simulations were performed at interactive frame rates.

In this section, the experimental results of simulating human feet are introduced. The experiment is divided into several parts. In the first part, we model the deformation of muscle as it is the core part to control human motions. We modelled the foot model when the toes were lifted in the second part. The third section replicated general foot gait motions. Lastly, other foot motions were simulated. The extensor digitorum longus and the extensor hallucis longus have set boundary conditions in the experiment of simulating muscle deformation. To illustrate the case of changing boundary conditions of foot motion, modeling the human foot during gait was also included in the experiment. In the gait experiment, the flexor digitorum brevis is included in the simulation. The contact area between the foot and the ground changes during a gait motion. This results in a change in the number of nodes with known displacement on the flexor digitorum brevis mesh's boundary.

Muscle Deformation

In the modeling of the anatomical foot, Figures 5 show the distortion of the extensor digitorum longus and extensor hallucis longus muscles. The wireframe models in blue color are the initial state of the muscles. The grey color represents the muscle and tendon models, and the skeleton is in brown color. When the toes are raised, the muscles deformed and shortened their length. The muscle bellies bulged when their lengths were shortened illustrating the elastic property of the muscle belly.

The BEM with linear boundary elements is used to deform the muscles in this experiment. The time required for the BEM's pre-computation and deformation operations, as well as the number of vertices and faces of the muscle models, were summarized in Table 1. The time required for the deformation process for muscles with defined boundary conditions is roughly the same as the mesh with a varying amount of known displacements. It took around 0.007s and 0.009s for deforming the muscles of the extensor hallucis longus and the extensor digitorum longus respectively. An experiment was carried out on the muscles of the extensor hallucis longus and extensor digitorum longus to observe if there was a link between the time required for deformation and the number of nodes with known displacement (Figures 6). The time required to compute deformation rises with the number of nodes with known displacement, as shown in the diagram. However, when a different number of nodes with known displacement were used, the time required for the pre-computation procedure was roughly the same, 30.201s and 19.137s for the muscles of the extensor hallucis longus and the extensor digitorum longus, respectively.

Table 1. Summary of the time required for the BEM's pre-computation and deformation procedures for the extensor hallucis longus and extensor digitorum longus muscles

Muscle Models	Number		Computation Time (seconds)	
	Vertices	Faces	Pre-computation	Deformation
extensor digitorum longus	287	570	30.209	0.009
extensor hallucis longus	248	492	19.136	0.007

Figure 5. Deformation of muscles corresponding to various foot toes movements.
The wireframe models in blue color are the initial state of the muscles. The grey
color represents the muscle and tendon models, and the skeleton is in brown color.
(Tang & Hui, 2007 and 2009)

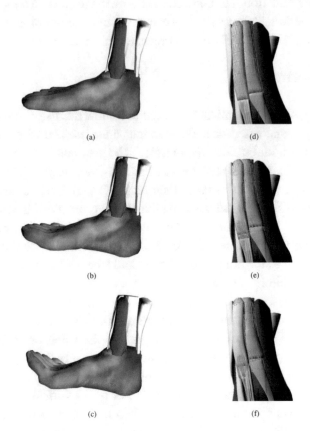

Modeling Toes Raising

When the toes were lifted, we used two primary musculotendons to visualize the
anatomy-based foot model. These muscles are the extensor digitorum longus and
the extensor hallucis longus. The majority of the extensor hallucis longus muscle
belly lies deep in the lower leg when the foot is flat on the floor, making the tendon
difficult to see. A actual foot stands flat on the floor in Figure 7(a). The muscle belly
shortens and the lower end of the muscle slides up, exposing the tendon, when the
toes are raised. The tendon can be seen running down the top of the foot. Figure
7(b) depicts a foot with its toes raised. We demonstrate our method by modeling
the extensor digitorum longus and the extensor hallucis longus, which are the
primary extensors (tendons) of the toes. Deformation of the tendons also appears

prominently on the skin surface at the joint's region. In addition, the extensors exist in different forms. The extensor hallucis longus is a single muscle with a single tendon that controls the big toe's mobility. The major extensor of the toes is the extensor digitorum longus. A single muscle belly is divided into four tendons in the distal phalanges of the second to fifth toes.

Figure 6. The number of nodes with known displacement and the computation time of the deformation process relationship for the muscles of: (a) the extensor hallucis longus and (b) the extensor digitorum longus

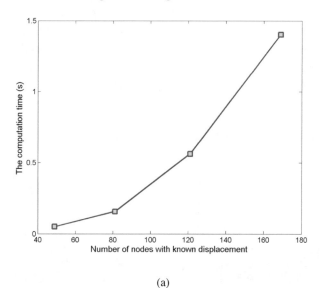

(a)

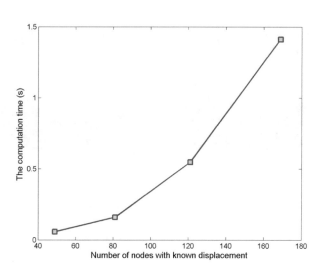

Figure 7. (a) A real foot is standing flat on the floor; (b) the toes are raised
(Tang & Hui, 2007 and 2009)

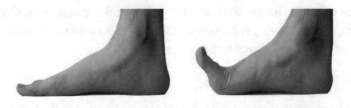

Experiments were conducted to examine the visual effects of geometry-based and physics-based tendon deformation during toe lifting. Figure 8 shows the side views of skin and tendon deformation with the physics-based approaches using the axial curves, and Figure 9 illustrates the close-up view. Figure 10 shows the comparison in different viewing angles. The results demonstrated that there is good visual realism using a physics-based approach compare with the real foot.

Figure 8. Foot modeling using the physics-based approach
(Tang & Hui, 2007 and 2009)

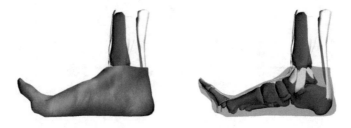

Figure 9. Foot modeling using physics-based approaches in a close-up view
(Tang & Hui, 2007 and 2009)

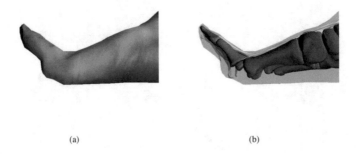

(a)   (b)

Figure 10. Foot modeling in different viewing angles
(*Tang & Hui, 2007 and 2009*)

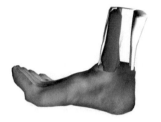 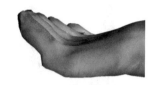

Modeling Gait Motion

An experimental system that simulates human foot gait motion was implemented. The deformation of the extensor digitorum longus and extensor hallucis longus muscles, as well as the deformation of foot tendons, are all part of the simulation. In addition, the muscle of the flexor digitorum brevis at the sole part of the foot is included in the simulation. The flexor digitorum brevis not only plays an important to support the shape of the foot during gait, but the situation of the changing boundary condition of the muscle can also be explored. The time required for modeling anatomical feet under changing boundary conditions can also be studied. Initial contact, midstance, forefoot contact, and toe-off are the four primary characteristics subphases of stance for the human foot (Figure 11). The flexor digitorum brevis was deformed using a varied number of nodes with known displacement depending on the distinctive subphases of stance and percentage of contact between the foot and the ground (Gefen, 2000). The three typical subphases of foot gait motion from midstance, forefoot contact, and toe-off were replicated in this experiment.

This experiment illustrates the deformation of the muscle of the flexor digitorum brevis during foot gait motion. The length of the muscle may fluctuate in this situation to maintain the geometry of the foot, and the number of nodes with known displacement changes during gait. The snapshots in the deformation of the flexor digitorum brevis of the foot during gait motion using the proposed physics-based approach are shown in Figure 12. At the subphases of the forefoot contact and toe-off, the length of the muscle is approximately 99% and 98% of the muscle length during midstance. The sole of the foot is fully in contact with the ground during the midstance subphases. The nodes at the bottom of the flexor digitorum brevis muscle are well known. During foot gait motion, however, the number of nodes with known displacement changes. As the foot moves forward, the muscle bends and the number of nodes with known displacement decreases.

Figure 11. Four characteristic subphases of foot gait motion
(Allard, 1995)

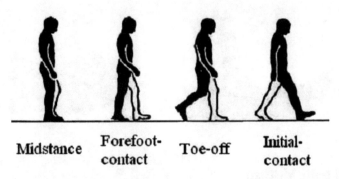

Table 2 illustrates the time required for the deformation processes of modeling the anatomical foot at different subphases of foot gait motion. The flexor digitorum brevis muscle is composed of 110 vertices and 216 faces. Pre-computation is required before to simulation. Setting up the mass-spring system and pre-computation of the BEM are both part of the pre-computation procedure. The muscles and tendons of the extensor digitorum longus, extensor hallucis longus, and flexor digitorum brevis were deformed in this experiment. Given the foot motions, the muscles and tendons are deformed accordingly. The muscle of the flexor digitorum brevis contains 110 vertices and 216 faces. The mass-spring system contains 46 springs.

The number of nodes in the flexor digitorum brevis with known displacement changes. At the midstance subphases, the muscle has the maximum number of nodes with documented displacement. It spends around 0.115s for the deformation process. However, as the number of nodes with known displacement drops from midstance to toe-off, the time required for the deformation process decreases. Table 2 summarized the total time required for modeling the foot during gait. The pre-computation step takes an average of 104.862 seconds.

Table 2. Summary of the time required for the deformation process for the muscle of the flexor digitorum brevis at different subphases of foot gait motion

	Number	Computation Time (seconds)
Subphases	Nodes with known displacement	Deformation
Midstance	51	0.056
Forefoot-contact	24	0.010
Toe-off	12	0.005

Figure 12. The snapshots in the deformation of the flexor digitorum brevis of the foot during gait motion

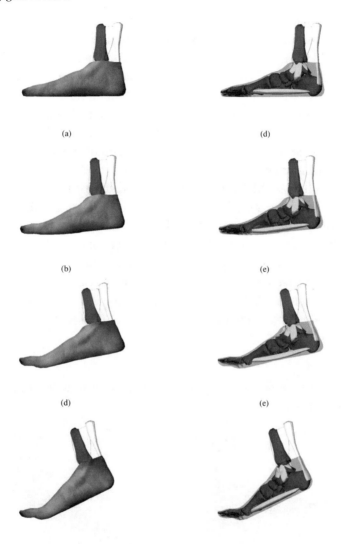

(a)　　　　　　　　　　(d)

(b)　　　　　　　　　　(e)

(d)　　　　　　　　　　(e)

Table 3. Summary of the time required for modeling the foot at different subphases of foot gait motion

	Computation Time (seconds)
Subphases	Deformation
Midstance	0.115
Forefoot-contact	0.083
Toe-off	0.067

Other Motions

This section illustrates the experimental results of the deformation of the Gastrocnemius muscle and the other foot motions. Figure 13 shows the comparison of the foot with and without deforming the Gastrocnemius muscle. Figure 14 illustrates the deformation of the Gastrocnemius muscle and its tendon using the BEM with linear boundary elements and the corresponding foot motions. During dorsiflexion and plantar flexion of the foot ankle, the gastrocnemius is the main muscle that elevates and lowers the foot heel. In this figure, the initial and deformed muscles are overlapped to compare the difference. The wireframe model in blue color is the initial state of the muscles. The grey color represents the deformed state. The model contains 410 vertices and 816 faces. The pre-computation phase takes 85.032 seconds to complete. The time required for the deformation process is 0.016 seconds with 44 known displacements. Figures 25 and 26 illustrate the result of modeling the foot with different foot motions and in the different viewing directions. Figure 15 compares the result of modeling the foot with and without deforming the tendons using the physics-based tendon deformation technique. In the figure, the foot and toes are raised. Tendon deformation is seen on the skin surface of the MTP and ankle areas for the foot. In Figure 16, the first toe of the foot is raised and inverted at the same time.

Figure 13. The foot with deforming the Gastrocnemius muscle when the foot heel is raised and lowered.

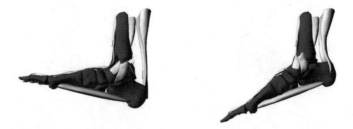

CONCLUSION

In this Chapter, a technique for modeling anatomical foot models is presented. For modeling muscle deformation, a BEM with linear boundary elements is used. Controlling the deformations of foot tendons is done using the axial deformation approach. Geometry-based and physics-based techniques are proposed to determine the shape of the axial curve that dictates tendons deformation. The geometry-based and physics-based methodologies are proposed to determine the shape of the axial curve that prescribes deformation of the tendons.

Figure 14. Deformation of the Gastrocnemius muscle when the foot heel is: (a) and (b) raised; (b) and (d) lowered. The initial and deformed muscles are overlapped. The wireframe model in blue color is the initial state of the muscle. The grey color represents the deformed muscle.

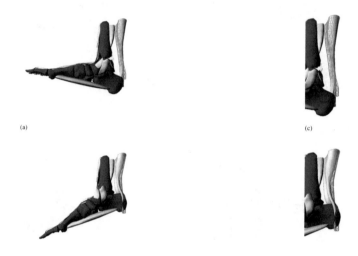

Experimental results on modeling anatomical foot models are successfully demonstrated. The extensor digitorum longus and the extensor hallucis longus, two primary foot musculotendon models, were deformed when the big toe was lifted to exhibit our experimental results. Using BEM with linear boundary elements for deforming muscle, interactive and realistic deformation can be achieved. To demonstrate the effect of tendons on skin layer deformation, several tests were carried out. The tendon emerged noticeably when the tendon was further expanded, according to the results of the experiments. Comparisons are made between the foot model with and without tendon distortion. In addition, tests are carried out to compare tendon deformation using geometry-based and physics-based techniques. There is also a demonstration of an experiment on modeling human foot gait motion under changing boundary conditions of the foot-deep muscle. The foot model is simulated in real-time in all of our studies. Despite the anatomy-based modelling approach is successfully demonstrated, the current results are mainly focused on the human food models. In the future, the works can be extended to the entire human body and demonstrate in various VR applications in real-time.

Figure 15. The foot with deforming the tendons when the foot and toes are raised. For the foot with tendon deformation, the tendons show on the skin surface of the MTP and ankle regions.

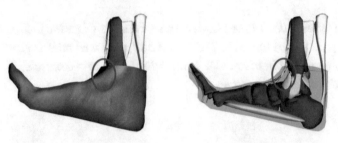

Figure 16. Snapshots of modeling the foot in different viewing angles when the first toe is raised and inverted.

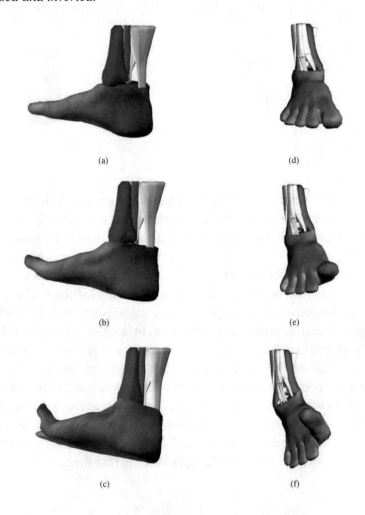

REFERENCES

Allard, P., Stokes, I. A. F., & Blanchi, J. P. (1995). *Three-dimensional analysis of human movement*. Human Kinetics.

Barcsay, J. (1973). *Anatomy for the artist*. Octopus Books.

Blemker, S. S., & Delp, S. L. (2005). Three-dimensional representation of complex muscle architectures and geometries. *Annals of Biomedical Engineering*, *33*(5), 661–673. doi:10.100710439-005-1433-7 PMID:15981866

Bro-Nielsen, M., & Cotin, S. (1996). Real-time volumetric deformable models for surgery simulation using finite elements and condensation. *Computer Graphics Forum*, *15*(3), 57–66. doi:10.1111/1467-8659.1530057

Bujalski, P., Martins, J., & Stirling, L. (2018). A Monte Carlo analysis of muscle force estimation sensitivity to muscle-tendon properties using a Hill-based muscle model. *Journal of Biomechanics*, *79*, 67–77. doi:10.1016/j.jbiomech.2018.07.045 PMID:30146173

Charles, J. P., Grant, B., D'Août, K., & Bates, K. T. (2021). Foot anatomy, walking energetics, and the evolution of human bipedalism. *Journal of Human Evolution*, *156*, 103014. doi:10.1016/j.jhevol.2021.103014 PMID:34023575

Choi, Y. K., Hui, K. C., & Tang, Y. M. (2007). Fitting a Polygon Mesh Through a Set of Curves. *Lecture Notes in Computer Science*, 4469.

Cotin, S., Delingette, H., & Ayache, N. (1999). Real-time elastic deformations of soft tissues for surgery simulation. *IEEE Transactions on Visualization and Computer Graphics*, *5*(1), 62–73. doi:10.1109/2945.764872

Delp, S. L., & Loan, J. P. (1995). A Graphics-based Software System to Develop and Analyze Models of Musculoskeletal Structures. *Computers in Biology and Medicine*, *25*(1), 21–34. doi:10.1016/0010-4825(95)98882-E PMID:7600758

Delp, S. L., Loan, J. P., Hoy, M. G., Zajac, F. E., Topp, E. L., & Rosen, J. M. (1990). An interactive graphics-based model of the lower extremity to study orthopaedic surgical procedures. *IEEE Transactions on Biomedical Engineering*, *37*(8), 757–767. doi:10.1109/10.102791 PMID:2210784

Desmyttere, G., Leteneur, S., Hajizadeh, M., Bleau, J., & Begon, M. (2020). Effect of 3D printed foot orthoses stiffness and design on foot kinematics and plantar pressures in healthy people. *Gait & Posture*, *81*, 247–253. doi:10.1016/j.gaitpost.2020.07.146 PMID:32818861

Gefen, A., Megido-Ravid, M., Itzchak, Y., & Arcan, M. (2000). Biomechanical Analysis of the Three-Dimensional Foot Structure During Gait - A Basic Tool for Clinical Applications. *Journal of Biomechanical Engineering, 122*(6), 630–639. doi:10.1115/1.1318904 PMID:11192385

Goldfinger, E. (1991). *Human anatomy for artists: the elements of form.* Oxford University Press.

Hashizume, M. (2021). Perspective for Future Medicine: Multidisciplinary Computational Anatomy-Based Medicine with Artificial Intelligence. *Cyborg and Bionic Systems.*

Hendriyani, Y., & Amrizal, V. A. (2019, November). The Comparison Between 3D Studio Max and Blender Based on Software Qualities. *Journal of Physics: Conference Series, 1387*(1), 012030. doi:10.1088/1742-6596/1387/1/012030

Hill, A. V. (1938). The heat of shortening and the dynamic constants of muscle. *Proceedings of the Royal Society of London. Series B, Biological Sciences, 126*(843), 136–195. doi:10.1098/rspb.1938.0050

Holowka, N. B., & Lieberman, D. E. (2018). Rethinking the evolution of the human foot: Insights from experimental research. *The Journal of Experimental Biology, 221*(17), jeb174425. doi:10.1242/jeb.174425 PMID:30190415

Hoy, M. G., Zajac, F. E., & Gordon, M. E. (1990). A musculoskeletal model of the human lower extremity: The effect of muscle, tendon, and moment arm on the moment-angle relationship of musculotendon actuators at the hip, knee, and ankle. *Journal of Biomechanics, 23*(2), 157–169. doi:10.1016/0021-9290(90)90349-8 PMID:2312520

Hui, K. C., & Leung, H. C. (2002). Virtual Sculpting and Deformable Volume Modelling. Proceedings of Information Visualisation, 664-669. doi:10.1109/IV.2002.1028846

Hui, K. C., & Wong, N. N. (2002). Hands on a virtually elastic object. *The Visual Computer, 18*(3), 150–163. doi:10.1007003710100120

James, D.L., & Pai, D.K. (1999). ArtDefo: Accurate Real Time Deformable Objects. *Proceedings of Computer Graphics*, 65-72.

Katsikadelis, J. T. (2002). *Boundary elements: theory and applications.* Elsevier.

Knudson, D. (2003). *Fundamentals of biomechanics.* Kluwer Academic/Plenum. doi:10.1007/978-1-4757-5298-4

Kobatake, H., & Masutani, Y. (2017). *Computational anatomy based on whole body imaging*. Springer. doi:10.1007/978-4-431-55976-4

Laclé, F., & Pronost, N. (2017). A scalable geometrical model for musculotendon units. *Computer Animation and Virtual Worlds*, *28*(1), e1684. doi:10.1002/cav.1684

Maganaris, C. N., Baltzopoulos, V., Ball, D., & Sargeant, A. J. (2001). In vivo specific tension of human skeletal muscle. *Journal of Applied Physiology*, *90*(3), 865–872. doi:10.1152/jappl.2001.90.3.865 PMID:11181594

Maier-Hein, L., Vedula, S. S., Speidel, S., Navab, N., Kikinis, R., Park, A., Eisenmann, M., Feussner, H., Forestier, G., Giannarou, S., Hashizume, M., Katic, D., Kenngott, H., Kranzfelder, M., Malpani, A., März, K., Neumuth, T., Padoy, N., Pugh, C., ... Jannin, P. (2017). Surgical data science for next-generation interventions. *Nature Biomedical Engineering*, *1*(9), 691–696. doi:10.103841551-017-0132-7 PMID:31015666

McGinnis, P. (1999). *Biomechanics of sport and exercise*. Human Kinetics.

McMahon, T. A. (1984). *Muscles, reflexes, and locomotion*. Princeton University Press. doi:10.1515/9780691221540

McNutt, E. J., Zipfel, B., & DeSilva, J. M. (2018). The evolution of the human foot. *Evolutionary Anthropology*, *27*(5), 197–217. doi:10.1002/evan.21713 PMID:30242943

Medeiros, D. M., & Martini, T. F. (2018). Chronic effect of different types of stretching on ankle dorsiflexion range of motion: Systematic review and meta-analysis. *The Foot*, *34*, 28–35. doi:10.1016/j.foot.2017.09.006 PMID:29223884

Mukund, K., & Subramaniam, S. (2020). Skeletal muscle: A review of molecular structure and function, in health and disease. *Wiley Interdisciplinary Reviews. Systems Biology and Medicine*, *12*(1), e1462. doi:10.1002/wsbm.1462 PMID:31407867

Rassier, D. E., MacIntosh, B. R., & Herzog, W. (1999). The length dependence of active force production in skeletal muscle. *Journal of Applied Physiology*, *86*(5), 1445–1457. doi:10.1152/jappl.1999.86.5.1445 PMID:10233103

Refai, M. I. M., Van Beijnum, B. J. F., Buurke, J. H., Saes, M., Bussmann, J. B., Meskers, C. G., . . . Veltink, P. H. (2019, July). Portable gait lab: Zero moment point for minimal sensing of gait. In *2019 41st Annual International Conference of the IEEE Engineering in Medicine and Biology Society (EMBC)* (pp. 2077-2081). IEEE.

Salathea, E. P., & Arangio, G. A. (2002). A Biomechanical Model of the Foot: The Role of Muscles, Tendons, and Ligaments. *Journal of Biomechanical Engineering*, *124*(3), 281–287. doi:10.1115/1.1468865 PMID:12071262

Sarver, D. C., Kharaz, Y. A., Sugg, K. B., Gumucio, J. P., Comerford, E., & Mendias, C. L. (2017). Sex differences in tendon structure and function. *Journal of Orthopaedic Research*, *35*(10), 2117–2126. doi:10.1002/jor.23516 PMID:28071813

Schoenfeld, B. J., Ogborn, D. I., Vigotsky, A. D., Franchi, M. V., & Krieger, J. W. (2017). Hypertrophic effects of concentric vs. eccentric muscle actions: A systematic review and meta-analysis. *Journal of Strength and Conditioning Research*, *31*(9), 2599–2608. doi:10.1519/JSC.0000000000001983 PMID:28486337

Sheppard, J. (1992). *Anatomy: a complete guide for artists*. Dover.

Tang, C. Y., Tsui, C. P., Tang, Y. M., Wei, L., Wong, C. T., Lam, K. W., Ip, W. Y., Lu, W. W., & Pang, M. Y. (2014). Voxel-based approach to generate entire human metacarpal bone with microscopic architecture for finite element analysis. *Bio-Medical Materials and Engineering*, *24*(2), 1469–1484. doi:10.3233/BME-130951 PMID:24642974

Tang, Y. M. (2010). Modeling skin deformation using boundary element method. *Computer-Aided Design and Applications*, *7*(1), 101–108. doi:10.3722/cadaps.2010.101-108

Tang, Y. M., & Ho, H. L. (2020). 3D Modeling and Computer Graphics in Virtual Reality. In *Mixed Reality and Three-Dimensional Computer Graphics*. Intech Open. doi:10.5772/intechopen.91443

Tang, Y. M., & Hui, K. C. (2007). The effect of tendons on foot skin deformation. *CAD Computer Aided Design*, *39*(7), 583–597. doi:10.1016/j.cad.2007.01.013

Tang, Y. M., & Hui, K. C. (2009). Simulating Tendon Motion with Axial Mass-spring System. *Computers & Graphics*, *33*(2), 162–172. doi:10.1016/j.cag.2009.01.002

Tang, Y. M., & Hui, K. C. (2011). Human foot modeling towards footwear design. *CAD Computer Aided Design*, *43*(12), 1841–1848. doi:10.1016/j.cad.2011.08.005

Tang, Y. M., Wu, Z. H., Liao, W. H., & Chan, K. M. (2010). A study of semi-rigid support on ankle supination sprain kinematics. *Scandinavian Journal of Medicine & Science in Sports*, *20*(6), 822–826. doi:10.1111/j.1600-0838.2009.00991.x PMID:19765241

Tang, Y. M., Zhou, A. F., & Hui, K. C. (2005). Comparison between FEM and BEM for Real-time Simulation. *Computer-Aided Design and Applications*, *2*(1-4), 421–430. doi:10.1080/16864360.2005.10738391

Tang, Y. M., Zhou, A. F., & Hui, K. C. (2006). Comparison of FEM and BEM for interactive object simulation. *CAD Computer Aided Design*, *38*(8), 874–886. doi:10.1016/j.cad.2006.04.014

Tieland, M., Trouwborst, I., & Clark, B. C. (2018). Skeletal muscle performance and ageing. *Journal of Cachexia, Sarcopenia and Muscle*, *9*(1), 3–19. doi:10.1002/jcsm.12238 PMID:29151281

Van Royen, A., Shahabpour, M., Al Jahed, D., Abid, W., Vanhoenacker, F., & De Maeseneer, M. (2020). *Injuries of the Ligaments and Tendons in Ankle and Foot.* Academic Press.

Xiang, Y., Arora, J. S., & Abdel-Malek, K. (2010). Physics-based modeling and simulation of human walking: A review of optimization-based and other approaches. *Structural and Multidisciplinary Optimization*, *42*(1), 1–23. doi:10.100700158-010-0496-8

Yamamoto, M., Shimatani, K., Hasegawa, M., & Kurita, Y. (2020). Effects of Varying Plantarflexion Stiffness of Ankle-Foot Orthosis on Achilles Tendon and Propulsion Force During Gait. *IEEE Transactions on Neural Systems and Rehabilitation Engineering*, *28*(10), 2194–2202. doi:10.1109/TNSRE.2020.3020564 PMID:32866100

Yano, H., Kasai, K., Saitou, H., & Iwata, H. (2003). Development of a gait rehabilitation system using a locomotion interface. *The Journal of Visualization and Computer Animation*, *14*(5), 243–252. doi:10.1002/vis.321

Zajac, F. E. (1989). Muscle and tendon: Properties, models, scaling and application to biomechanics and motor control. *Critical Reviews in Biomedical Engineering*, *17*, 359–411. PMID:2676342

Zajac, F. E., Topp, E. L., & Stevenson, P. J. (1986) A dimensionless musculotendon model. *Proceedings IEEE Engineering in Medicine and Biology*.

Zhang, X., Pauel, R., Deschamps, K., Jonkers, I., & Vanwanseele, B. (2019). Differences in foot muscle morphology and foot kinematics between symptomatic and asymptomatic pronated feet. *Scandinavian Journal of Medicine & Science in Sports*, *29*(11), 1766–1773. doi:10.1111ms.13512 PMID:31278774

Zhou, A. F., Hui, K. C., Tang, Y. M., & Wang, C. C. L. (2006). An Accelerated BEM Approach for the Simulation of Deformable Objects. *Computer-Aided Design and Applications*, *3*(6), 761–769. doi:10.1080/16864360.2006.10738429

Chapter 8
Prototyping VR Training Tools for Healthcare With Off-the-Shelf CGI:
A Case Study

Tomasz Zawadzki
Arkin University of Creative Arts and Design, Cyprus

Slawomir Nikiel
University of Zielona Gora, Poland

Gareth W. Young
Trinity College Dublin, Ireland

EXECUTIVE SUMMARY

Cloud computing, big data, wearables, the internet of things, artificial intelligence, robotics, and virtual reality (VR), when seamlessly combined, will create the healthcare of the future. In the presented study, the authors aim to provide tools and methodologies to efficiently create 3D virtual learning environments (VLEs) to immerse participants in 360^0, six degrees of freedom (6DoF) patient examination simulations. Furthermore, the authors will discuss specific methods and features to improve visual realism in VR, such as post-processing effects (ambient occlusion, bloom, depth of field, anti-aliasing), texturing (normal maps, transparent, and reflective materials), and realistic lighting (spotlights and custom lights). The presented VLE creation techniques will be used as a testbed for medical simulation, created using the Unity game engine.

DOI: 10.4018/978-1-7998-8790-4.ch008

INTRODUCTION

Over the last decade, constantly decreasing computer hardware and software costs and increasing processor speeds have made computer simulations more popular in the classroom. Furthermore, Virtual Reality (VR) and Augmented Reality (AR) platforms are rapidly maturing. As technological capabilities have grown, the applied uses of such technologies for education and training have also become more accessible. In particular, VR enables the user to submerge themselves into a virtual environment fully. As a result, VR can be used in training situations that would be too dangerous to have users participate in the physical world (Stansfield et al., 2005). VR training dramatically reduces risks and improves logistics by (re-)creating virtual environments where staff and operators can practice realistic simulated critical situations or scenarios. XR (Extended Reality) combines real and virtual environments where the interaction between humans and machines is generated by wearables or computer technology. In other words, XR is an umbrella term that captures all augmented, virtual, and mixed reality together (Mann et al., 2018). In this paper, we will focus on VR as a subset of XR technology in healthcare only.

Moreover, Sulbaran and Baker (2000) have shown that learners enjoy VR training more than other traditional training methods and can retain the knowledge gained longer than acquired using different ways. Recent studies by Baukal and Ausburn (2013) show that the retention rates for VR learning reach over 75% compared to only 10% for reading and less than 50% for lecture-style education. In VR, trainees typically wear head-mounted displays (HMDs) with six degrees of freedom (6DoF) and wireless controllers for navigation and interaction, with more recent developments facilitating full hand tracking. Instructors can initiate immersive scenarios depicting any of a series of emergencies. Trainees can be graded, and they lose points whenever they create incorrect actions or make unjustified decisions that would lead to injuries in the real world. Therefore, VR can effectively build knowledge and understanding in the classroom (Young et al., 2020).

Researchers have proposed a virtual system to help prepare miners for dangerous situations that could not be addressed through traditional training methods (Kizil & Joy, 2001; James et al., 2013). VR has been used to train emergency first responders and their commanders (Li et al., 2005). VR has also been used in fire-hazard training systems (Smith & Ericson, 2009). Researchers have created various virtual fires where school children were asked to respond to the situations. However, using purely synthetic VR, trainees performed virtual, rather than actual, fire hazards. This researcher's approach has found that virtual learning environments (VLEs) offer significantly less risk to trainees (Tate et al., 1997). Further studies have shown that VR systems can effectively isolate trainees from dangerous threats during highly critical skills training. Thus, VR gained-skills training has the great potential to reduce risk, increase acceptance, and improve effectiveness over classic training methods alone (Fan et al., 2011).

The perceived reality of the experienced virtual scene is crucial to immerse the user in the content. Currently, readily available modeling technologies, like CGI tools, create new standards and demands. Computer games are filled with virtual humans that are visually pleasing but highly unrealistic. Evaluation of perceived information is more often based on emotional than rational aspects; if the authors create a simulation that looks more like a game, then there is a risk that the user won't take it seriously. Prior studies have focused on communicating key learning concepts, while others focused on creating general "sandboxes" that freely allowed trainees to explore pre-defined VLEs. Recent research has also focused on developing more realistic lifelike scenes and humans in VLEs (see digital humans) ("Digital humans," n.d.).

The main goal of visualization is to bring an understanding of data. The task is to present highly complex information most comprehensively and legibly. When considering 3D, the visualization process mainly focuses on understanding spatial relations and recognizing a particular physical object or phenomenon. The most natural way to convey this information is to build a three-dimensional model or evoke the sense of presence in a specific place with 360-degree panoramic images. Virtual visualization might be the next stage in developing visualization systems, and 3-dimensional computer graphics is currently the market standard even on mobile devices. The adequate definition says virtual reality is applying information technology to create an interactive 3-dimensional world effect, in which every object has presence property. It is possible to create single objects, digital humans-avatars, virtual buildings, or even whole virtual cities. Unfortunately, most visualizations depict static models with none or only simplified atmospheric/light/material effects (weather, light, skin textures) and often with limited or no environmental context (pedestrians-humanoids and foliage). Animation and narratives help to bring some life to VR. Digital narratives techniques have been successfully adapted to history, architecture, and journalism. This approach, along with virtual humans, can form a breakthrough solution. We must remember that avatars are processed in the brain like real people, and players can recognize varying levels of familiarity in avatar faces. Hence, social norms such as interpersonal distance are maintained when interacting with avatars.

The current research proposes to combine findings from several research areas and, based upon these findings, design a VR medical-examination training system for teaching MD students and support personnel in hospital environments. The current project is meant to serve as a testbed for a larger, more comprehensive long-term research project aiming to use interactive VR to provide practical high-risk-critical training for medical staff. The analysis of computer games (Mütterlein et al., 2018) shows that the interaction with humanoids (and other users) can significantly affect the user's psyche through the emotional charge.

Virtual reality has become increasingly used for medical-therapeutic purposes. The therapeutic potential of VR technology has already been experimentally tested, ranging from physical rehabilitation (Levin et al., 2015) through rehabilitation of violent offenders (Seinfeld et al., 2018) to the treatment of people experiencing or at risk of psychosis (Rus-Calafell et al., 2018). VR applications also include pain management (Matamala-Gomez et al., 2019), anxiety disorders, and phobias (Freeman et al., 2017). The potential of VR for training purposes in several areas, including medicine, surgery, and disaster response, is also gaining popularity (Spiegel, 2018; Vehtari et al., 2019). It is reasonable then to suppose that more realism in VR training scenarios will increase their effectiveness.

Alongside the prevalence of high-speed data processing computers, it has become easier to construct immersive 3D scene interactivity (from elements of VR game engines). Integration of virtual information within photorealistic or cinematic quality scenes will recreate critical situations with lifelike fidelity. It creates a possibility of displaying additional information about an examined patient and guarantees much more realistic experiences than pictures, films, or 3D images displayed on a screen.

One of the crucial features of our approach to VR is immersion, which enhances users' situated experience. The sensation of being there no longer necessitates a physical presence (Flower, 2018). In healthcare, it is vital to get VR to the level as realistic and detailed as possible, especially when there are plans to perform very complicated operations in a virtual environment. It has been found that presence and interactivity contribute to immersion by using a flow-based conceptualization of immersion. Likewise, interactivity contributes to "presence," and "immersion" influences satisfaction with a VR experience, indicating that a flow-based conceptualization of immersion is a suitable predictor in VR contexts (Mütterlein, 2018). In our case, the authors will focus on developing various graphical enhancements, such as post-processing, texturing, and lighting. Techniques such as ambient occlusion lighting, where enclosing spaces receive less ambient light, virtual endoscopy is an excellent example of ambient occlusion. It provides a more realistic representation of the 3D geometry than standard Phong lighting. Depth of field and bloom effects can be utilized in healthcare to produce virtual cinematic experiences, while anti-aliasing improves the overall quality and presence within VR. Texturing techniques (especially using normal maps) and reflective materials can create photorealistic scenes and medical training simulations. Real-time lighting is also essential for fully immersed VR experiences.

The presented research is organized as follows. First, the background of VR and immersive environments are discussed. Then, the design of an interactive VR training system and visual scene enhancing is described. A discussion of the issues encountered during the creation of the system is then given. Finally, concluding remarks are presented.

AN APPLICATION - VR MEDICAL-EXAMINATION TRAINING SYSTEM (VR METS)

Unity Game Engine

The VR Medical-Examination Training System (VR METS) was created in the Unity game engine. Unity software can run on multiple platforms Windows, Linux, Mac, with online and offline modes (Che Mat et al., 2014). In our case, we focused on the Windows platform only. Unity supports multiple XR application development, and in our case, VR METS focused on VR only. In the future, our project can be expanded to AR or MR.

The outlined process was started by importing the Vive Input Utility (VIU) plugin to the engine. The VIVE Input Utility is a toolkit for developing VR experiences in Unity, especially for the VIVE/VIVE Pro, and targeting many platforms from a joint code base, including Oculus Rift, Rift S Go, Quest, and Google Daydream.

Our solution was based on a single camera as implemented in ViveCameraRig (Figure 1.). Using two cameras: one for the left eye and the second for the right eye as available in other VR packages (SteamVR). Sometimes other Unity post-processing effects packages and VR packages may cause conflict problems.

Figure 1. Vive input utility - ViveCameraRig

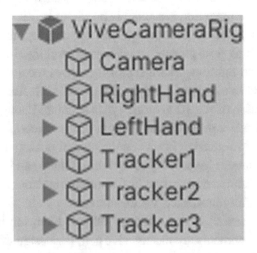

In this chapter, we have focused on six special effects, four of them were created using a post-processing package: ambient occlusion (AO), depth of field (DoF), bloom (BL), and anti-aliasing (AA) to smooth the corners and improve visual quality; the rest are related to other effects, such as reflection probe (RP) to enhance reflections and improve texture, and normal map (NM).

The next step was to import the post-processing package from Package Manager in Unity (Figure 2.).

Figure 2. Package manager – post-processing effects

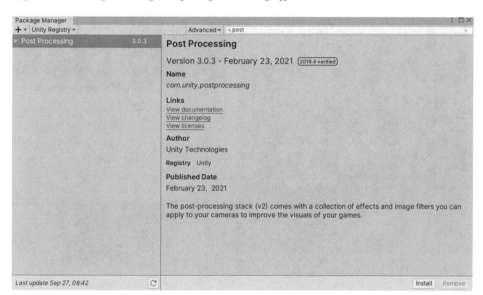

The imported post-processing package included additional features: post-processing Profile, post-process Layer, and post-process Volume. First, we had to create the post-processing Profile for each effect: ambient occlusion, depth of field, and bloom, in an area called – Project (where the project hierarchy and project files we located) (Figure 3.).

The next step was to create Layers for each special effect in the VR camera, add a post-processing Layer, and select all results to be displayed (Figure 4.). The rendering path was set to Deferred.

Anti-aliasing was embedded in the post-processing Layer and could be controlled independently (Figure 5.) There was no need to create an additional post-processing Profile for it as it was already embedded.

Figure 3. Creating post-processing profiles – steps

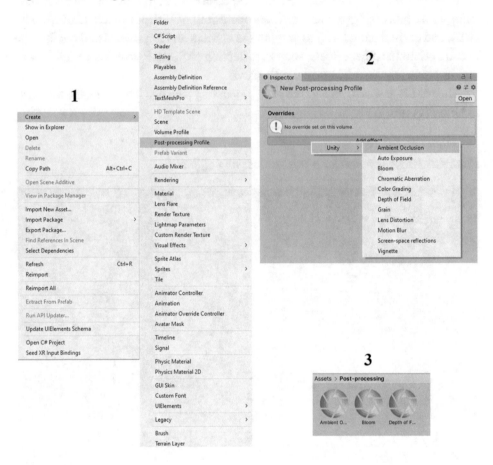

Figure 4. VR camera - creating post-processing layers

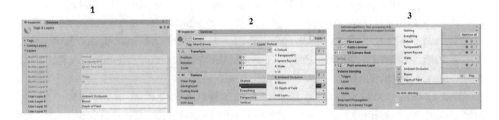

The last step was to create an empty game object and add Volume to it to control each special effect separately (Figure 6.).

Figure 5. Anti-aliasing

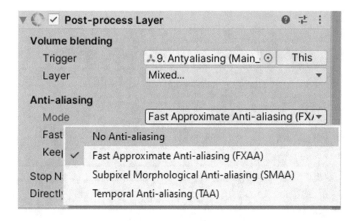

Figure 6. Post-processing volumes and parameters for DoF, AO, BL effects

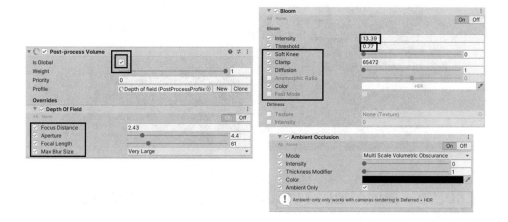

Other effects in the scene were created using standard Unity components. Set up started from Type - Real-time and Every frame refresh mode. A reflection probe was created using the reflection probe component from the "Lights" setting to improve reflections in the background. This effect was controlled by intensity, box projection, resolution, and HDR parameters (Figure 7.).

The texture's visual quality was enhanced using the Normal Map technique, which imitated a flat texture bump map effect (Figure 8.).

Figure 7. Reflection probe

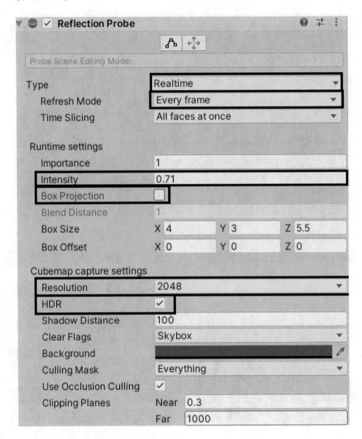

RESULTS – ENHANCING VISUAL QUALITY IN VR METS

Scene realism is an essential aspect of creating VR training systems that might be used for healthcare. Among various approaches, manipulating visual effects to achieve a higher level of visual realism was widely adopted. For instance, additional details of the textures were added to control visual realism (Davis et al., 2015; Jaeger and Mourant, 2001) or allowing users to watch scenes with different altitudes (Kingdon et al., 2001; Watanabe et al., 2008). Besides influencing the visual aspect of virtual environments, there are other important factors. One of them is manipulating visual realism by cognition. Golding et al., 2012 created two VR scenes with different levels of visual realism triggered by the change of the camera (up-right or inverted). While the up-right scene was assigned to a higher realism state, the inverted stage was set to a lower level of graphical realism, and the inverted world was unknown to most users.

Figure 8. Normal map texture creation – stages

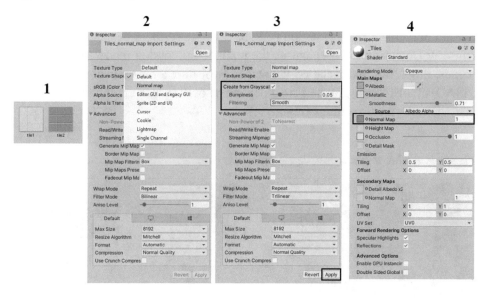

Unfortunately, higher visual fidelity in VR did not correlate with a better user experience and can generate a more motion sickness effect. Finding a golden mean between visual realism and user experience is still a difficult task in VR. Users who experienced better immersion and higher graphic realism showed a higher-level discomfort. This unexpected result may come from a sensory mismatch between visual and vestibular information. In the study, most participants could passively navigate in a virtual scene and received some limited vestibular details while sitting in their seats (Davis et al., 2015; Jaeger et al., 2001; Kingdon et al., 2001). This asymmetric interaction can exacerbate the conflict between sensory information. In other words, as the stimulus gets closer to reality, the user is more immersed in VR and expects atrial input signals corresponding to visual stimulation. However, users cannot obtain such vestibular information, so the conflict and VR disease also worsen.

Alongside the prevalence of high-speed data processing computers, it has become easier to construct immersive 3D scenes using interactivity (virtual reality elements). Combining virtual information with the photorealistic (or cinematic) quality will re-create critical situations with lifelike fidelity. It creates a possibility of displaying additional information about an examined patient and guarantees much more realistic experiences than pictures, films, or 3D images displayed on a screen.

Ambient Occlusion is a post-processing effect that approximates crevice shadows, simulating what happens in natural environments by darkening creases, holes, intersections, and surfaces close to each other. This approach gives a more realistic appearance to objects where ambient light is blocked out or occluded. The quality of computer rendering and perception realism largely depends on the shading method used to implement the interaction of light with the surfaces of objects in a stage. Ambient Occlusion (AO) enhances the realistic impression rendered objects and scenes. Properties that make up the screen Real-time ambient occlusion in space (SSAO) of interest the graphics are independent of the scene's complexity and fully operational dynamic settings (Figure 9.).

Figure 9. Ambient occlusion: left – off, right - on

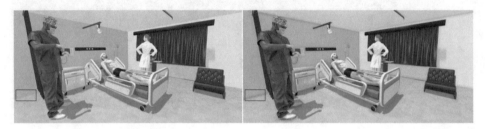

Depth of field (DOF) is the distance between the nearest and the farthest objects that are in acceptably sharp focus in an image. The depth of field can be calculated based on focal length, distance to subject, the acceptable circle of confusion size, and aperture (Figure 10.).

Figure 10. Depth of field: left – off, right - on

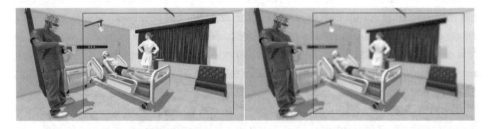

Bloom is an effect used to recreate the imaging artifact of actual cameras. The result creates streaks of light that extend from the border of bright areas of the image, creating the illusion of very bright light overwhelming the camera or the eye registering the scene (Figure 11.).

Figure 11. Bloom: left – off, right - on

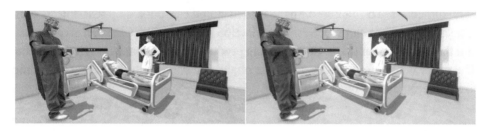

Normal mapping is a <u>texture mapping</u> technique used for faking the lighting of bumps and dents – an implementation of <u>bump mapping</u>. It is used to add details without using more <u>polygons</u> (Figure 12.).

Figure 12. Normal map: left – off, right - on

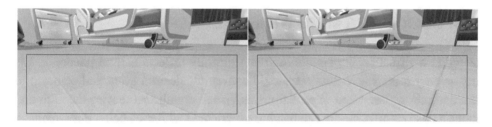

Post-processing anti-aliasing, each pixel is slightly blurry after rendering. The GPU determines where the edge of the polygon is by comparing the color contrast between each of the two pixels - two similar pixels indicate that they are part of the same polygon. Pixels are blurred in proportion to their difference (Figure 13.).

Figure 13. Anti-aliasing: left – off, right - on

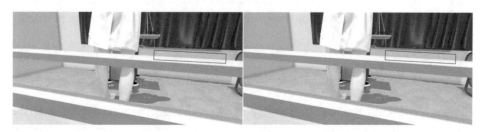

A reflection probe is like a camera that captures a spherical view of its surroundings in all directions. The captured image is then stored as a cube map that objects with reflective materials can use. Several reflection probes can be used in a given scene, and things can be set to use the cube map produced by the nearest reflection probe. The result is that the reflections on the object can change convincingly according to its environment (Figure 14.).

Figure 14. Reflection probe: left – off, right – on

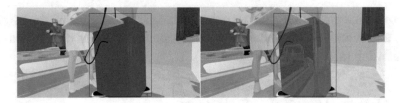

DISCUSSION – VR METS OTHER KEY ASPECTS

Creating a virtual reality simulation that faithfully reflects natural phenomena is not an easy task. The virtual set should convey the desired event and conform to the designer's vision and expectations as visual stimuli. Moreover, the film and game industries offer new user engaging experiences with even better photorealistic three-dimensional (3D) graphics, surrounding sound, and complex interaction. This method induces increasing demand for better non-entertaining visualizations for a more expansive (VR-game-educated) audience. Different approaches were considered, exploiting a range of technological solutions that challenged the production of the real-plus-virtual performance. The main goal was to provide the best technical and narrative quality possible with available means. The technologies used in the projects included stereoscopic 360 environments depicting hospital examination scenes and HMDs untracked and with user tracking. We should consider/solve the following issues from the authors' experience and available scientific resources confirming observations, and we should consider/solve the following problems when preparing virtual simulations.

Uncanny Valley

Generally speaking, the "uncanny valley" is a hypothesized relationship between the degree of an object's resemblance to reality (in a particular case – to the human being) and the observer's emotional response to such an object. In the field of aesthetics, the uncanny valley is defined to be "a term used in the scientific hypothesis, according to which a robot, drawing or computer animation that looks or functions similar (but not identical) to a human, causes unpleasant feelings or even disgust in observers" (MacDorman, 2006). The uncanny valley concept was defined early in the 70s of the 20th century when the first humanoid robots were constructed. The more the constructed humanoids resembled humans, the more they were accepted by human users, but it worked only up to a point where robots with an external appearance very close to human beings turned out to be very discomforting or even scary because of the small, elusive details disclosing their artificiality. That moment was called the uncanny valley. The uncanny valley denotes an observable dip in the human affinity for the replica, a relation that otherwise increases with the replica's visual and behavioral reality.

Nowadays, examples of the uncanny valley hypothesis can be found mainly in robotics, computer graphics/virtual reality, and lifelike dolls. With the proliferation of virtual reality and highly realistic cinematic/photorealistic computer animation, the uncanny valley has been referred more and more to reaction to the authenticity of artificial stimuli as it approaches indistinguishability from reality. The uncanny valley hypothesis predicts that virtual objects appearing almost real will risk eliciting eerie feelings in the viewers. What happens next after crossing the uncanny valley? According to some researchers, we go straight to the perfect simulation indistinguishable from reality, but another opinion assumes other scenarios. A very high acceptance of an almost ideal medium is followed by a drastic decline to the second valley of singularities (Mitchell, 2019). Such a situation usually occurs in some horror-themed VR environments, e.g., when we encounter a "virtual" precipice. The VR user is fully aware that they experience computer simulation, but the body/subconsciousness reacts with an atavistic fear of taking a step into the "chasm." Also, radical alterations of avatar behavior and actions cause uncanny valley and are rejected by testers (Padrao et al., 2016).

The recent development of improved hand tracking also introduced specific uncanny situations related to virtual hands and direct manipulation: jitter defined as misalignment between the virtual hands and user's actual hands, so-called "drift" is the feeling that the user is moving in the virtual world, even while they standstill. Virtual objects appear to move around for no reason because of a constant offset of where the VR headset/computer thinks the user's hand is compared to its actual location. This incongruence is usually caused by insufficient lighting or too much light coming into the headset. Grotesque Teleports are situations when a part of the virtual hands or whole virtual hands appear completely disjointed somewhere else in the virtual environment, thus breaking the immersion. In virtual reality, one does not watch someone else having an experience (as in the movies). The VR user is not in control of the character (as in computer games). In virtual reality, the VR user is part of the medium, which personally experiences all sensory experiences.

The so-called "second uncanny valley" exists in the transitional period between the suspension of unbelief and the inability to suspend faith in the incident, which is not taken seriously as the surrounding "real-life" reality. Moving on further, one can reach a perfect simulation utterly indistinguishable from real life.

An example of this may be seen in human faces generated by the GANN artificial intelligence; they are neither beautiful nor ugly, they are ordinary, and although there are no such people physically, we are entirely unable to distinguish them from photos of real people (Karras, 2018). To avoid the uncanny valley side effect, we can stick to the artificial-looking scene (particularly the humanoids), preserving visual clues to perceive three-dimensional environments fully. As far as hand tracking and direct manipulation are considered, to avoid jitter, virtual hands are represented in abstract ways, like with shapes, clouds, or sparkles in some applications. This design is made to hide the jitter effect, so users don't pick up on any obvious jittering.

Scale/ Homuncular Flexibility

VR users can accept substantial structural transformations to their virtual bodies, temporarily altering self-body perception (Normand et al., 2011, Yee et al., 2009; Slater et al., 2010). This effect was first observed in the early 1980s and was dubbed Homuncular Flexibility (Lanier, 2006). Some formal studies of Homuncular Flexibility have confirmed the earlier, informal observations (Won et al., 2015a). One example of this effect is that participants embodied in differently shaped avatars can overestimate their body size (Piryankova et al., 2014). It can be felt to be changed after using VR in the first weeks. People previously thought to be larger seemed smaller, and the VR user's size seemed larger. Other studied examples are that adults can have the illusion of having a child body (Banakou et al., 2013) or a black body (Peck et al., 2013; Banakou et al., 2016). Such experiences change the attitude of participants; for example, parents may change their behavior toward their children (Hamilton-Giachritsis et al., 2018), white people may become less biased against black (Maister et al., 2015), or domestic violence offenders may improve upon their recognition of fear in women after being virtually embodied as a woman subject to abuse by a virtual man (Seinfeld et al., 2018). Most of the currently available scientific research has explored positive benefits, but there is a risk of homonuclear feasibility or more dangerous body dystrophia where a virtual body/avatar may seem to be much more attractive than a physical body.

Reality Dissociation

In VR optics, despite the perception of depth, the user's eyes focus on the approximately two-meter artificial focal plane created by the lenses (for Oculus VR headsets).

This optical effect causes a temporary disassociation, which develops the eyes' difficulty focusing correctly in real life and will generally disappear after a few days. Adjusting time will vary for different users, but it may cause a disconnect in viewing the world after experiencing VR (general feeling of lightheadedness) vs. how one usually does. We can think of it akin to how looking at a static image for a reasonably long period will cause an afterimage effect thanks to the nerves involved becoming overexerted (same for other sensory nerves and muscles). That effect can be limited by careful use of focus. We can either build a virtual environment with the essential information placed in the focal plane or slightly blur objects of secondary value (props, background), forcing viewer eyes to concentrate on the focal plane. More prolonged exposure to VR HMD may infer behavior in real life. VR users who move through the virtual environment with the joystick/controller sometimes have to make the conscious effort/thought to move around in real life. VR experiences with limited user movement or sitting down (or standing still in one place) usually have less of the reality dissociation side effect.

Cybersickness

VIMS (Visually Induced Motion Sickness) is the broad term the encompasses simulation sickness, or cybersickness is an effect of a mismatch among visual, vestibular, and proprioceptive senses that occurs with changes in the motion of the user. Slowing down or stopping, turning while moving or stepping are all forms of movements that may induce VIMS. The VR rendering engine uses some software tricks (e.g., predictive tracking, TimeWarp) to shield the user from the effects of latency, but it is not always practical. To minimize the VIMS VR simulation, viewing the environment from a stationary position should be avoided. This perspective is the most comfortable in virtual reality, then. When moving through the environment is required, users are most comfortable moving through virtual environments interactively, with 6DoF, and at a constant velocity (humans walk at an average rate of 1.5 m/s). If one moves in virtual reality, they need to pick up the pace of stomping so that the brain starts making mistakes, and then nausea will be dramatically reduced. VR researchers should, therefore, make use of careful design considerations when creating character locomotion (Lewis-Evans, 2018).

Perception of Time

Virtual reality is a highly immersive experience that engages users in various ways. Some researchers have found that virtual reality interaction creates an effect called "time compression," where the time goes by faster than in real life (Mullen, 2021). Prior studies of time perception in virtual reality have often used surveys asking participants about their experiences after the fact. The current research team wanted to integrate a time-keeping task into the virtual reality experience to capture what was happening at the moment. The actual amount of time that had passed when each participant stopped the incident was recorded, and this revealed a gap between VR participants' perception of time and the actual time. The time gap was approximately 30 percent longer than in the classical desktop version of the simulation. That time compression effect was observed among test participants who played the game in virtual reality first. The paper concluded this was because participants judged time in the second round on whatever initial time estimates they made during the first round, regardless of format (Mullen, 2021). Some researchers struggle to discover why virtual reality seems to contribute to time compression. According to Mullen, one possible explanation is that a VR user has less body awareness. Future experiments to test this theory could bring new insights to help designers maximize benefits and minimize side effects from time compression. The result of time compression could be beneficial in some situations, for instance, enduring an unpleasant medical treatment or long and repetitive training, but in other circumstances, it could also have harmful consequences.

Stereopsis

The nature of human vision is highly complex, and understanding the very heart of seeing things involves research both in physiology and psychology of perception (Gombrich 1999, Gombrich 2001). Humans are accustomed to viewing the world through two eyes. Two-eyed vision provides extra cues to estimate image depth. Stereopsis or binocular vision enables humans to measure distance with eye convergence and stereoscopic vision. Eye convergence is a measure of the eyes' optical axes when fixating on some point in the space. In reality, the convergence angle for distant views is near zero, and for closer objects, optical axes converge to keep the center of visual interest positioned over the two sensitive foveae (Walius, 1962). The range of the convergence angle depends upon the physiological abilities of the observer. Within the high-acuity foveal region, depth perception is fading at 100-150 m. At that distance, motion parallax and perspective become much more helpful to estimate distance. Perception of distant and closer objects depends on accommodation as well. The mechanism of accommodation provides clear vision by tensioning or relaxing the ciliary muscle attached to the periphery of crystalline lenses. With age, the lenses become less flexible and result in a person focusing at a constant distance.

Bela Julesz proved that stereo perception was independent of object recognition (Walius, 1962). When two identical patterns of random dots are viewed through a stereoscope, they are perceived without the sensation of depth. However, it was shown that if a portion of one pattern was displaced horizontally, the stereogram tricked the brain into believing that a 3D structure was observed. The brain uses that displacement or disparity between the two stereoscopic images called parallax (see below) to measure depth. The first attempts to create stereoscopic images were described in 1832 by Charles Wheatstone, who invented the stereoscope. The idea was perfected by Sir David Brewster (Vince, 1995). The Brewster's stereoscope consists of two pictures and a couple of mirrors redirecting and separating views for the left and right eye of the observer.

Currently, VR Head Mounted Displays work in precisely the same way. The parallax controls the depth of view, the difference between the left and the right eye determining the distance we perceive. Generally, it is possible to obtain greater variability in image depth with the more significant Field of View. When the parallax is equal to zero, we see objects "on the screen," so the distance between the virtual and real image is the same. In the case of HMDs, the perceived screen distance is determined by so-called focal distance or infinity optics (dependent on the set of lenses), and it ranges from 2 meters (Oculus Rift/Quest) to 7 meters (military-grade HMDs). Negative parallax makes the objects "pop up" from the screen/focal distance and the effect that can give eye strain when observed for a longer time. Positive parallax puts things farther behind the screen and seems to be more comfortable for the viewer. Depth perception from stereopsis is susceptible up close but quickly diminishes along with distance. Mountains that are miles apart in the space will provide almost the same sense of depth as two objects' inches apart on the desk distanced one meter from the observer.

Increasing the distance between the virtual cameras can enhance the understanding of depth from stereopsis but may result in unintended side effects. It may force users to converge their eyes more than usual, which could lead to eye strain. Moreover, it can give rise to perceptual anomalies and discomfort if one fails to scale head motion equally with eye separation. The optics of the Oculus HMD make it most comfortable to view objects that fall within a range of 0.75 to 3.5 meters from the VR user's eyes. The virtual things users will look at for extended periods (such as menus and avatars) should fall in that range. One must remember that perception of the stereoscopic space is relative, and the sharpest image is guaranteed only with the zero parallaxes (focal distance of the HMD). Moreover, to obtain immersion, one does not have to rely entirely on the stereoscopic 3D effect to provide depth to virtual content; proper lighting, delicate texture, motion parallax (the way objects appear to move concerning each other when the user moves), and other visual features are equally (if not more) important to conveying depth and space to the user.

Stereo Blindness

To obtain stereoscopic sensation, the human observer needs to adjust their vision. For some people, this is sometimes hard or even impossible and approx. 10% of the human population cannot obtain stereoscopic 3D sensation. The so-called stereo-blinded people perceive two overlapping images. Even for the average observer, when viewing stereoscopic images, they may induce eye strain and other neuro-psychological side effects after some time. The reason is that the observer must force the eyes to stare in parallel (as for distant views) while focusing on relatively close print, thus fighting the stimuli to converge eyes on objects recognized as close ones. However, there are some (yet not clinically tested) opinions that people who have been stereo-blind their entire lives and using VR regularly can cure it (also outside of VR). There is probably some retraining of the brain, but the science behind it is not well understood.

Depth of Field

Each three-dimensional scene created in visual reality has a maximum usable depth to develop effective and "user-friendly" 3D stereography. If the virtual production is to have captions, this should be taken into account when working out the total depth budget. This depth budget may be calculated as a percentage between the left and right eyes separation concerning screen width. We need to remember that the sharpest image is guaranteed only with zero parallaxes (placed in the focal distance of the HMD). When visual objects are placed too far in front of the focal length of HMD and too far behind the focal distance of HMD at the same time (too much depth), the viewer will not be able to 'fuse' the stereo 3D image.

Ghosting

If we provide two versions of the same virtual scene, however, one set is slightly different from the other it is called ghosting. The rendering of these scenes into the left/right eyes takes two different environments and pretends they're one. For example, in one eye, a room looks new and full of life, wherein the other is old, and the furniture looks slightly deteriorated. Everything is kept precisely in the same position and shape, so the viewer's eyes would still get a perception of 3D and will process the scene, but perhaps having these two slight changes of images. These issues could be an effect of a glitch in visual stimulation (e.g., wrongly constructed reflection probe) or turn to be a perfect tool for representing a whole new VFX possible only in fully immersive virtual reality. These could be ghosts, madness, drugs, deja vu, alternate realities representing things that the character can see but other people in the game or simulation. Several VFX can be used to model the simulation scene to avoid ghosting, including the ambient occlusion, bloom, and normal mapping. Generally, the images presented to each eye should differ only in terms of viewpoint; post-processing effects (e.g., light distortion, bloom) must be applied to both eyes consistently and correctly rendered in z-depth to create an adequately fused image.

Retinal Rivalry

This side effect is very similar to the ghosting mentioned above, considering specific /pixel size visual disparities. When something appears only in one eye, the viewer very often cannot reconcile the images. This effect can occur in reflections, aliasing, glints, lens flares & motion artifacts. One needs to close one eye, then the other, to see the differences between the eyes. Bright, thin objects/images, particularly in the periphery, can create noticeable display flicker and retinal rivalry for sensitive users. To avoid retinal rivalry, darker colors, normal mapping, anti-aliasing, and carefully adjusted reflection probe techniques can be used.

Screen Door Effect

Visible pixelation (often referred to as the "Screen Door Effect" or SDE) of the perceived image in HMD results from low quality of hardware display. The pixel density of the display matrix is a dominant factor in SDE. However, the pixel configuration also matters, as does the type of used lenses either. Looking at what is displayed on the VR head-mounted display screen, one will notice that the frame's shape is distorted and somewhat rounded rather than square. This alteration is because the lenses then distort that to the viewer's eyes, giving the appearance of a regular image. What is seen through the center of the lenses will be a reasonably decent resolution, but what is seen as the gaze is moved away from the center is that things become a little less crisp. The image contents at the peripheral view are displayed with a lower pixel density. One can consider supersampling or anti-aliasing to remedy low apparent resolution. Another solution is to use high-end HMDs like Varjo or Pixmax to provide display resolutions that eliminate the screen door effect.

CONCLUSION AND FUTURE WORK

At the forefront of emergent technologies that can reshape the world of healthcare are VR and AR. Putting doctors and patients into a VLE enables education and healthcare to improve its current performance and become even more efficient. VR has many benefits in terms of security and training. It is particularly possible to simulate critical or highly uncomfortable situations for doctors/nurses and supporting personnel, helping them know how to react in real-world cases. Before being used in examination and intervention applications, MD students can be virtually immersed in their future work environment and be trained in various instances. And since new technologies like the Oculus Rift and the HTC Vive keep track of things like how your head moves in space, it is possible to use that data to give trainers insight into what trainees are paying attention to in VR. Immersive technology is changing the way organizations train their people. The virtual training of medical staff facilitates a set of acceptable solutions characterized by different configurations of real-life scenarios that guarantee timely completion of interventions with a minimum total cost of the training process. This approach makes it possible to benefit in the service of the efficiency of the healthcare.

Immersive learning and training platforms more commonly apply multimodal design elements, such as avatars and anthropomorphic virtual agents, impacting students' motivational outcomes and delivering novel forms of visually enriched embodied communication (Rasimah et al., 2011). Previous research has highlighted tendencies, such as gender-specific preferences for exergames and the familiarity effect when engaging with XR technology (Buchem et al., 2021). Furthermore, simulation training in VR is advantageous for medical professionals (Tsai et al., 2021; Shah et al., 2021). However, due to the small number of case studies and lack of comprehensive comparisons between VR and conventional medical interventions, contemporary studies lack a solid foundation for comparing the physical world with the digital (Safikhani et al., 2021). Therefore, additional student-user-focused studies are needed to evaluate the impact of the VR environments' technological and design aspects, as introduced in this chapter.

The VR experiences described in this chapter are based upon the simulation of a domain-specific environment, the virtual operating theatre, a doctor's office, etc., with visual enhancements made via the introduction of various graphical effects. In general, XR simulations (and VR as a subset) are becoming more widely adopted in medical education as they offer low-risk exposure for students to clinical environments and situate the requisite knowledge and skills for clinical teaching. Although the authoring of VR/XR medical education spaces, from a user-experience perspective, rests upon other modalities, such as 6DoF movement, 3D assets, interaction, and the modalities of the platform (Antoniou et al., 2021), the visual components of the reconstruction remain fundamental. Therefore, by incorporating realistic VR/XR simulations and training into student programs, the platform offers novel opportunities for educators to provide personalized domain-specific instruction to prepare students for the many complexities of patient care, treatment, and well-being.

The global COVID-19 pandemic has introduced new social distancing measures and lockdown protocols that have had an immense impact on medical students' lives, affecting their instruction in many ways. Research has shown that the pandemic has chiefly affected the younger populations (ages 18-25), who have developed symptoms of post-traumatic stress disorder (PTSD), anxiety, depression, and other signs of emotional distress (Office of National Statistics UK, 2021). In addition, remote learning has been introduced to protect students and staff, creating an additional barrier for students who require further support. The introduction of realistic VR environments and social VR can perhaps alleviate these negative impacts in future remote learning and social distancing educational contexts.

ACKNOWLEDGMENT

This publication has partially emanated from research conducted with the financial support of Science Foundation Ireland (SFI) under Grant Number 15/RP/2776.

REFERENCES

Antoniou, P. E., Chondrokostas, E., Bratsas, C., Filippidis, P. M., & Bamidis, P. D. (2021). A Medical Ontology Informed User Experience Taxonomy to Support Co-creative Workflows for Authoring Mixed Reality Medical Education Spaces. *7th International Conference of the Immersive Learning Research Network*, 1-9.

Banakou, D., Groten, R., & Slater, M. (2013). Illusory ownership of a virtual child body causes overestimation of object sizes and implicit attitude changes. *Proceedings of the National Academy of Sciences of the United States of America*, *110*(31), 110. doi:10.1073/pnas.1306779110 PMID:23858436

Banakou, D., Pd, H., & Slater, M. (2016). Virtual embodiment of white people in a black virtual body leads to a sustained reduction in their implicit racial bias. *Frontiers in Human Neuroscience*, *10*, 601. doi:10.3389/fnhum.2016.00601 PMID:27965555

Baukal, C. E., Ausburn, F. B., & Ausburn, L. J. (2013). A Proposed Multimedia Cone of Abstraction: Updating a Classic Instructional Design Theory. *Journal of Educational Technology*, *9*(4), 15–24.

Buchem, I., Vorwerg, S., Stamm, O., Hildebrand, K., & Bialek, Y. (2021). Gamification in Mixed-Reality Exergames for Older Adult Patients in a Mobile Immersive Diagnostic Center: A Pilot Study in the BewARe Project. *7th International Conference of the Immersive Learning Research Network (iLRN)*, 1-9.

Che Mat, R., Shariff, A. R. M., Nasir Zulkifli, A., Shafry Mohd Rahim, M., & Hafiz Mahayudin, M. (2014). Using game engine for 3D terrain visualisation of GIS data: A review. *IOP Conference Series. Earth and Environmental Science*, *20*, 1. doi:10.1088/1755-1315/20/1/012037

Davis, S., Nesbitt, K., & Nalivaiko, E. (2015). Comparing the onset of cybersickness using the Oculus Rift and two virtual roller coasters. *Proceedings of the 11th Australasian Conference on Interactive Entertainment*, 3-14.

Dickey, P. J., Eger, T., Frayne, R., Delgado, G., & Ji, X. (2013). Research Using Virtual Reality: Mobile Machinery Safety in the 21st Century. *Minerals (Basel)*, *3*(2), 145–164. doi:10.3390/min3020145

Fan, X., Yang, R., Wu, D., & Ma, D. (2011). Virtual Assembly Environment for Product Design Evaluation and Workplace Planning. In D. Ma, X. Fan, J. Gausemeier, & M. Grafe (Eds.), *Virtual Reality & Augmented Reality in Industry*. Springer. doi:10.1007/978-3-642-17376-9_9

Flower, C. (2015). Virtual reality and learning: Where is the pedagogy? *British Journal of Educational Technology*, *46*(2), 412–422. doi:10.1111/bjet.12135

Freeman, D., Reeve, S., Robinson, A., Ehlers, A., Clark, D., Spanlang, B., & Slater, M. (2017). Virtual reality in the assessment, understanding, and treatment of mental health disorders. *Psychological Medicine*, *47*(14), 2393–2400. doi:10.1017/S003329171700040X PMID:28325167

Gombrich, E. H. (1999). *The Image and the Eye*. Phaidon Press Ltd.

Gombrich, E. H. (2001). *Art and Illusion*. Princeton Univ. Press.

Hamilton-Giachritsis, C., Banakou, D., Garcia Quiroga, M., Giachritsis, C., & Slater, M. (2018). Reducing risk and improving maternal perspective-taking and empathy using virtual embodiment. *Scientific Reports*, *8*(1), 2975. doi:10.103841598-018-21036-2 PMID:29445183

Hodges, L. (2001). Treating Psychological and Physical Disorders with VR. *IEEE Computer Graphics and Applications*, 25–33.

Jaeger, B. K., & Mourant, R. R. (2001). Comparison of simulator sickness using static and dynamic walking simulators. *Proceedings of the Human Factors and Ergonomics Society Annual Meeting*, *45*(27), 1896–1900. doi:10.1177/154193120104502709

Karras, T. (2018). *A Style-Based Generator Architecture for Generative Adversarial Network, Neural and Evolutionary Computing*. Cornell University.

Kingdon, K. S., Stanney, K. M., & Kennedy, R. S. (2001). Extreme responses to virtual environment exposure. *Proceedings of the Human Factors and Ergonomics Society Annual Meeting*, *45*(27), 1906–1910. doi:10.1177/154193120104502711

Kizil, M. S., & Joy, J. (2001). *What can virtual reality do for safety?* St University of Queensland.

Lanier, J. (2006). *Homuncular flexibility. In Edge*. The World Question Center.

Levin, M. F., Weiss, P. L., & Keshner, E. A. (2015). Emergence of virtual reality as a tool for upper limb rehabilitation: Incorporation of motor control and motor learning principles. *Physical Therapy*, *95*(3), 415–425. doi:10.2522/ptj.20130579 PMID:25212522

Lewis-Evans, B. (2018). A short guide to user testing for simulation sickness in Virtual Reality. In *Games User Research*. Oxford University Press.

Li, L., Zhang, M., Xu, F., & Liu, S. (2005) ERT-VR: An immersive virtual reality system for emergency rescue. Virtual Reality, 194–197. doi:10.100710055-004-0149-6

MacDorman, K., & Ishiguro, H. (2006). The uncanny advantage of using androids in social and cognitive science research. *Interaction Studies: Social Behaviour and Communication in Biological and Artificial Systems*, *7*(3), 297–337. doi:10.1075/is.7.3.03mac

Maister, L., Slater, M., Sanchez-Vives, M. V., & Tsakiris, M. (2015). Changing bodies changes minds: Owning another body affects social cognition. *Trends in Cognitive Sciences*, *19*(1), 6–12. doi:10.1016/j.tics.2014.11.001 PMID:25524273

Mann, S., Furness, T., Yuan, Y., Iorio, J., & Wang, Z. (2018). *All Reality: Virtual, Augmented, Mixed (X), Mediated (X,Y), and Multimediated Reality*. CoRR. abs/1804.08386.

Matamala-Gomez, M., Donegan, T., Bottiroli, S., Sandrini, G., Sanchez-Vives, M. V., & Tassorelli, C. (2019). Immersive virtual reality and virtual embodiment for pain relief. *Frontiers in Human Neuroscience*, *13*, 279. doi:10.3389/fnhum.2019.00279 PMID:31551731

MitchellB. (2019). https://medium.com/@bryanmitchell_67448/there-is-a-second-valley-past-the-uncanny-valley-22d2ea193e0

Mullen, G., & Davidenko, N. (2021, May). Time Compression in Virtual Reality. *Timing & Time Perception (Leiden, Netherlands)*, *9*(4), 377–392. doi:10.1163/22134468-bja10034

Mütterlein, J. (2018). *The Three Pillars of Virtual Reality?* Investigating the Roles of Immersion, Presence, and Interactivity. doi:10.24251/HICSS.2018.174

Normand, J. M., Giannopoulos, E., Spanlang, B., & Slater, M. (2011). Multisensory stimulation can induce an illusion of larger belly size in immersive virtual reality. *PLoS One, 6*(1), e16128. doi:10.1371/journal.pone.0016128 PMID:21283823

Office of National Statistics UK. (2021). *Dataset — Coronavirus and depression in adults in Great Britain.* https://www.ons.gov.uk/peoplepopulationandcommunity/wellbeing/datasets/coronavirusanddepressioninadultsingreatbritain

Padrao, G., Gonzalez-Franco, M., Sanchez-Vives, M. V., Slater, M., & Rodriguez-Fornells, A. (2016). Violating body movement semantics: neural signatures of self-generated and external-generated errors. *Neuroimage, 124*(Pt A), 174–156.

Peck, T. C., Seinfeld, S., Aglioti, S. M., & Slater, M. (2013). Putting yourself in the skin of a black avatar reduces implicit racial bias. *Consciousness and Cognition, 22*(3), 779–787. doi:10.1016/j.concog.2013.04.016 PMID:23727712

Piryankova, I. V., Wong, H. Y., Linkenauger, S. A., Stinson, C., Longo, M. R., Bülthoff, H. H., & Mohler, B. J. (2014). Owning an overweight or underweight body: Distinguishing the physical, experienced and virtual body. *PLoS One, 9*(8), e103428. doi:10.1371/journal.pone.0103428 PMID:25083784

Rasimah, C. M. Y., Ahmad, A., & Zaman, H. B. (2011). Evaluation of user acceptance of mixed reality technology. *Australasian Journal of Educational Technology, 27*(8). Advance online publication. doi:10.14742/ajet.899

Rus-Calafell, M., Garety, P., Sason, E., Craig, T. J., & Valmaggia, L. R. (2018). Virtual reality in the assessment and treatment of psychosis: A systematic review of its utility, acceptability and effectiveness. *Psychological Medicine, 48*(3), 362–391. doi:10.1017/S0033291717001945 PMID:28735593

Safikhani, S., Pirker, J., & Wriessnegger, S. C. (2021). Virtual Reality Applications for the Treatment of Anxiety and Mental Disorders. *2021 7th International Conference of the Immersive Learning Research Network (iLRN)*, 1-8.

Seinfeld, S., Arroyo-Palacios, J., Iruretagoyena, G., Hortensius, R., Zapata, L. E., Borland, D., de Gelder, B., Slater, M., & Sanchez-Vives, M. V. (2018). Offenders become the victim in virtual reality: Impact of changing perspective in domestic violence. *Scientific Reports, 8*(1), 2692. doi:10.103841598-018-19987-7 PMID:29426819

Shah, M., Siebert-Evenstone, A., Eagan, B., & Holthaus, R. (2021). Modeling Educator Use of Virtual Reality Simulations in Nursing Education Using Epistemic Network Analysis. *2021 7th International Conference of the Immersive Learning Research Network (iLRN)*, 1-8.

Slater, M., Spanlang, B., Sanchez-Vives, M. V., & Blanke, O. (2010). First person experience of body transfer in virtual reality. *PLoS One*, *5*(5), 5. doi:10.1371/journal.pone.0010564 PMID:20485681

Smith, S., & Ericson, E. (2009). Using immersive game-based virtual reality to teach fire-safety skills to children. *Virtual Reality (Waltham Cross)*, *13*(2), 87–99. doi:10.100710055-009-0113-6

Spiegel, J. S. (2018). The ethics of virtual reality technology: Social hazards and public policy recommendations. *Science and Engineering Ethics*, *24*(5), 1537–1550. doi:10.100711948-017-9979-y PMID:28942536

Stansfield, S., Shawver, D., Rogers, D., & Hightower, R. (2005). Mission visualization for planning and training. *IEEE Computer Graphics and Applications*, 12–14.

Sulbaran, T., & Baker, N. C. (2000). Enhancing engineering education through distributed virtual reality. ASEE/IEEE frontiers in education conference, 3–18. doi:10.1109/FIE.2000.896621

Tate, D. L., Silbert, L., & King, T. (1997) Virtual environments for shipboard firefighting training. In *Proceedings of the IEEE 1997 virtual reality international annual symposium*. IEEE Computer Society Press. 10.1109/VRAIS.1997.583045

Tsai, Y. C., Lin, G. L., & Cheng, C. C. (2021). Work-in-Progress-Development of Immersive Nursing Skills Learning System and Evaluation of Learning Effectiveness. *2021 7th International Conference of the Immersive Learning Research Network (iLRN)*, 1-3.

Vehtari, A., Simpson, D. P., Yao, Y., & Gelman, A. (2019). Limitations of bayesian leave-one-out cross-validation for model selection. *Computational Brain & Behavior*, *2*(1), 22–27. doi:10.100742113-018-0020-6 PMID:30906917

Vince, J. (1995). *Virtual Reality Systems*. Wesley Publishing Company.

Walius, N. A. (1962). *Stereoscopy*. Russian Academy of Science. (in Russian)

Watanabe, H., & Ujike, H. (2008). The activity of ISO/Study Group on "Image Safety" and three biological effects. *Proceedings of the 2008 Second International Symposium on Universal Communication*, 210– 214. 10.1109/ISUC.2008.11

Won, A. S., Bailenson, J., Lee, J., & Lanier, J. (2015). Homuncular flexibility in virtual reality. *J. Comput. Commun*, *20*, 241–259.

Yee, N., Bailenson, J. N., & Ducheneaut, N. (2009). The Proteus effect: Implications of transformed digital self-representation on online and offline behavior. *Communication Research*, *36*(2), 285–312. doi:10.1177/0093650208330254

Young, G. W., Stehle, S., Walsh, B. Y., & Tiri, E. (2020). Exploring Virtual Reality in the Higher Education Classroom: Using VR to Build Knowledge and Understanding. *Journal of Universal Computer Science*, *26*(8), 904–928. doi:10.3897/jucs.2020.049

Chapter 9
Cross Reality in Crisis Management

Mian Yan
School of Intelligent Systems Science and Engineering, Jinan University, China

Alex Pak Ki Kwok
School of Intelligent Systems Science and Engineering, Jinan University, Hong Kong, China

Cheng Yao Wang
Department of Electrical Engineering, City University of Hong Kong, Hong Kong, China

Xin Lian
School of Computer Science and Technology, Xi'an Jiaotong University, China

Can Biao Zhuang
School of Intelligent Systems Science and Engineering, Jinan University, China

Chang Gao
School of Intelligent Systems Science and Engineering, Jinan University, China

Ying Ting Huang
School of Intelligent Systems Science and Engineering, Jinan University, China

EXECUTIVE SUMMARY

The continuous technological advancement of computer simulation, display technology, and the internet of things leads to the opportunities to use cross-reality (XR) technologies in crisis management. XR emphasizes the compositions of different concepts in reality-virtuality continuum under a shared online virtual world, including virtual reality (VR), augmented reality (AR), and mixed reality

DOI: 10.4018/978-1-7998-8790-4.ch009

(MR). It is touted as a promising tool to facilitate crisis management strategies in different stages, including prevention, onsite management, and recovery. This research contributes to the field of research in VR, XR, and crisis management (an essential component of healthcare) in the following four ways: (1) It proposes an idea to apply XR in crisis management. (2) It proposes a framework to connect VR, AR, and MR serving one purpose. (3) It presents a qualitative study to examine the user perception of the XR-based crisis management method. (4) It brings out the challenges and opportunities of using XR in crisis management.

INTRODUCTION

Emergency and disasters can strike anytime, damaging infrastructures and inflicting human casualties. Therefore, it is essential for every stakeholder, including firefighters, police, first-aiders, healthcare staff in the emergency department, and emergency response engineers, to respond to the incidents systematically and efficiently. To achieve this, the readiness and the efficient collaboration of the emergency response teams in responding to crises, such as fire and earthquake, are critical. Normally, organizations would develop emergency response procedures and disaster management plans to guide their crisis response teams to settle the crisis. A big assumption behind these plans is that every individual could follow the guidelines and react correctly under stress. However, human history told us that this assumption is not valid (Kwok et al., 2020). In particular, Robert and Lajtha (2002) specified that "the key to effective crisis management lies not so much with the writing of detailed manuals (that have a low likelihood of being used, and an even lower likelihood of being useful)". Also, it is not surprising that humans would make mistakes during emergency incidents, leading to more severe consequences. Therefore, organizations should provide regular training and practical onsite guidance to their emergency response teams to equip each staff with the capabilities, flexibility, and confidence to handle sudden and unexpected events (Robert & Lajtha, 2002).

Crisis management is the actions that are taken to prevent or lessen the impact of a crisis. Crisis management involves three phases: pre-crisis (preparation), crisis response, and post-crisis (recovery) (Coombs & Laufer, 2018). Each phase requires tight and rapid coordination among different stakeholders and departments. For this reason, the use of cross reality (XR) concept, which emphasizes the collaboration of virtual reality (VR), mixed reality (MR), and augmented reality (AR) under a shared online virtual world (Paradiso & Landay, 2009), in the crisis management training can produce a marked effect in the following aspects:

- VR technology can provide an immersive environment for emergency response staff to familiarise themselves with their roles and responsibilities (e.g., Smolentsev et al., 2017).
- AR technology can provide emergency response staff with onsite guidance on the rescue plan and the best rescue routes (e.g., Tsai et al., 2012).
- MR technology can show emergency response engineers the present damage situation and then offer them guidance for assessing, repairing, and rebuilding the infrastructures to restore the situation to normal (e.g., Espíndola et al., 2013).

Because of these reasons, this chapter studied the possibilities of using XR technology in crisis management. It should contribute to the field of research in VR, XR, and crisis management (an essential component of healthcare) in the following four ways:

- The potential of using XR technology in crisis management has not yet been exploited. This study is novel in proposing a framework to adopt XR technology in crisis management.
- It is one of the few studies which connects VR, AR, and MR for one purpose: to manage the crisis.
- It presents a study to examine the user perception of the XR-based crisis management method.
- It discusses the challenges of using XR in crisis management based on the study results and provides insights for the management to better use the technology.

BACKGROUND

The Development of VR, AR, and MR Technology

Recent advancements in immersive technologies have introduced the world to three fascinating terms: VR, AR, and MR. While these three terms often describe media that changes users' perception of reality, their difference is significant and worth explaining. In 1994, Milgram et al. (1995) proposed a concept called Reality-Virtuality Continuum, as displayed in Figure 1. They highlighted the underlining differences among various computer display systems alongside the level of reality. The reality-virtuality continuum is the ancestor of the term: MR.

Figure 1. Reality-virtuality continuum.
Source: (Milgram et al., 1995)

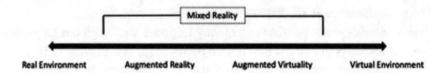

The reality-virtuality continuum treats the real environment and virtual environment as two consecutive ends. At the far left, the real environment is made up entirely of real objects. AR is placed next to the real environment. It refers to the idea that the display incorporates digital information into the real-world scene. On the opposite side of the continuum, the virtual environment, by contrast, is a world which only consists of virtual objects. VR is often regarded as this case. In contrast to AR, Augmented Virtuality (AV), next to the virtual environment, refers to the idea that the display of a virtual environment is augmented through real objects. The remaining term MR refers to the area between the two extremes, where the real and virtual worlds are mixed. Milgram and Kishino (1994) noted that the advancement of display technologies would eventually blur the definition of the terms: AR and AV, making them hard to be distinguished. However, the term: MR would remain valid for describing the middle area of the real and virtual environment. In the rest of this section, each taxonomy of display technologies is introduced in detail.

Virtual Reality

VR is a technology that involves an interactive 3D model that looks very similar to the real world (Kanade et al., 1997). The first VR device named Sensorama was invented by Morton Heilig in 1957 (Milgram & Kishino, 1994). For more than 50 years after its invention, VR is still regarded as an emerging technology. With VR, users can fully immerse themselves into a 3D virtual world, walk freely inside, and interact with the virtual objects or characters to complete tasks that would be otherwise difficult to be carried out in the real world (Brooks, 1999). In general, VR has the following three characteristics (Burdea & Langrana, 1992) (Figure 2):

- **Immersion:** VR gives users a feeling of being physically present in an artificial virtual world (Smolentsev et al., 2017).
- **Interaction:** VR allows users to interact with the virtual environment and objects more naturally than flat graphic interactions (Sathia Bhama et al., 2020).

- **Imagination:** VR technology enables users to visit a whole new world built from imagination. Users can explore the world actively through perceptual knowledge.

Figure 2. Virtual reality triangle: immersion-interaction-imagination.
Source: *(Burdea & Langrana, 1992)*

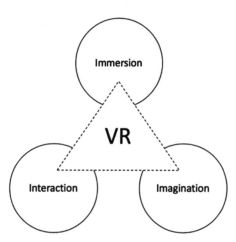

Due to these characteristics, VR was proven to be useful in many fields, such as medical, military, and education. In the medical field, VR could fill the shortcomings of traditional medical education (Park, 2018), which is based on apprenticeship and hands-on training in operation rooms. With VR, untrained doctors could gain confidence and support by repeating their surgery skills in front of a virtual human body model in a controlled environment without affecting the actual patients (Yiannakopoulou et al., 2015; Zhou et al., 2019). Surgeons could also repeatedly simulate the operation using a 3D virtual model and develop the best surgical plan for complex surgical procedures (Kenngott et al., 2021). In the military field, VR could facilitate the design process of advanced weapons to display complex concepts and functions of a product. Engineers could test and adjust the product design based on the prototype (Kerttula & Tokkonen, 2001). VR could also be used for large-scale military exercises. Bhagat et al. (2016) developed a 3D interactive VR system for military live firing training. They claimed that virtual training outperformed traditional live firing training in terms of learning motivation and learning outcomes. In the education field, VR could stimulate students' learning interest and engagement in the class for its ability to present interactive 3D virtual objects in front of the students (Liu et al., 2017). As such, students could take an active part in the learning activity. Edwards et al. (2019) designed a VR-based learning application for chemistry education. They claimed that VR is advantageous to increase the students' engagement, motivation, and interest in the class.

Augmented Reality

AR is a technology that enhances users' perception of the physical world by superimposing virtual elements onto the actual environment (Azuma, 1997; Li et al., 2017). AR devices need to calculate the camera images' position and angle in real-time to achieve this function (Lee, 2019). The difference between AR and VR is noticeable. VR replaces the real world, whereas AR complements it (Zhou et al., 2008). Azuma (1997) noted that AR has the following three properties:

- Integrates the real and virtual environment
- Natural and real-time human-computer interaction
- Registered in 3-D

In the last decade, the use of AR in the medicine, retail, and tourism industry increased dramatically due to its potentials in overlaying digital information in real environments. Medicine is one of the earliest application fields of AR technology. AR was used in medical training, patient diagnosis, and surgical treatment (Li et al., 2017). AR could assist doctors in patient diagnosis and rehabilitation by providing them with digital images and critical information intuitively and naturally (Negrillo-Cárdenas et al., 2020). For example, Hemanth et al. (2020) explored the possibilities to diagnose heart diseases using an AR-supported mobile application. They claimed that the application is a helpful tool for doctors and specialists in related fields. Besides, AR could reshape customer shopping experiences in the retail industry. Retail is one of the emerging areas for AR research (Alhalabi & Lytras, 2019). AR could improve their shopping experience by letting customers make better buying decisions. AR could allow customers to try on shoes virtually before buying them (Dacko, 2017). It could also provide customers with a new way to try out new makeup by merging customers' makeup images and their body reflection in the mirror (Martínez et al., 2014). AR could also help customers to find their products interactively. For example, AR could lead customers toward where the desired product is located (Cruz et al., 2019). With AR, customers could enjoy the pleasure of shopping, even without leaving home. Indeed, AR could also effectively enhance people's travel experience. In the tourism industry, AR could provide visitors with extra information about the destinations (Torres-Ruiz et al., 2020). Shin et al. (2010) proposed an AR-based application that could intelligently guide visitors moving around the art galleries. They commented that their application could prevent visitors from getting lost and let visitors receive more information about the artifacts, thereby improving their engagement in the art galleries.

Mixed Reality

MR is a technology where AR and VR meet (Milgram & Kishino, 1994). It aims at merging the real space and virtual space to produce a new visual environment where physical and virtual entities coexist and interact in real-time (Lifton et al., 2009). MR is different from AR in the sense that AR superimposes straightforward digital content on top of the actual world. In contrast, MR projects 3D computer-generated content that is spatially aware and responsive. Traditionally, MR refers to all display technologies that fall into the middle of the reality-virtuality continuum (Milgram et al., 1995). According to Milgram et al. (1995), both AR and AV could be considered as MR. MR should also include the following three properties, as shown in Figure 3 (Milgram & Kishino, 1994; Milgram et al., 1995):

- The extent of world knowledge: It refers to spatiality. A model of the physical world is constructed in the computer such that the computer can know precisely the positions and locations of the physical objects.
- Reproduction Fidelity: It refers to the quality of the computer graphics rendering and realism of the actual world. The fidelity of MR is high such that users cannot distinguish between the virtual world and the real world.
- The extent of Presence Metaphor: It refers to how users feel immersed or present in the displayed scene. MR devices can alter users' sense of place and presence.

Figure 3. The MR classification space
(Milgram et al., 1995)

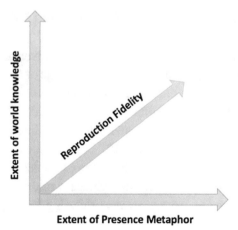

Extent of Presence Metaphor

Milgram and Kishino (Milgram & Kishino, 1994) suggested six MR examples that fulfill their definition:

- Monitor-based (non-immersive) video displays.
- Video-based head-mounted displays.
- Optical see-through head-mounted displays.
- Video see-through HMD.
- Completely immersive AV systems to which video "reality" is added.
- Partially immersive AV systems in which real physical objects exist in the virtual scene.

Unlike the relatively long application history of VR and AR, MR technology is still making its way into the mainstream. Although researchers have controversial views on whether Microsoft's Hololens belongs to MR, Microsoft's Hololens is indeed a well-known example of an existing, commercially available MR device. On the one hand, Hololens is a useful tool for guiding clinical interventions (Vassallo et al., 2017). On the other hand, Hololens is helpful in controlling industrial manipulators (Puljiz et al., 2019). Puljiz et al. (2019) pointed out that the built-in hand tracking and positioning functions of Hololens could make the calculation of the hands' position relative to the robot feasible and smoothen the interaction between the users and the robots. Besides Hololens, Espíndola et al. (2013) also proposed an approach called CARMMI to improve maintenance management using MR. CARMMI was able to provide information about failure components to operators in the maintenance tasks through MR. El Ammari and Hammad (2019) also developed a collaborative BIM-based MR approach for facility management. In their framework, multisource facilities information, BIM models, and feature-based tracking were integrated into an MR setting. Managers could hence deliver visual instructions to onsite workers from their offices.

Cross Reality – A Combination of AR, MR, and VR

While the term: XR is sometimes regarded as a universal term of immersive technologies (Joyce, 2018), XR emphasizes the linkage of the actual world and the virtual world via the collaboration of a broad spectrum of display technologies, including VR, AR, and MR (Zarraonandia et al., 2019). With XR, users from different levels of "reality" (VR, AR, and MR) could interact and collaborate to complete complex tasks (Reilly et al., 2010).

ShadowLab (Lifton et al., 2009) is one of the examples of XR applications that fulfill this definition. It is a system that links the real world and the virtual world. The system captured information from the real world using light, sound, and movement sensors to drive the phenomena in the virtual world and projected virtual phenomena into the real world through distributed displays. Real and virtual visitors could see and collaborate to carry out tasks simultaneously using VR and AR technology (Lifton et al., 2009). Davies et al. (2013)'s application is another example of XR applications. Davies et al. (2013) introduced an XR system that could help students explore cultural heritages onsite with instant access to background information and revisit the virtual representation of the cultural heritages in the classroom or at home.

Zarraonandia et al. (2019) also explored the possibilities of XR serious games designed for purposes other than entertainment. Their system could allow geographically distant people to interact and collaborate to solve a problem using VR, AR, and MR devices. Specifically, VR was used to create an immersive feeling and a first-person learning perspective for users far away from sites (Smolentsev et al., 2017). In contrast, AR was used to augment physical objects for users on sites (Kim et al., 2018). Zarraonandia et al. (2019) commented that XR technology enables teachers to create training games that can be performed in real space and cyberspace simultaneously.

The Applications of VR, AR, and MR in Crisis Management

When a crisis occurs, it is the responsibility of the emergency response teams to take prompt actions to minimize the number of deaths and injuries and restore the situation. However, crises are often physiologically and psychologically demanding. It is not surprising that humans would act wrongly during emergencies. These mistakes, if not well managed, could lead to more severe results. Examples of common mistakes include inadequate situation assessment, erroneous judgments, blind allegiance to the procedures, adverse reaction under stress, unclear roles resulting in tasks falling through the cracks, and miscommunication (Crichton & Flin, 2004; Rouse et al., 1992). Therefore, the importance of preparation and onsite management is widely recognized in the domain of emergency management (Coombs & Laufer, 2018). Crisis management is an area where VR, AR, and MR technology could help. In the rest of this section, the development of the VR, AR, and MR technology in crisis management is discussed in detail.

Virtual Reality in Crisis Management

Regular training is widely recognized in the domain of emergency management (Beroggi et al., 1995). However, emergency drills in the real environment consume many human, material, and financial resources, making organizations hesitate to conduct emergency drills frequently (Kwok et al., 2019). Prasolova-Førland et al. (2017) also commented that using field tests as training modules to simulate emergencies and prepare for crises could be expensive, dangerous, inflexible to adapt to different scenarios, and difficult to replicate. Without frequent training, it is questionable whether the emergency response staff can make a rapid, effective, and appropriate response to the situation during an emergency. VR technology could help in this area. There is a lengthy application history of VR in emergency preparedness training.

Beroggi et al. (1995) drew attention to the possibility of using VR for emergency management. They commented that VR could support problem-solving and decision-making during an emergency. Later, Smith and Trenholme (2009) noticed that it could be hard and inconvenient to conduct realistic fire evacuation drills in modern buildings, so they adopted VR technology to support virtual drills in 3D virtual buildings. Xu et al. (2014) also developed a rational VR-based fire training simulator taking complete account of the various aspects of smoke hazards. Using their simulator, trainees could experience realistic but non-threatening fire scenarios such that trainees could learn how to find the safest path for evacuation or rescue. Williams-Bell et al. (2015) noted that VR could stimulate the physical and psychological stresses of the search and rescue task. Hence, it could train firefighters to make the right decision under pressure. Kwok et al. (2019) also applied VR and discrete event simulation techniques to develop a hazard simulation system with the capability to recreate large-scale and multi-agency emergency incidents for crisis training.

Compared to large-scale real-life exercises, VR retains a considerable cost advantage. Hence, the VR-based virtual drill is increasingly recognized. Also, as VR-based virtual drill is highly engaging, promoting greater knowledge transfer (Hsu et al., 2013), increasingly more emergency preparedness training based on VR is implemented (Ferguson et al., 2020).

Augmented Reality in Crisis Management

Rapid response and decision-making are critical for reducing causalities and loss (Ahmad et al., 2014). Unfortunately, humans often make mistakes under stress. Therefore, it is essential to provide real-time guidance to the emergency response staff. Due to the ability to superimpose digital information on users' views, AR can be used for evacuation and supporting collaboration among the emergency response teams.

Tsai et al. (2012) constructed an application called Mobile Escape Guidelines, which employed AR technology on mobile devices to provide users essential geographic information and escape guidelines. Their system could show the escape routes on top of users' viewpoints such that users could follow the instruction to escape from accident sites quickly. Sebillo et al. (2016) also developed an AR application to enhance the training efficacy for onsite emergency drills. Their application aimed at making emergency response staff feel confident with the emergency protocol by reproducing emergency scenarios using AR. Via the AR mobile interface, trainees could receive real-time instructions from trainers. On the other hand, trainers could modify the training tasks base on the data collected from the drills. Sebillo et al. (2016) commented that AR is a low-cost tool for conducting highly realistic exercises in the real environment. Itamiya et al. (2019) created an AR smartphone application to provide people with an immersive experience for disaster awareness during peacetime. The application could superimpose disasters such as floods, debris, and fire smoke on the actual surroundings. They claimed that the application helped improve people's crisis awareness.

To this end, AR can provide emergency responders with decision support and escape routes guidance.

Mixed Reality in Crisis Management

While MR could be applied to many domains, such as manufacturing and education, Microsoft listed crisis management as one of HoloLens' major application areas and promoted research in this field (Asgary, 2017). Gaining the advantages from MR technology, emergency response staff could see 3D geographic information from a depth-spatial-persistence perspective (Wang et al., 2018). There are several examples of successful MR applications in crisis management.

Li and Zuo (2021) established an MR-based underground mine emergency escape system. They showed that the system could effectively help underground mine workers during an emergency evacuation. Sharma et al. (2019) proposed an MR 3D visualization system to facilitate the communication among emergency response teams about the emergency using 3D building models and floor plans. They highlighted MR's ability to show detailed geographic information in a 3D form, such that emergency response teams could plan the best route together for rescue and evacuation. Asgary et al. (2019) also developed an MR application to visualize different volcanic phenomena for emergency management training. They viewed that MR had enormous potential to assist in disaster and crisis management because it could help emergency response teams understand the situation straightforwardly by reading the 3D models. Other similar research includes (Stigall et al., 2018). It aimed at offering users an enthralling-visuals evacuation experience to escape from dangers in case of emergency.

In summary, MR balances the advantages of AR and VR. Unlike AR, which only overlays straightforward digital content onto users' views, MR does more in letting users feel depth spatial persistence (Sharma et al., 2019). Therefore, MR can provide users with a more realistic onsite experience to facilitate their communication and decision-making.

CONCEPT OF CROSS REALITY IN CRISIS MANAGEMENT

XR is, by nature, a shared online virtual world in which users can interact with each other, virtual objects, and real-world information using VR, AR, and MR technology. Paradiso and Landay (2009) further regarded XR as: "Sensor networks can tunnel dense real-world information into virtual worlds, where this data is interpreted and displayed to dispersed users. Interaction of virtual participants can incarnate into the physical world through a plenitude of diverse displays and actuators." Such a concept is similar to the idea of Digital Twin, an increasingly popular concept for intelligent manufacturing.

Digital Twin emphasizes the integration of the physical and cyberspace (Chhetri et al., 2004). It aims at creating a digital replica of physical entities to facilitate the decision-making process (Saddik, 2018). Such a digital replica is not a static one but is a mirror of the physical object. The digital replica updates and changes as their physical counterparts change. Tao et al. (2019) pointed out the benefits of using Digital Twin in manufacturing: "Digital twin enables designers to fully customize, easily compare and effectively assess. Designers can better understand customer requirements through data and information about customer reviews and usage habits. Moreover, they can compare the performance of virtual products under different circumstances to ensure the inconsistency between the actual behavior and the desired actual of the manufactured product is decreased to the minimum." With the advancement of the internet of things, data from the real world is more accessible. With the data, a digital simulation model that mirrors the physical world can be easily constructed. If a disaster occurs in the real world, the same damage should be simulated at once in the virtual world. Because of the mirror characteristic of simulation model, the computer can instantly examine the disaster situation, for example, the spread of fire and number of injuries, and provide the emergency response teams with a clear picture about the disaster situations. Figure 4 shows the concept of the use of XR technology in crisis management. VR, AR, and MR technology can facilitate crisis management in the following three ways:

- Virtual Reality: Provide a virtual environment for drills and exercises.
- Augmented Reality: Provide onsite staff with clear guidance for search and rescue.
- Mixed Reality: Provide engineers with clear instructions for recovery.

Figure 4. Concept of XR in crisis management

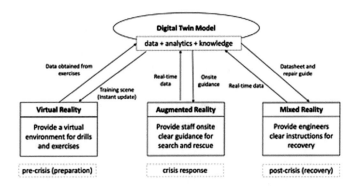

Virtual Reality (Preparation)

Regular training is essential to ensure that the crisis response staff can perform their duties rapidly and correctly. Hence, organizations from time to time conduct emergency drills to keep their teams well prepared for crises. However, emergency drills usually require considerable human and material resources to make the drill vivid and genuine. It may also disturb the normal operations of the organizations. Hence, many organizations are not willing to conduct emergency drills frequently. These restrictions eventually limit the number of opportunities for the crisis response staff to learn and practice the organizations' emergency procedures.

Given that VR technology can give users an immersive experience of being physically present in an artificial virtual world, it can be adopted as a training tool. The crisis response staff can experience the simulated disaster and get familiar with the emergency procedures in the virtual environment. The virtual copy of the actual system that was built according to the architectural floor plan can be downloaded from the server. As the simulation model is a digital replica of the actual system, it matches the physical attributes of the real system. Hence, the simulation model can instantaneously react to the actions taken by the crisis response staff and evaluate the spread of disaster. Since the emergency drills are performed in a virtual environment that the computer can keep tracking the location and actions of each staff, the whole crisis management strategy and the performance of each team can be recorded and uploaded to the server via the network for further analysis. Besides, the nearby motion tracking sensors and cameras can also help track the staff's motions and emotions. Hence, data regarding occupational safety and health can also be collected. All these data are helpful for data scientists and crisis management researchers to optimize deployments for peak efficiency, examine their crisis management plans, and protect the safety of the crisis response staff.

Augmented Reality (Response)

The duty to implement the emergency plans lies with the crisis response staff onsite, who need to face a tremendously complex, hazardous, and stressful environment. Hence, it is not surprising that the staff would make mistakes during emergency incidents. Therefore, clear and concise onsite guidance is essential to ensure that prompt and efficient actions are taken during an emergency.

Given that AR technology can superimpose computer-generated information on users' views of the physical world across various sensory modalities such as visual, auditory, and haptic, it can act as a remote guidance tool to instruct onsite staff to execute the emergency protocols during an emergency. The AR device can assist rescue teams in rapidly reporting the most up-to-date information via the internet to the server. As a digital twin system is built in the server using data gathered from VR training and real-time input from sensors such as video cameras on the emergency scene, the digital twin model can instantaneously compute, reflect, and even foresee the event occurring. Hence, an intelligent planning system can be formed to cope with the changing situation to improve efficiency and reduce risks. For example, the computer can calculate the best rescue paths for the crisis response teams and navigate them using AR technology (Berger & Lo, 2015).

Mixed Reality (Recovery)

Disaster and crisis may damage properties and infrastructures, bringing public health, environmental and infrastructural problems. In the post-crisis phase, the emergency should have been settled by the emergency response teams. Therefore, the focal point of the attention should be shifted to recovery. As the digital geometries of the real world before the crisis is stored on the server, the computer can easily compare the information between the virtual and physical environment and tell damage condition of the actual system. Information about the damage condition can be shown to the engineers and technicians via MR. MR can mix the real and virtual world to generate a new environment where physical and virtual entities can coexist and interact in real-time (Milgram & Kishino, 1994). Hence, it can help emergency response engineers and technicians to understand complex information and get an insight into the complex repair tasks in a straightforward view. 3D models of the infrastructures can be downloaded from the server. Technicians can get the information they need for carrying out the repair tasks from the model, such as datasheet and step-by-step repair scenarios. They can also contact the engineers for assistance via video conference. In the video conference, the engineers can view what the technician is seeing and guide the technicians using holographic pointers.

FEASIBILITY OF THE CONCEPT

A qualitative study was conducted to explore the feasibility of the concept. The study aimed to examine and comprehend people's attitudes on using XR for crisis management and explore the factors impacting their sentiments and possible attitudes. As the study was exploratory in nature, a qualitative study was suitable for gathering this sort of information (Alwidyan et al., 2020; Berg & Lune, 2012).

Participants and Study Procedures

This study adhered to the American Psychological Association's Code of Ethics and was approved by the Institutional Review Board at the authors' institution. Each subject provided informed consent before the experiment began. The informed consent form involved three major parts: (1) disclosure - informing subjects about the study's background and providing them with the information necessary to make an autonomous decision; (2) capacity - stating the subject's capacity to comprehend the information presented and make a reasonable judgment about the possible consequences of their decision; (3) voluntariness - emphasizing the decision's voluntary nature (Shah et al., 2021). The participants were recruited from a local university through a convenient sample and snowball sampling technique, which involved posting invitations in WeChat groups, encouraging group members to participate, and spreading the information to other groups. This form of recruiting is frequently employed in qualitative research (Naderifar et al., 2017). Inclusion criteria for enrollment were: (1) 18-year-old or above, (2) had the normal or corrected-to-normal vision, and (3) had prior knowledge or experience in management (e.g., studied management-related subjects).

In the study, the participants were asked to watch a video clip about conducting an XR-based emergency drill in a public transportation scenario. The five-minute video clip showcased a prototype system and demonstrated how XR technology could be used for crisis management. After that, the participants were allowed to experience part of the prototype system. For example, they were placed in a virtual metro station with an electric fire. They were trained to evacuate the passengers and recover the situation. Figure 5 shows the screenshots of the virtual emergency drill environment. After that, the subjects were required to fill in a survey about their demographic information, followed by two open-ended questions exploring their perceived facilitators and barriers to using XR in crisis management. Textual data concerning the use of the XR technologies were recorded by asking participants: "What was your overall experience with crisis management using XR technologies?" and "Do you think you would react the same as you have practiced in the virtual environment had it been a real emergency incident?"

Figure 5. Screenshot of the virtual emergency drill environment

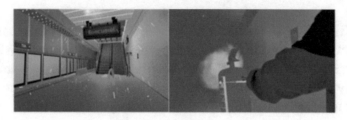

Data Analysis

This study used an inductive content analysis approach to examine the people's opinions of using XR for crisis management, with the goal of categorizing their viewpoints into themes and sub-themes. Content analysis refers to "a research method for the subject interpretation of the content of text data through the systematic classification process of coding and identifying themes and patterns" (Hsieh & Shannon, 2005). It is a systematic categorization procedure that involves coding and detecting themes and patterns. It is a method that is frequently used in qualitative research to extract themes and subthemes (underlying elements) from people's opinions (e.g., Alwidyan et al., 2020; Omura et al., 2020; Yari et al., 2019; Zhu et al., 2020). Therefore, this study used content analysis to analyze the data.

In detail, two researchers repeatedly read all the textual data to verify the completeness and accuracy and get a comprehensive understanding of the contents and contexts of participants' responses. When they read through the textual data, they examined the meanings of participants' opinions, highlighted key statements, created labels for the statements, and formed themes and sub-themes by grouping similar ideas. Data examination, labeling, and grouping were performed independently by the two researchers. They and a third researcher met to compare and contrast the coding schemes, reconcile any discrepancies, and determine the final themes and sub-themes. The frequencies were counted to examine whether a sub-theme is common.

After finishing the analysis, the researchers recontacted some subjects, questioning them about the themes and findings to confirm the results' credibility and integrity. The participants said they were unsurprised by these findings, suggesting that these themes were consistent with their views (Alwidyan et al., 2020).

Results

A total of 100 subjects (male:female = 1:0.49; age: 18-24) were enrolled in this study. They all reported that they had information technology experience and management knowledge or experience (e.g., studied management-related subjects). Three themes emerged related to facilitators and barriers to the adoption of XR technology in crisis management. They were human attributes, technology characteristics, and factors associated with interactions between humans and technology. Ten sub-themes pertinent to the above-mentioned themes were generated including prior experience, training, equipment and facilities, application-specific scenario design, cost, telepresence, perceived ease of use, perceived usefulness, perceived enjoyment, and physical adaptability. Table 1 and Table 2 present the emerged themes, sub-themes, and their associated sample quotes from the textual data for participants' perceived facilitators and barriers, respectively. As shown in Table 3, 310 interview statements were derived, among which 230 (74.2%) were related to facilitators, and 80 (25.8%) were related to barriers. In general, perceived usefulness (n=115, 50%) and telepresence (n=50, 21.7%) were the most-mentioned two factors that facilitate individual's adoption of XR in crisis management; application-specific scenario design (n=42, 52.5%) and equipment and facilities (n=11, 13.75%) were the most-mentioned two factors that impede individual's adoption of XR technology in crisis management.

Table 1. Factors that facilitate the use of XR in crisis management

Themes	Sub-themes	Sample Quotes From the Textual Data
Human attributes	Prior experience	"I have some prior experience in using VR technologies so that I can get familiar with it (VR-based drill) quickly."
	Training	"The instructions and explanations before using the technology are important (in using it)."
Technology characteristics	Application-specific scenario design	"With the scenario design, people can feel more immersive in this virtual environment than in a real training system." "The situation of an emergency incident was perfectly stimulated. I feel immersive in it (the training scenario)."
	Cost	"The training can be conducted regardless of the limitation of space, saving many resources." "It (VR-based drill) helps to save quite a lot of manpower and material resources."
Factors associated with interactions between humans and technology	Telepresence	"The visual experience was good due to the telepresence of the technology."
	Perceived ease of use	"The manipulate of the equipment was quite easy." "I think it (the XR technology) is very easy to understand and use."
	Perceived usefulness	"The immersive crisis management training method allowed me to gain valuable experience and skills that are helpful in preparing for a real crisis." "It (VR-based drill) will be beneficial to us when we encounter such (emergency) situations in the future."
	Perceived enjoyment	"(The concept of using) XR-based crisis management method is novel and interesting, which drives me to explore."

Table 2. Factors that impede the use of XR in crisis management

Themes	Sub-themes	Sample Quotes From the Textual Data
Human attributes	Prior experience	"Because I never used such systems before, it was not easy for me to use them." "It seems that the (XR-based) crisis management training does not provide much benefit. Maybe it's just because this is the first time I use this kind of technology."
	Training	"I just need more practice to get familiar with it." "I need some guidance before using the system because I'm not familiar with VR technologies."
Technology characteristics	Equipment and facilities	"The use of operating handles of the VR equipment was not comfortable and sensitive." "I feel that the quality of the displayed images (in the VR equipment) was not enough; the resolution needs to be increased."
	Application-specific scenario design	"I think that the scenario needs more details, such as when using the fire extinguisher and the ringing the alarm bells. The lack of these details makes me hardly feel it is real." "(In the scenario), individuals' emotions and facial expressions were not well simulated so that the alarms and emergency incident barely bring me the sense of moral panic."
	Cost	"The cost of this set of equipment should be very high so that the public cannot widely use it at this time point."
Factors associated with interactions between humans and technology	Telepresence	"I feel that the virtual environment was way too unrealistic. I just can't convince myself that I was actually conducting a real emergency drill."
	Perceived ease of use	"There were some delays when interacting with the VR system, and this made it a bit hard to use."
	Perceived usefulness	"I may learn some countermeasures from it (VR-based drill) when encountering emergencies, but they may not be practical." "There are many uncertainties in a real emergency that generates a lot of chaos, the simulations in the XR system may not be useful."
	Physical adaptability	"My first impression of this XR system was physical discomfort." "It (the head-mounted display) brought me some eye fatigue. This made me a little bit uncomfortable."

Discussion and Implications

Based on the data collected from the participants, adopting XR in crisis management system contains the following advantages:

- As shown in Table 3, perceived usefulness, which refers to the XR-based crisis management training that can provide users with relevant knowledge and skills about how to react to emergencies, was the most prominent facilitator that drives people's intention to use XR for crisis management training. As one subject reported, *"the immersive crisis management training method allowed me to gain valuable experience and skills that are helpful in preparing for a real crisis."* Using the XR-based crisis management training allows people to experience simulating emergency drills, conduct practices, and be prepared in advance.

- Telepresence was another mostly mentioned facilitator that helps develop people's positive attitudes towards using XR technologies in crisis management training. As one subject said, *"the visual experience was good due to the telepresence of the technology."* Hence, XR-based crisis management training is considered novel to most users and can provide them with a sense of telepresence when simulating emergency drills, which, in turn, promotes individual's acceptance and adoption of XR in crisis management.

Table 3. The frequency of factors identified by interviewers

Themes	Sub-themes	Frequency			Percentage
		Facilitators (n=230)	Barriers (n=80)	Total (n=310)	
Human attributes	Prior experience	2	4	6	1.9
	Training	1	2	3	1.0
Technology characteristics	Equipment and facilities	0	11	11	3.5
	Application-specific scenario design	9	42	51	16.5
	Cost	15	3	18	5.8
Factors associated with interactions between humans and technology	Telepresence	50	8	58	18.7
	Perceived ease of use	20	1	21	6.8
	Perceived usefulness	115	2	117	37.7
	Perceived enjoyment	18	0	18	5.8
	Physical adaptability	0	7	7	2.3

In the meantime, the XR system should address the following problems to make it more feasible and acceptable:

- It is suggested that more realistic interactive scenarios should be designed. As one subject reported, *"I think that the scenario needs more details, such as when using the fire extinguisher and the ringing the alarm bells. The lack of these details makes me hardly feel it is real."* This implies that the details of the scene design would affect users' perception of the authenticity of the XR system, which may affect the effectiveness of crisis management training. Therefore, XR systems should be designed and developed as detailed, realistic, and diversified as possible to ensure the effectiveness of emergency training.

- Regarding equipment and facilities, it is of great importance that the resolution of the displayed virtual reality image should be improved to enhance the authenticity and credibility of the XR system. As one subject mentioned, *"I feel that the quality of the displayed images (in the VR equipment) was not enough; the resolution needs to be increased."* Besides, the design of XR equipment should be considered from the perspective of human factors engineering. As one subject said, *"the use of operating handles of the VR equipment was not comfortable and sensitive."* Thus, those facilities and equipment should be designed in a more user-friendly way to reduce the discomfort, dizziness, and eye fatigue caused by the XR system.

Limitations

This study has several limitations. To begin, over 80% of subjects stated that they had no prior VR or emergency experience. This demographic background may affect how they comprehend the concept, as prior experience is a factor in facilitating new technology acceptance. However, as VR, AR, and MR are still developing technologies, this demographic sample should be regarded as normal. The results should reflect the actual situation when an organization wishes to implement XR. Second, this research was a pilot study designed to understand better how potential users embraced the concept of using XR for crisis management. As a result, the stated outcomes may be influenced by participants' impressions of the video presentation and prototype content. As a result, additional quantitative studies with a bigger sample size should be conducted.

CONCLUSION

Crisis management is an essential organizational function. It is critical to conduct damage control and recovery. The recent advances in information and communication technologies, computer graphics, sensor technologies, and display technologies have powered the possibility to adopt XR in crisis management. This chapter has introduced the latest development of XR technology, particularly in crisis management, proposed a framework that integrated VR, AR, and MR for crisis management, and presented a study that examined the user perception of the XR-based crisis management method. Based on the study, it has also discussed the way and challenges of adopting XR technology. This chapter is valuable to the field of research in virtual reality and crisis management as it showed how to adopt XR technology in crisis management and provided management insights on how potential users would think about the technology.

ACKNOWLEDGMENT

This work was supported by the National Natural Science Foundation of China [grant numbers 71904062 and 72001091]; Guangdong Basic and Applied Basic Research Foundation [grant numbers 2020A1515110889]; Fundamental Research Funds for the Central Universities of China [grant numbers 21618317 and 21619320]; Department of Natural Resources of Guangdong Province [grant numbers [2020]071]; and National Key R&D Program of China [grant numbers 2019YFB1705401].

REFERENCES

Ahmad, N., Ali, Q., Crowley, H., & Pinho, R. (2014). Earthquake loss estimation of residential buildings in Pakistan. *Natural Hazards*, *73*(3), 1889–1955. doi:10.100711069-014-1174-8

Alhalabi, W., & Lytras, M. D. (2019). Editorial for special issue on Virtual Reality and Augmented Reality. *Virtual Reality (Waltham Cross)*, *23*(3), 215–216. doi:10.100710055-019-00398-6

Alwidyan, M. T., Trainor, J. E., & Bissell, R. A. (2020). Responding to natural disasters vs. disease outbreaks: Do emergency medical service providers have different views? *International Journal of Disaster Risk Reduction*, *44*, 101440. doi:10.1016/j.ijdrr.2019.101440 PMID:32363141

Asgary, A. (2017). Holodisaster: Leveraging Microsoft HoloLens in Disaster and Emergency Management. *IAEM Bulletin*, 20-21.

Asgary, A., Bonadonna, C., & Frischknecht, C. (2019). Simulation and Visualization of Volcanic Phenomena Using Microsoft Hololens: Case of Vulcano Island (Italy). *IEEE Transactions on Engineering Management*, 1–9. doi:10.1109/TEM.2019.2932291

Azuma, R. T. (1997). A Survey of Augmented Reality. *Presence*, *6*(4), 355–385. doi:10.1162/pres.1997.6.4.355

Berger, J., & Lo, N. (2015). An innovative multi-agent search-and-rescue path planning approach. *Computers & Operations Research*, *53*, 24–31. doi:10.1016/j.cor.2014.06.016

Beroggi, G. E. G., Waisel, L., & Wallace, W. A. (1995). Employing virtual reality to support decision making in emergency management. *Safety Science*, *20*(1), 79–88. doi:10.1016/0925-7535(94)00068-E

Bhagat, K. K., Liou, W.-K., & Chang, C.-Y. (2016). A cost-effective interactive 3D virtual reality system applied to military live firing training. *Virtual Reality (Waltham Cross)*, *20*(2), 127–140. doi:10.100710055-016-0284-x

Brooks, F. P. (1999). What's real about virtual reality? *IEEE Computer Graphics and Applications*, *19*(6), 16–27. doi:10.1109/38.799723

Burdea, G., & Langrana, N. (1992). Virtual force feedback: Lessons, challenges, future applications. *Winter Annual Meeting of the American Society of Mechanical Engineers*.

Chhetri, M. B., Krishnaswamy, S., & Loke, S. W. (2004). Smart Virtual Counterparts for Learning Communities. In C. Bussler, S.-k. Hong, W. Jun, R. Kaschek, Kinshuk, S. Krishnaswamy, S. W. Loke, D. Oberle, D. Richards, A. Sharma, Y. Sure, & B. Thalheim (Eds.), Web Information Systems – WISE 2004 Workshops. Berlin: Academic Press.

Coombs, W. T., & Laufer, D. (2018). Global Crisis Management – Current Research and Future Directions. *Journal of International Management*, *24*(3), 199–203. doi:10.1016/j.intman.2017.12.003

Crichton, M. T., & Flin, R. (2004). Identifying and training non-technical skills of nuclear emergency response teams. *Annals of Nuclear Energy*, *31*(12), 1317–1330. doi:10.1016/j.anucene.2004.03.011

Cruz, E., Orts-Escolano, S., Gomez-Donoso, F., Rizo, C., Rangel, J. C., Mora, H., & Cazorla, M. (2019). An augmented reality application for improving shopping experience in large retail stores. *Virtual Reality (Waltham Cross)*, *23*(3), 281–291. doi:10.100710055-018-0338-3

Dacko, S. G. (2017). Enabling smart retail settings via mobile augmented reality shopping apps. *Technological Forecasting and Social Change*, *124*, 243–256. doi:10.1016/j.techfore.2016.09.032

Davies, C., Miller, A., & Allison, C. (2013). Mobile Cross Reality for cultural heritage. *2013 Digital Heritage International Congress (DigitalHeritage)*.

Edwards, B. I., Bielawski, K. S., Prada, R., & Cheok, A. D. (2019). Haptic virtual reality and immersive learning for enhanced organic chemistry instruction. *Virtual Reality (Waltham Cross)*, *23*(4), 363–373.

El Ammari, K., & Hammad, A. (2019). Remote interactive collaboration in facilities management using BIM-based mixed reality. *Automation in Construction*, *107*, 102940. doi:10.1016/j.autcon.2019.102940

Espíndola, D. B., Fumagalli, L., Garetti, M., Pereira, C. E., Botelho, S. S. C., & Ventura Henriques, R. (2013). A model-based approach for data integration to improve maintenance management by mixed reality. *Computers in Industry*, *64*(4), 376–391. doi:10.1016/j.compind.2013.01.002

Ferguson, C., van den Broek, E. L., & van Oostendorp, H. (2020). On the role of interaction mode and story structure in virtual reality serious games. *Computers & Education*, *143*, 103671. doi:10.1016/j.compedu.2019.103671

Hemanth, J. D., Kose, U., Deperlioglu, O., & de Albuquerque, V. H. C. (2020). An augmented reality-supported mobile application for diagnosis of heart diseases. *The Journal of Supercomputing*, *76*(2), 1242–1267. doi:10.100711227-018-2483-6

Hsieh, H.-F., & Shannon, S. E. (2005). Three approaches to qualitative content analysis. *Qualitative Health Research*, *15*(9), 1277–1288. doi:10.1177/1049732305276687 PMID:16204405

Hsu, E. B., Li, Y., Bayram, J. D., Levinson, D., Yang, S., & Monahan, C. (2013). State of virtual reality based disaster preparedness and response training. *PLoS Currents, 5*.

Itamiya, T., Tohara, H., & Nasuda, Y. (2019). Augmented Reality Floods and Smoke Smartphone App Disaster Scope utilizing Real-time Occlusion. *2019 IEEE Conference on Virtual Reality and 3D User Interfaces (VR)*.

Joyce, K. (2018). *AR, VR, MR, RR, XR: A Glossary To The Acronyms Of The Future*. Retrieved 28 Dec 2019 from https://www.vrfocus.com/2017/05/ar-vr-mr-rr-xr-a-glossary-to-the-acronyms-of-the-future/

Kanade, T., Rander, P., & Narayanan, P. J. (1997). Virtualized reality: Constructing virtual worlds from real scenes. *IEEE MultiMedia*, *4*(1), 34–47. doi:10.1109/93.580394

Kenngott, H. G., Pfeiffer, M., Preukschas, A. A., Bettscheider, L., Wise, P. A., Wagner, M., Speidel, S., Huber, M., Nickel, F., Mehrabi, A., & Müller-Stich, B. P. (2021). IMHOTEP: Cross-professional evaluation of a three-dimensional virtual reality system for interactive surgical operation planning, tumor board discussion and immersive training for complex liver surgery in a head-mounted display. *Surgical Endoscopy*. Advance online publication. doi:10.100700464-020-08246-4 PMID:33475848

Kerttula, M., & Tokkonen, T. (2001). Virtual design of multiengineering electronics systems. *Computer*, *34*(11), 71–79. doi:10.1109/2.963447

Kim, Y., Hong, S., & Kim, G. J. (2018). Augmented reality-based remote coaching for fast-paced physical task. *Virtual Reality (Waltham Cross)*, 22(1), 25–36. doi:10.100710055-017-0315-2

Kwok, P. K., Yan, M., Chan, B. K. P., & Lau, H. Y. K. (2019). Crisis management training using discrete-event simulation and virtual reality techniques. *Computers & Industrial Engineering*, 135, 711–722. doi:10.1016/j.cie.2019.06.035

Kwok, P. K., Yan, M., Qu, T., & Lau, H. Y. K. (2020). User acceptance of virtual reality technology for practicing digital twin-based crisis management. *International Journal of Computer Integrated Manufacturing*, 1–14. doi:10.1080/095119 2X.2020.1803502

Lee, H. (2019). Real-time manufacturing modeling and simulation framework using augmented reality and stochastic network analysis. *Virtual Reality (Waltham Cross)*, 23(1), 85–99. doi:10.100710055-018-0343-6

Li, J., & Zuo, M. (2021). Emergency Rescue Training System for Earthquakes Based on Immersive Technology. *2021 IEEE 5th Advanced Information Technology, Electronic and Automation Control Conference (IAEAC)*.

Li, Q., Huang, C., Lv, S., Li, Z., Chen, Y., & Ma, L. (2017). An Human-Computer Interactive Augmented Reality System for Coronary Artery Diagnosis Planning and Training. [PubMed]. *Journal of Medical Systems*, 41(10), 159. doi:10.100710916-017-0805-5

Lifton, J., Laibowitz, M., Harry, D., Gong, N., Mittal, M., & Paradiso, J. A. (2009). Metaphor and Manifestation Cross-Reality with Ubiquitous Sensor/Actuator Networks. *IEEE Pervasive Computing*, 8(3), 24–33. doi:10.1109/MPRV.2009.49

Liu, D., Bhagat, K. K., Gao, Y., Chang, T.-W., & Huang, R. (2017). The Potentials and Trends of Virtual Reality in Education. In D. Liu, C. Dede, R. Huang, & J. Richards (Eds.), *Virtual, Augmented, and Mixed Realities in Education* (pp. 105–130). Springer Singapore. doi:10.1007/978-981-10-5490-7_7

Martínez, H., Skournetou, D., Hyppölä, J., Laukkanen, S., & Heikkilä, A. (2014). Drivers and bottlenecks in the adoption of augmented reality applications. *Journal ISSN*, 2368, 5956. doi:10.11159/jmta.2014.004

Milgram, P., & Kishino, F. (1994). A taxonomy of mixed reality visual displays. *IEICE Transactions on Information and Systems*, 77(12), 1321–1329.

Milgram, P., Takemura, H., Utsumi, A., & Kishino, F. (1995). *Augmented reality: A class of displays on the reality-virtuality continuum.* Telemanipulator and Telepresence Technologies.

Naderifar, M., Goli, H., & Ghaljaei, F. (2017). Snowball Sampling: A Purposeful Method of Sampling in Qualitative Research. *Strides in Development of Medical Education, 14*(3).

Negrillo-Cárdenas, J., Jiménez-Pérez, J.-R., & Feito, F. R. (2020). The role of virtual and augmented reality in orthopedic trauma surgery: From diagnosis to rehabilitation. *Computer Methods and Programs in Biomedicine*, *191*, 105407. doi:10.1016/j.cmpb.2020.105407 PMID:32120088

Omura, M., Stone, T. E., Petrini, M. A., & Cao, R. (2020). Nurses' health beliefs about paper face masks in Japan, Australia and China: A qualitative descriptive study. *International Nursing Review*, *67*(3), 341–351. doi:10.1111/inr.12607 PMID:32686094

Paradiso, J. A., & Landay, J. A. (2009). Guest Editors' Introduction: Cross-Reality Environments. *IEEE Pervasive Computing*, *8*(3), 14–15. doi:10.1109/MPRV.2009.47

Park, J. (2018). Emotional reactions to the 3D virtual body and future willingness: The effects of self-esteem and social physique anxiety. *Virtual Reality (Waltham Cross)*, *22*(1), 1–11. doi:10.100710055-017-0314-3

Prasolova-Førland, E., Molka-Danielsen, J., Fominykh, M., & Lamb, K. (2017). Active learning modules for multi-professional emergency management training in virtual reality. *2017 IEEE 6th International Conference on Teaching, Assessment, and Learning for Engineering (TALE).*

Puljiz, D., Stöhr, E., Riesterer, K. S., Hein, B., & Kröger, T. (2019). *General Hand Guidance Framework using Microsoft HoloLens.* arXiv preprint arXiv:1908.04692.

Reilly, D. F., Rouzati, H., Wu, A., Hwang, J. Y., Brudvik, J., & Edwards, W. K. (2010). TwinSpace: an infrastructure for cross-reality team spaces. *Proceedings of the 23nd annual ACM symposium on User interface software and technology.* 10.1145/1866029.1866050

Reski, N., & Alissandrakis, A. (2020). Open data exploration in virtual reality: A comparative study of input technology. *Virtual Reality*, *24*(1), 1–22. doi:10.100710055-019-00378-w

Robert, B., & Lajtha, C. (2002). A New Approach to Crisis Management. *Journal of Contingencies and Crisis Management*, *10*(4), 181–191. doi:10.1111/1468-5973.00195

Rouse, W. B., Cannon-Bowers, J. A., & Salas, E. (1992). The role of mental models in team performance in complex systems. *IEEE Transactions on Systems, Man, and Cybernetics*, *22*(6), 1296–1308. doi:10.1109/21.199457

Saddik, A. E. (2018). Digital Twins: The Convergence of Multimedia Technologies. *IEEE MultiMedia*, *25*(2), 87–92. doi:10.1109/MMUL.2018.023121167

Sathia Bhama, P. R. K., Hariharasubramanian, V., Mythili, O. P., & Ramachandran, M. (2020). Users' domain knowledge prediction in e-learning with speech-interfaced augmented and virtual reality contents. *Virtual Reality (Waltham Cross)*, *24*(1), 163–173. doi:10.100710055-017-0321-4

Sebillo, M., Vitiello, G., Paolino, L., & Ginige, A. (2016). Training emergency responders through augmented reality mobile interfaces. *Multimedia Tools and Applications*, *75*(16), 9609–9622. doi:10.100711042-015-2955-0

Shah, P. R., Grewal, U. S., & Hamad, H. (2021). *Informed Consent*. StatPearls.

Sharma, S., Bodempudi, S. T., Scribner, D., Grynovicki, J., & Grazaitis, P. (2019). Emergency Response Using HoloLens for Building Evacuation. In Virtual, Augmented and Mixed Reality. Multimodal Interaction. doi:10.1007/978-3-030-21607-8_23

Shin, C., Kim, H., Kang, C., Jang, Y., Choi, A., & Woo, W. (2010). Unified Context-Aware Augmented Reality Application Framework for User-Driven Tour Guides. *2010 International Symposium on Ubiquitous Virtual Reality*.

Smith, S. P., & Trenholme, D. (2009). Rapid prototyping a virtual fire drill environment using computer game technology. *Fire Safety Journal*, *44*(4), 559–569.

Smolentsev, A., Cornick, J. E., & Blascovich, J. (2017). Using a preamble to increase presence in digital virtual environments. *Virtual Reality*, *21*(3), 153–164. doi:10.100710055-017-0305-4

Stigall, J., Bodempudi, S. T., Sharma, S., Scribner, D., Grynovicki, J., & Grazaitis, P. (2018). *Building Evacuation using Microsoft HoloLens*. Academic Press.

Tao, F., Sui, F., Liu, A., Qi, Q., Zhang, M., Song, B., Guo, Z., Lu, S. C. Y., & Nee, A. Y. C. (2019). Digital twin-driven product design framework. *International Journal of Production Research*, *57*(12), 3935–3953. doi:10.1080/00207543.2018.1443229

Torres-Ruiz, M., Mata, F., Zagal, R., Guzmán, G., Quintero, R., & Moreno-Ibarra, M. (2020). A recommender system to generate museum itineraries applying augmented reality and social-sensor mining techniques. *Virtual Reality*, *24*(1), 175–189. doi:10.100710055-018-0366-z

Tsai, M.-K., Lee, Y.-C., Lu, C.-H., Chen, M.-H., Chou, T.-Y., & Yau, N.-J. (2012). Integrating geographical information and augmented reality techniques for mobile escape guidelines on nuclear accident sites. *Journal of Environmental Radioactivity*, *109*, 36–44. doi:10.1016/j.jenvrad.2011.12.025 PMID:22260929

Vassallo, R., Rankin, A., Chen, E. C., & Peters, T. M. (2017). *Hologram stability evaluation for Microsoft HoloLens. Medical Imaging 2017: Image Perception.* Observer Performance, and Technology Assessment.

Wang, W., Wu, X., Chen, G., & Chen, Z. (2018). Holo3DGIS: Leveraging Microsoft HoloLens in 3D Geographic Information. *ISPRS International Journal of Geo-Information*, *7*(2), 60.

Williams-Bell, F. M., Kapralos, B., Hogue, A., Murphy, B. M., & Weckman, E. J. (2015). Using Serious Games and Virtual Simulation for Training in the Fire Service: A Review. *Fire Technology*, *51*(3), 553–584. doi:10.100710694-014-0398-1

Xu, Z., Lu, X. Z., Guan, H., Chen, C., & Ren, A. Z. (2014). A virtual reality based fire training simulator with smoke hazard assessment capacity. *Advances in Engineering Software*, *68*, 1–8. doi:10.1016/j.advengsoft.2013.10.004

Yari, A., Ardalan, A., Ostadtaghizadeh, A., Zarezadeh, Y., Boubakran, M. S., Bidarpoor, F., & Rahimiforoushani, A. (2019). Underlying factors affecting death due to flood in Iran: A qualitative content analysis. *International Journal of Disaster Risk Reduction*, *40*, 101258. doi:10.1016/j.ijdrr.2019.101258

Yiannakopoulou, E., Nikiteas, N., Perrea, D., & Tsigris, C. (2015). Virtual reality simulators and training in laparoscopic surgery. *International Journal of Surgery*, *13*, 60–64. doi:10.1016/j.ijsu.2014.11.014 PMID:25463761

Zarraonandia, T., Díaz, P., Santos, A., Montero, Á., & Aedo, I. (2019). A Toolkit for Creating Cross-Reality Serious Games. In M. Gentile, M. Allegra, & H. Söbke (Eds.), Games and Learning Alliance. doi:10.1007/978-3-030-11548-7_28

Zhou, F., Duh, H. B.-L., & Billinghurst, M. (2008). Trends in augmented reality tracking, interaction and display: A review of ten years of ISMAR. *Proceedings of the 7th IEEE/ACM international symposium on mixed and augmented reality.*

Zhou, Z., Jiang, S., Yang, Z., & Zhou, L. (2019). Personalized planning and training system for brachytherapy based on virtual reality. *Virtual Reality (Waltham Cross)*, *23*(4), 347–361. doi:10.100710055-018-0350-7

Zhu, R., Lucas, G. M., Becerik-Gerber, B., & Southers, E. G. (2020). Building preparedness in response to active shooter incidents: Results of focus group interviews. *International Journal of Disaster Risk Reduction*, *48*, 101617. doi:10.1016/j.ijdrr.2020.101617

Chapter 10
Demystifying Augmented Reality (AR) in Marketing From the E-Commerce Perspective

Farzad Sabetzadeh
City University of Macau, China

Yusong Wang
City University of Macau, China

EXECUTIVE SUMMARY

Augmented reality (AR) technology has been widely used in various business applications in the past five years. Since the beginning of 2020, with the COVID-19 pandemic and its impact on various industries, AR has become one of the technologies that have significantly reduced physical interactions between buyers and sellers. This chapter reflects its finding in fours areas: 1) eCommerce mobile AR apps can allow customers to better interact with products virtually. 2) AR facilitates customer shopping journey in three stages of purchasing, namely before-purchase, purchase, and after-purchase stages. 3) Design and develop mobile AR apps with two features of virtuality and interactivity to the extent that enables customers to favor AR apps to the offline shopping experience in a sustainable trend. 4) Online retailers can utilize their AR apps to predict target customers' preferences, hence giving them effective promotions to motivate them to buy their preferred products online.

DOI: 10.4018/978-1-7998-8790-4.ch010

INTRODUCTION

Augmented reality (AR), by definition, is a technology that overlays virtual things in the physical world through an AR headset or by utilizing a phone or tablet's camera (Marr, 2018). AR can also be defined as a set of technologies that combines actual circumstances with computer-produced virtual objects (Azuma, 1997; Fan, Chai, Deng, & Dong, 2020; Lamantia, 2009), which improve and augment reality by adding it with real-time interaction (Qin, Peak, & Prybutok, 2021). Investigating the history of the development of AR, it can be divided into three stages: (1) Early dedication to catch people's attention; (2) Adopters try it in-house; (3) and expansion in number of users (Javornik, 2016). In stage 1, the first AR technology was invented in 1968 by Ivan Sutherland, a computer scientist at Harvard University, who created a head-mounted display system based on AR technology. Since then, many institutions have developed AR furthermore to testify its application in different sectors. After 40 years, the commercial application of AR firstly came out in 2008, which was used for advertising by German agencies, and other companies have gradually adopted AR technology in their businesses (Javornik, 2016). In stage 2, AR technology was more developed in advance and was adopted by more commercial industries. It was engaged in various platforms but more focused on mobile apps. Customers gained more value from companies that adopted AR technology in this period (Javornik, 2016), next in stage 3, AR was further engaged in the societal aspect, and its application on tourism was wider.

Potential customers usually would like to try their desired items in the retail market before buying them (Smart Insights, 2020). For instance, in physical stores, cosmetics samples, fitting rooms, automobile test drives, and other similar notions are set up, aiming to allow customers to try their desired goods to enhance the possibility of their purchasing (Smart Insights, 2020). However, in the online retailing market, or eCommerce, customers, cannot touch and experience the goods they would like to buy, personally, because it is wholly transacted online and virtually (KHURANA, 2019). One disadvantage of eCommerce compared to physical selling is that customers cannot try (the samples of) their desired products before making a purchase decision (Ferreira, 2019). Moving into the importance of eCommerce, the sales of the global eCommerce retailing industry increased dramatically from USD 1,336 billion in 2014 to USD 4,280 billion in 2020 (Sabanoglu, 2021). In addition, the sales of eCommerce occupy the global retail sales also enhanced significantly from 7.4% in 2015 to 18% in 2020 (Coppola, 2021). At the end of 2020, it even took nearly 16% (USD 672 billion) of the total retail sales (USD 4,226 trillion) in China (M., 2020). Based on the data, it can be concluded that the role of eCommerce in the retail market was gradually coming into effect, meaning it contributes to the world economy much more and could not be ignored. It is meaningful to think of solutions to mitigate this drawback of eCommerce, thus improving its function of facilitating the global economy.

Based on the above situation identified, the purpose and goal of this research is that by adopting AR technology in the e-Commerce market, online retailers can present and market their goods virtually, making customers try and know more about products before purchase, and ultimately increasing the sales revenues and profits compared to the normal operations that do not use AR technology.

BACKGROUND

Augmented Reality (AR)

AR is a technology that allows people to interact with brands that have been digitally improved the vision (van Esch et al., 2019), causing the pleasure and information being delivered to buyers (Romano, Sands, & Pallant, 2020). AR is becoming an empirical interface for digital marketing technologies that seamlessly mix interactive virtual objects with people's views of the actual (real) surroundings (Chylinski et al., 2020). Through AR, physical surroundings are overlayed with computer-produced elements (Filed, 2020). By using AR, adopters can see and hear the physical worlds they are surrounded by, attached with virtual tridimensional content and accompanying sounds. It is being used to supplement the physical world rather than a substitute (Ozturkcan, 2020). In eCommerce circumstance, it is applied to a website or smartphone as a mobile app which allows consumers to try goods virtually by projecting the object through a phone's camera (Kim & Forsythe, 2008; Pantano & Gandini, 2017).

Adopting AR in Marketing

Applying AR technology in marketing makes retailers and brands show their products, accessories, and customization virtually, allowing buyers to visualize these products before purchasing (Pantano & Servidio, 2012). It is a term called Augmented Reality Marketing (ARM) that concentrates on producing, communicating, and allocating digital affordances (cues) in a real world to support and enhance customer behaviors (decision-making) and experiences (Chylinski et al., 2020; Heller, Chylinski, de Ruyter, Mahr, & Keeling, 2019; Poushneh & Vasquez-Parraga, 2017). As a marketing strategy and practice, AR makes businesses provide carefully created in-store experiences to mobile apps in smartphones by providing a more engaged and interactive experience (Cehovin & Ruban, 2017; Swilley, 2016). When AR is utilized for brand awareness which makes a company's clients and customers learn their products and services in a novel way, that is AR marketing (ANVIL, 2020). ANVIL (ANVIL, 2020) also claims that applying AR is invaluable for a business's brand recognition, and its customer activity can be enhanced a lot.

The Problem of the eCommerce Industry

By Lightspeed (Lightspeed, 2021), one obvious drawback of the eCommerce industry is that customer's in-store engagement is scarce compared to offline retailing. It argues that customers would like to speak out their demands and concerns with a salesperson in a physical store, which is more helpful and efficient than comparing and selecting products by themselves (Lightspeed, 2021). Besides, only pictures and videos regarding the products and their information which are showed online are insufficient. Customers still need to touch (feel the textile), smell (the odor), and even try (whether it fits or not) those products before they purchase them (Lightspeed, 2021). Dasha (M., 2020) also mentioned that not all goods are suitable for sale online because they are hard to select to make sure they suit shoppers well, such as high-heels, formal attire, and other luxuries.

The Problem of Using AR in eCommerce

From statistics, the AR industry is predicted to be USD 135.22 billion in 2022, with an estimated revenue of around USD 120 billion in 2020 and USD 68 billion in 2019, indicating it is a trend to use it as a marketing tool (Filed, 2020). However, the huge benefits it brings make many businesses follow the fashion blindly, thus cannot implementing their campaign effectively because AR deviates customers' attention from useful products information. Customers only focus on those entertainment elements (Hasa, 2020). In addition, organizations do not consider a customer's perspective when using AR, which means a comprehensive customer experience and journey analysis is lacking (Collins, 2020; Halan, 2020). Corporations can improve the value delivered to customers by providing them a satisfied and desired shopping experience through an effective and meaningful interaction, which ultimately derives from purchase actions (Collins, 2020). That is what businesses need to think of clearly. From this point of view, the final purpose of using AR is primarily to increase sales by providing value to customers, which is significant.

How Does AR Help to Enhance the Customer Experience in eCommerce

As this article explained previously, AR is a technology that improves the physical environment through computer-created virtual objects (ANVIL, 2020). It can employ a new layer of the message which is showed on not transparent plastic or glass screen over an existing object, which is gained, demonstrated, and manipulated through a smartphone, PC, or tablet that is leveraged by optical and sensory systems (ANVIL, 2020). Thus, AR can be engaged in software applications (apps) in mobile devices such as phones and tablet platforms, which is called mobile-based AR (Makarov, 2020). To deliver a qualified augmented experience, in mobile-based AR, good function of mobile devices' processing power, camera lenses, and internet availability are simultaneously required, ultimately achieving a type of projection-based AR which regards projecting and overlaying virtual content on real objects or surfaces directly, based on the users' surroundings (Collins, 2020; Makarov, 2020). In addition, mobile AR apps are relatively more accessible for both customers and businesses to obtain and use, as it is engaged in widely adopted smartphones and tablets that allow two entities to view the AR objects through the devices' screen as a hologram (Makarov, 2020). Moreover, thanks to the two standardized AR software development tools (SDKs) of ARKit and ARCore which was developed by Apple and Google respectively, were launched in 2017, mobile AR apps' creation was democratized and the number of AR facilitated mobile devices was nearly doubled, tripling the amount of active mobile AR users in one year and a half (Makarov, 2020). Conclusively speaking, large use of smartphones, cost reduction, mobility enhancement, and capability of AR, which provides empirical value converted AR from laboratory testing into business practices (Rese, Baier, Geyer-Schulz, & Schreiber, 2017). From the above facts, AR has a relatively mature ecosystem, and it is convenient to be adopted in business, creating an opportunity for eCommerce retailers to develop their own mobile AR apps to show their products.

Besides, AR apps enable users to overlay desired images in a 3D virtual space, and consumers can move into the room (ANVIL, 2020). In this way, users can rotate, add, put, remove, and position virtual digital images generated by AR, whatever they want, to achieve compelling interactivity (ANVIL, 2020). One category of AR experiences that mobile AR apps can deliver is named surface-based world effect, meaning there is an AR object created that can move on an ensured surface, for instance, a desk or the tiles (Hasa, 2020). Marek (Hasa, 2020) explained that what the IKEA Place app provides represents the surface-based AR experience because customers can put any IKEA furniture they like anywhere on a surface of the physical world. From this point of view, in eCommerce, online shoppers can interact with projected products effectively by using mobile AR apps. To summarize, by adopting AR technology, eCommerce's disadvantage of lack of physical products interaction can be reduced to some extent. Besides the proof of technology (AR)'s function itself, the previous study also gives us insights regarding the benefits AR could bring to marketing businesses and customers.

In the customer decision-making process, AR technologies facilitate consumers to make decisions because they enhance customer enjoyment and eliminate uncertainty when choosing products (Hoyer, Kroschke, Schmitt, Kraume, & Shankar, 2020). Mobile AR apps give contextual messages and visualization to consumers before the purchasing stage, thus improving their shopping experience in the buying period and enhancing possible after-purchase services (Qin et al., 2021). Because AR can impact involvement, decision-making and improve experiences, its benefits are valuable to retailers and consumers (Huang & Liao, 2015; Huang & Liu, 2014). Customers are supported with specific product information when retailers adopt AR, assisting customers' choice-making (Oh, Yoon, & Shyu, 2008). AR has a vast potential to heighten online service feelings by improving the functional and happiness-oriented values and purchase experiences (Hilken, de Ruyter, Chylinski, Mahr, & Keeling, 2017; Jones, Reynolds, & Arnold, 2006). Therefore, due to the additional value provided by mobile AR apps in online retailing, consumers' desire to purchase will be facilitated dramatically (Poushneh & Vasquez-Parraga, 2017). From an internal operations perspective, one advantage AR brings to retailers is the chance to try virtually, which increases their transformation and rate of return (Dacko, 2017). Applying AR in marketing increases customer satisfaction, and loyalty increases a lot and more repetitive buying behaviors and affirmative evaluation (McLean & Wilson, 2019). Engaging AR in mobile devices makes customers better align their buying decisions to the specific aim of shopping (van Esch et al., 2019). AR technologies enable customers to try on clothes virtually, look and seek various colors and sizes, and possibly post pictures of their desired goods on social media (Beck & Crié, 2018). With an ability to interact with chosen items, customers are more confident to make decisions (Suh & Lee, 2005). AR can enhance the number of choices customers face, but it can also prevent them from selection overload and alternatives confusion to some degree (Garaus, Wagner, & Kummer, 2015). Moreover, website articles have generally explained other advantages of using AR in the retail market to both customers and retailers.

By using AR, both online and offline retailers can (1) improve customer's shopping experience; (2) enhance engagement of the customer; (2) fill the gap between online and offline purchasing; (4) and increase shoppers' buying confidence as much as possible (Makarov, 2021). AR makes online retailers provide customers a more personal, interactive, and involving shopping experience, which changes the way they select and purchase (citrusbits, n.d.). Citrusbits' editor (citrusbits, n.d.) also argues that one tendency in the eCommerce industry is that if people can be involved in AR technology during their shopping experiences, 70% of them will become more loyal to the brand, and 40% of them would like to spend more on the item they desired. Many big corporations like L'Oreal, Nike, and Adidas have already adopted AR to connect more with customers, aiming to obtain a competitive advantage (Zhang, 2019). Specifically, using AR as a strategy enhanced Sephora's brand reputation both physically and digitally, increasing its sales significantly (Zhang, 2019). More and more companies are implementing AR to achieve their marketing goals, thus facilitating brand value and increasing customer involvement (PAINE, 2018; Zhang, 2019). Zhang (Zhang, 2019) claimed that eCommerce businesses could provide customization and personalization services to consumers by leveraging AR technologies, and customers can save their time by using AR to try various items virtually.

To conclude, both literature and website articles have validated the effectiveness and usefulness of using AR in eCommerce, as this technology brings many advantages to both buyers (customers) and sellers (retailers), which further proves that AR could be used as a solution to settle down no interaction weakness in online retail. However, the problem of using AR in eCommerce mentioned above need to be solved or mitigated by exploring how AR improves customer shopping experiences and provides value in detail, from a customer's perspective, rather than talking about its benefits generally and barely, which is helpful to earn profits for businesses. The main part of this article below will focus on this point and specifically put up solutions to that AR application problem.

Research Design and Method

There are two main research questions to answer:

1. How to allow customers to interact with products by using AR in eCommerce?
2. How to facilitate customers' shopping experience efficiently and precisely to enhance sales by using AR in eCommerce?

From the previous analysis, the two purposes of this research are: by using AR in eCommerce to (1) make customers interact with their desired products online; (2) facilitate customers' shopping experiences efficiently and precisely to ultimately enhance sales.

Wholly based on description rather than numbers, qualitative research will be conducted in this study by collecting and using secondary material data from previous research, website articles, papers, and other sorts of things, which is explained as follows:

As for the first research purpose, it can be achieved by illustrating the functionality of AR technology and how it can be engaged in the apps of mobile devices. The explanation relies on before AR studies.

As for the second research purpose, to provide value to customers by enhancing their shopping experiences meaningfully, a specific analysis of how AR influences customer shopping journey in the before-purchase, purchase, and after-purchase stages need to be demonstrated (Romano et al., 2020), which is also based on previous research. In addition, from a customer decision-making perspective, how to design characteristics of mobile AR apps properly to make customers affect and continue to use that AR app, which potentially enhances their willingness to make a purchase decision (Qin et al., 2021) can be explained at the same time. It is also from another literature as secondary data. A predictive function is realized here as eCommerce businesses can use their AR apps to collect users' data, predict their preferences, thus providing them effective promotion incentives to enhance the purchase possibility of the targets (servreality, 2020).

When all the above two research aims are achieved, integrating them together, a Balanced Scorecard Model can be adopted to justify the AR solutions for two eCommerce problems. Because AR as a technology is an intangible asset owned by the company, which could bring constant long-term values compared to tangible assets (Daglar, 2020), with an ineffective deployment of that intangible asset, management may lose opportunities to formulate a powerful strategy to enhance company's competitiveness (SIMONS, 2018). Luckily, a balanced scorecard is developed to permit managers to determine forward-looking indicators that connect intangible assets, measuring whether intended goals are achieved by leveraging intangible assets (SIMONS, 2018). It is based on four perspectives: (1) financial aspect, (2) customer aspect, (3) internal business aspect, (4) learning and growth aspect (Qiu, 2020). Because of the causality among the four dimensions, the financial aspect is positioned at the top (SIMONS, 2018), indicating it is the final goal because making money is the priority for a business.

By adopting AR, how that technology benefits online retailers and customers from those four perspectives will be explored in this research, as the function of the balanced scorecard is to provide a framework to measure and justify the effectiveness of the derived AR solutions.

RESEARCH ANALYSIS

How to Allow Customers to Interact With Products by Using AR in eCommerce?

The literature defines AR as a set of technologies that integrate real circumstances with computer-produced virtual objects (Azuma, 1997; Fan et al., 2020; Lamantia, 2009), which improve and augment reality by adding real-time interaction (Qin et al., 2021). By using AR, adopters can see and hear the physical worlds they are surrounded by, attached with virtual tridimensional content and accompanying sounds. It is being used to supplement the physical world rather than a substitute (Ozturkcan, 2020). Based on the primary function of AR technology, those computer-created virtual objects could be virtual products that are sold online by eCommerce retailers, which are projected and overlayed on the physical worlds that customers are surrounded. Also, those virtually online-sold items can be showed on a smartphone, PC, or tablet's not transparent plastic or glass screen through its camera lenses and sensory systems (ANVIL, 2020). From this point, AR can be engaged in software applications (apps) in mobile devices, which is called mobile-based AR (Makarov, 2020). Moreover, two standardized AR SDKs make mobile AR app development easier for eCommerce retailers and allow customers to learn and adopt mobile-based AR fast and conveniently (Makarov, 2020). Ultimately, customers can rotate, add, put, remove, and position AR-generated virtual products whatever they want, on real surroundings in real-time through mobile devices, achieving compelling interactivity (ANVIL, 2020; Qin et al., 2021).

To conclude, because AR is relatively mature, it can be engaged in mobile devices apps that online retailers develop. Customers can download this AR app to virtually project, visualize, and try products online, satisfying their need of trying it before purchase. In this way, the first research purpose of interactivity is realized.

How to Facilitate Customers' Shopping Experience Efficiently and Precisely to Enhance Sales by Using AR in eCommerce?

To analyze how AR facilitates customers' online shopping experience specifically, based on a previous paper concerning how AR affects customers journey of purchase in the before-purchase, purchase, and after-purchase three stages, Romano et al. (Romano et al., 2020) found that: 1) before the purchase: a) AR makes customers consider and virtually try-on more type of products, particularly in design and styles; b) AR helps customers to tighten their intended selection from consideration set that is formed in the process a); c) AR eliminates customers' brand perception, which is a benefit to novel and developing brands but is a drawback to existing brands. Next, the author (Romano et al., 2020) revealed that: 2) during the purchase: a) AR enables customers to experience how the desired goods would look like when being worn on combinedly, from an aesthetic perspective; b) AR gives customers a sense of playfulness and enjoyment; however, it could be imbalanced between enjoyment value and usefulness value provided by AR; besides, that benefit AR brings might be unsustainable. Finally, 3) after the purchase, the writer (Romano et al., 2020) claimed that: a) AR strengthens customers' confidence regarding the choice they made; b) under the condition of high purchase confidence, AR amplifies the gap between the perceived products and actual one customers get.

The above literature explores the influence of AR in three customer purchase journeys in their shopping experience in detail, putting up how AR facilitates customers' shopping experience, which brings values to customers and retailers as well how AR distracts customers' shopping experience, which has a negative impact to both customers and eCommerce retailers (Romano et al., 2020). It could be used as a reference that provides eCommerce insights regarding how to implement AR strategies well to efficiently enhance customers' shopping experiences and what to do with AR to prevent its reverse effects on value provided. Therefore, the part of facilitating the shopping experience in the second research purpose is achieved. However, the other part of increasing sales by enhancing customers' shopping experience in the second research purpose was not mentioned in the above literature. Other literature potentially solves this problem to some extent.

To analyze how customers specifically make purchase decisions with the help of mobile AR apps from a customer perspective, Qin et al. (Qin et al., 2021) conducted research on how AR apps' features ultimately influence customers' affection and action towards them that AR app. The theoretical foundation of their study is S (stimulus) –O (organism) -R (response) customer decision-making framework, which indicates circumstances' different aspects (stimulus) drives out cognitive and emotional customer states (organism), which finally contributes to an acceptance or a rejection action (response) (Garaus et al., 2015; Mehrabian & Russell, 1974). In the SOR theory, besides the interaction factor (with an external environment), the user's feelings (experiences) are considered. Other than AR technology alone, which provides a layer of virtuality over reality(interaction), how the user perceives and reacts to that interaction (Response) is equally important. Based on AR, the stimulus is the features of AR apps that play a role as stimuli that affects customer experiences internally (Zhao, Wang, & Sun, 2020). Qin's paper (Qin et al., 2021) refers to two AR app features: interactivity and virtuality. Organism in this situation is the response of internal customer judgment when using AR technologies (Mehrabian & Russell, 1974). Qin's paper (Qin et al., 2021) refers to four reactions of hedonic, utilitarian, informativeness, and ease of use. The response is the customers' reactions and actions towards AR apps psychologically (Mehrabian & Russell, 1974). In Qin's paper (Qin et al., 2021), refers to customers' attitudes and behavioral purposes towards AR apps. Engaging stimulus, organism, and response three aspects together, an AR-focused relationship is derived as below:

Conducting research, Qin (Qin et al., 2021) found that: (1) interactivity positively affects hedonic, utilitarian, informativeness, and ease of use; (2) virtuality decides hedonic, utilitarian, and informativeness; (3) attitude is significantly influenced by hedonic, utilitarian, and informativeness; (4) attitude determines behavioral intentions. It is visualized by the figure below:

Figure 1. S-O-R framework based on mobile AR apps
(Qin et al., 2021)

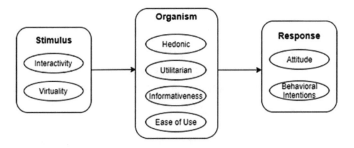

Figure 2. Causality of different factors in the S-O-R framework
(Qin et al., 2021)

Learning and growth perspective	
How AR achieves	**Measures**
Talent people required to develop apps	Human capital
IT system built to facilitate database	Infrastructure capital
Need: • Strong leadership • Customer-oriented corporate culture	Organization capital

The findings of this research ensured that the excellent function on interactivity and virtuality two mobile AR apps features could make customers affect and form a positive attitude towards that AR app they use, ultimately enhancing their frequency to use it, which means people would use it continuously (Qin et al., 2021). However, there is no support for a guaranteed, and transparent relationship between a positive attitude and actual purchase behaviors exists. It could be used as a reference that provides eCommerce retailers with how to design and develop that two AR apps features (virtuality & interactivity) properly to psychologically enhance customers' favor regarding retailers' AR apps, which ultimately increases their frequency of using business' AR apps. Customer data in this way can be collected through business' AR apps to allow eCommerce retailers predict each target customer's preferences, driving out effective promotion incentives, which can potentially facilitate customers' purchasing behaviors and ultimately enhance sales (servreality, 2020). Moreover, from common sense, developing AR apps with well-functional interactivity and virtuality can improve customers' shopping experience. From this perspective, the other part of increasing sales and enhancing customers' shopping experience through interactivity in the second research purpose is simultaneously realized.

Validation of Analysis on How to Facilitate Customers' Shopping Experience Using Balanced Scorecard Approach

The above two AR solutions to the second research question or research problem identified and analyzed are not separate and repellent; on the contrary, they can be used together to achieve a synergy effect. The first study mainly concentrates on how AR can facilitate customers' online shopping journeys (Romano et al., 2020). Whereas the second previous study primarily focuses on how to design characteristics of mobile AR apps to enhance customer experience and increase sales furtherly at the same time (Qin et al., 2021). Applying two AR solutions into a real eCommerce environment, an eCommerce business can develop its own mobile AR app relatively quickly (based on analysis to Q1) to allow customers to interact with virtual products and enable them to try them on before purchase. During this stage of mobile AR app development, the eCommerce business must consider designing the AR technology properly to realize the best virtuality and interactivity functions and features of that mobile AR app. After that, under the condition of a well-functioned mobile AR app, by being adopted by customers, AR facilitates customer purchase journey in three stages, therefore enhancing their shopping experience better and providing more value to them. As customers favor and use that AR app continuously to get an enjoyable shopping experience through interaction, with promotion motivation provided according to prediction, an increasing sale could be obtained. Engaging the application of AR solutions to a real eCommerce situation into Balanced Scorecard (BSC), this article will explain it based on BSC's four perspectives as follows (Figure 3):

1. Customer perspective: this dimension measures whether customers can get satisfaction from products and services provided by the company and a good experience from the company (Qiu, 2020; SIMONS, 2018). In this case, by using AR apps, a) customers can conveniently interact with virtual products, thus obtaining a playful and pleasant sense when purchasing (Qin et al., 2021; Romano et al., 2020). Based on this, customers' good experience with

eCommerce is realized. b) customers can virtually try on more goods and get rich information regarding the product they desire before purchase (Qin et al., 2021; Romano et al., 2020), which improves their online shopping experience. c) during the purchase, customers can easily view how the desired items combinedly look like (Romano et al., 2020), thus enhancing their satisfaction regarding the goods sold online. d) after the purchase, customers' decision-making confidence is higher (Romano et al., 2020), which also increases their shopping experience.

2.   Internal business perspective: this dimension measures whether internal organizational processes such as innovation, operations, customers management (marketing and sales) can bring value and satisfaction to customers, finally helping the business achieve desired financial performance (Qiu, 2020; SIMONS, 2018). In this case, by using AR apps, a) eCommerce retailers can set up a feedback sending function in that AR app, aiming to collect customers' perceptions regarding the products they interact with (Qin et al., 2021), which makes retailers know how to improve existing goods and if it is feasible to innovate new items. b) eCommerce retailers can utilize AR technologies to bring virtual goods and visualize them to online shoppers (market) conveniently (Romano et al., 2020), hence realizing efficient operations. c) online retailers can predict customers' preferences by collecting their data through the app. By doing so, customized promotion incentives are provided to different shoppers, attracting and retaining customers by making them search for their favorite products again, achieving good customer management practices.

3.   Learning and growth perspective: this dimension measures whether corporations can formulate strategies and leverage talent and infrastructure resources to constantly obtain organizational goals (Qiu, 2020; SIMONS, 2018). In this case, to use AR apps, a) eCommerce business needs to recruit talent who can design and develop AR apps with efficient interactivity and virtuality functions and characteristics (Qin et al., 2021), aiming to provide a satisfactory interactive experience to customers. In this way, human capital resources are acquired. b) a reliable information system must be built, which forms a database used to store customers' feedback and digital reserve information regarding those products engaged in AR apps. From this sense, infrastructure capital resources are formulated. c) eCommerce retailers are supposed to create strong leadership to ensure employees can make AR apps function well and can handle customers' feedback (demands, suggestions, and problems) in time. In addition, a customer-oriented corporate culture is suggested be implemented, aiming to provide customers good shopping experiences constantly (SIMONS, 2018). By doing so, organizational capital resources are gained.

4.   Financial perspective: this dimension measures whether businesses can achieve economic gain that benefits stakeholders and investors and enhances company value. In this case, as customers favor and use that AR app continuously to get an enjoyable shopping experience through interaction, with promotion motivation provided according to prediction, an increasing sale could be obtained (servreality, 2020). Besides, the other three BSC dimensions analyzed above can also prove that AR solutions can ultimately help companies achieve financial goals.

Because benefits brought by AR solutions satisfy all the measurements from four BSC perspectives, AR solutions in analysis to Q2 are fully proved based on this approach. It is showed in the diagram below:

Figure 3. AR solutions based balanced scorecard model

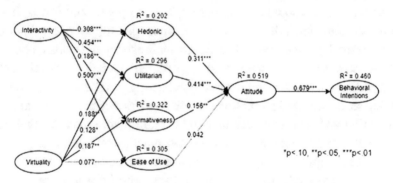

Figure 4. Customer from Figure 3

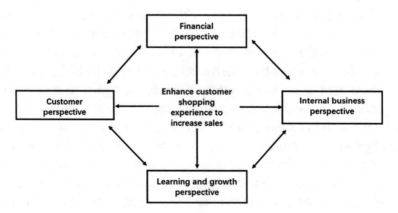

Figure 5. Internal business from Figure 3

Customer perspective	
How AR achieves	Measures
• Interactivity • Playful and pleasant sense • More products available • Rich products information • Confident decision made	Good shopping experience
Virtually view how goods look like combinedly	Products satisfaction

Figure 6. Learning and growth from Figure 3

Internal business perspective	
How AR achieves	Measures
Feedback collection through apps	Innovation
Bring virtual products to customers (market)	Operations
Predict customer preferences to post customized promotion	Customers management

Figure 7. Financial from Figure 3

Financial perspective	
How AR achieves	Measures
• Use AR apps frequently • Satisfactory shopping experience • Promotion (added)	Economic gains
Effects from other BSC perspectives	

DISCUSSION

Discussion on AR Technologies

Another definition of AR put-up by IAB (Internet Advertising Bureau, 2017) is an experience that leverages a camera to alter or improve the physical environment from users' view. That experience can be based on an app or website, whereas being engaged in an app is more typical in contemporary society (Internet Advertising Bureau, 2017). Another comment towards AR: "experiences brought by AR are a novel approach to generate context and increase experiences over the content and attributes that come from real surroundings such as position or recognized picture and item (Internet Advertising Bureau, 2017)." That AR description reflects the function of AR and the previous literature on AR can be engaged in mobile devices such as phones and tablet platforms, which is called mobile-based AR (Makarov, 2020). Moreover, sensors and cameras are pretty developed, built in mobile devices to help AR apps realize their functions (ANVIL, 2020). In this way, people can adopt AR only through built-in cameras in their smartphones. Therefore, AR is highly portable and can be used easily. No high skills are required. In addition, based on the theory of the technological development curve (Schilling, 2020), the Gartner Hype Cycle website (Panetta, 2018) has derived a graph to show the development stage of various emerging technologies in 2018 (Figure 8). It indicates that AR was at the "trough of disillusionment" stage in 2018, indicating it was heading to the mature phase (Panetta, 2018). From this point of view, AR is feasible and mature enough to be applied in other areas.

Figure 8. AR in Gartner Hype Cycle in 2018
(Panetta, 2018)

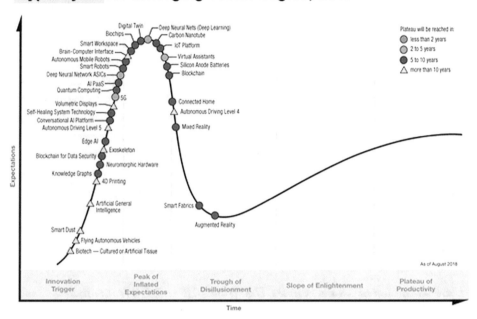

Hype Cycle for Emerging Technologies, 2018

What is more, two AR enablers (ARCore & ARKit) play the role of SDK to allow AR to be adopted widely (Makarov, 2020). In detail, ARKit is an AR developer platform for iOS systems launched by Apple in 2017 (Apple Developer Documentation, 2021). In contrast, ARCore is an AR developer platform for Android systems launched by Google in 2018 (Google: ARCore, 2020). Combined with supported camera and sensor technologies that can be built in mobile devices (ANVIL, 2020), AR's ecosystem is established, providing opportunities for many companies to access and apply this technology in their businesses. From this point of view, AR is suitable to be applied in business domain.

According to data, the number of AR users in America increased rapidly from 37.6 million in 2017 to 68.7 million in 2019, estimated to reach 77.7 million and 85.0 million in 2020 and 2021, respectively (Figure 9) (Petrock, 2019). Moreover, at the beginning of 2019, 95% of iPhones supported AR through ARKit, and ARCore was compatible with more than 50% of devices power by both Android and iOS systems (Interactive Advertising Bureau, 2019; Zibreg, 2019). There were over 500 million devices engaged with AR (Ramella, 2018). Over 200 AR apps are provided through Google Play, and more than 2,000 AR apps are offered by App

Store (Ramella, 2018). These statistics further prove and feasibility and suitability of AR technologies.

However, there are some limitations regarding AR technology itself. One is that developing AR apps is costly and can be taxed technologically, which becomes an entry barrier for many small-to-medium enterprises (SMEs) (servreality, 2020). Another AR limitation is based on the limitation of Big Data. AR requires retrieving and generating digital information from the network to realize its function, causing a potential privacy concern to many customer adopters (servreality, 2020). Furthermore, that limitation also is resulted from AR's function of capturing the personal environment in real life. It is a worry whether businesses will utilize their AR apps to collect customers' private information for immoral purposes (servreality, 2020). Finally, accuracy limitation might be the biggest problem of AR (Sabetzadeh, 2021). Whether AR can overlay virtual objects smartly and accurately to make users sense their distance from the items and the size of the visualized products by comparing them to the real items in users' physical surroundings sometimes is not functional. These limitations could be lessened to some extent as other technologies that support AR become more mature, enhancing AR technologies significantly.

Figure 9. Amount of AR users in the U.S. from 2017 to 2020 (estimated)
(Petrock, 2019)

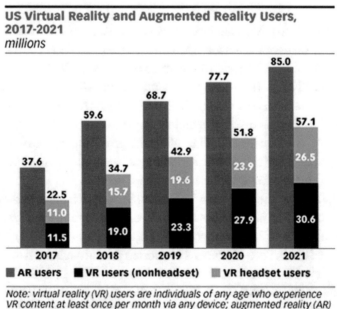

US Virtual Reality and Augmented Reality Users, 2017-2021
millions

Note: virtual reality (VR) users are individuals of any age who experience VR content at least once per month via any device; augmented reality (AR) users are individuals of any age who experience AR content at least once per month via any device
Source: eMarketer, March 2019
245839   www.eMarketer.com

Discussion on eCommerce Problems

From the previous literature review, one obvious drawback of eCommerce is the lack of physical interactivity experience provided to customers, such as smell, feel, and try-on products (Lightspeed, 2021). In addition, if online shoppers have any problems or doubts during the shopping experience, they cannot communicate with and ask a real salesperson directly. That is another weakness of eCommerce (Lightspeed, 2021). From common sense, when customers feel unsure about their intended products, their purchase desire would be significantly damaged because people typically have a risk aversion phycology. When the goods delivered are not suitable to the shoppers or deviate from their expectations, customers will claim a return and refund service, which is very complicated and time-consuming. Therefore, customers would not buy that product, and the retailer's sales revenue is potentially reduced. However, as the sales of eCommerce occupied the total retail market more and more in recent years and sales revenue increased significantly (Coppola, 2021; Sabanoglu, 2021), eCommerce's important position cannot be ignored. It brings huge economic value to society. From this point of view, adopting AR technology to solve or mitigate the negative impacts of eCommerce problems is necessary, which aims to achieve an effective (result-enhanced) influence.

After identifying AR can help customers interact with online retailers' products, many eCommerce businesses blindly adopt that technology without thinking about bringing a good and practical shopping experience to customers through AR (Hasa, 2020). That is the next problem after solving the problem of eCommerce's disadvantage by using AR, and that second eCommerce problem is about the inefficient application of AR. Because many theories regarding the function of AR only validate the aspect of technological push, from a customer perspective, how AR in detail facilitates shopper's online experience scientifically is not considered and researched by eCommerce retailers, making AR implementation not efficient (Collins, 2020; Halan, 2020). That is to say, the aspect of market pull is not fully understood and analyzed by online businesses. Even though customers can interact with virtual products by using AR, if their shopping experience is not satisfactory, they are not impressed by the products they interact with, which cannot enable them to buy the goods. Therefore, online retailers cannot achieve increased sales goals. However, as the last paragraph explained, eCommerce is becoming more critical in recent years, and it is significant to facilitate social economy (Coppola, 2021; Sabanoglu, 2021). To do this, how to provide a satisfactory and efficient customer shopping experience is essential, which aims to achieve an efficient (process-enhanced) influence.

Discussion on Application of AR to eCommerce

Mainly based on the content discussed in 4.1 part, 1) two AR SDKs (ARCore & ARKit) which are launched by two dominant smartphone operation systems providers, 2) advanced sensory systems, cameras, and processing power technologies combinedly form and provide an ecosystem for AR, which allows it to be built in smartphone apps (ANVIL, 2020; Makarov, 2020). It also proves that AR is highly compatible; for instance, at the beginning of 2019, 95% of both ARKit and ARCore based AR was consistent with more than 50% devices power by both Android and iOS systems (Interactive Advertising Bureau, 2019; Zibreg, 2019), which is also mentioned before. Based on this view, AR can be applied in eCommerce based on the following processes: 1) online retailers utilize AR SDK to develop their own mobile AR apps. 2) After customers download the business's AR apps through App Store or Google Play, 3) they can leverage their smartphone's cameras to project virtual products into the real world, thus interacting with them (try it online). 4) If shoppers favor the product they interacted with, they make an order and pay for the item. The function of the smartphone's cameras in the third process is powered by sensory systems, camera lenses, and processing capability, which are built-in mobile devices. That is the whole process of how AR is applied in eCommerce.

In addition, some other external factors also facilitate AR to be applied in eCommerce. According to the Statista website (Statista, 2020), the smartphone adoption rate in Asia Pacific Region was 64% in 2019, which was expected to reach 81% in 2025 (Figure 10), indicating that the coverage rate of smartphones in Asia is very high, which further facilitates the AR adoption rate in Asia. A large number of customers can access eCommerce's AR apps through smartphones. Moreover, the fast network development ensures a stable and high Internet speed which supports and enables AR apps to function well (Eha, 2013). While projecting virtual content into the physical world, AR apps need data from the cloud (Internet) to retrieve and generate those digital objects. Thus the rapid advancement of the telecom industry supports this app requires a lot (O'Farrell, 2019). All these factors help form a more integrated ecosystem for AR, enhancing its possibility to be applied in the eCommerce area.

To summarize, both internal AR's development itself and compatibility and external ecosystem (network) factors can prove that AR can be adopted in the eCommerce business, helping online retailers achieve their ultimate financial goals. However, its application also has limitations. By using AR, customers can only virtually see products and try them on. They cannot further touch the materials and smell the odor of their desired items. For example, by smelling different perfumes' odor, customers can obtain a natural feeling towards the scent and compare and distinguish scents easily. In this way, customers get a good shopping experience,

Figure 10. Smartphone adoption rate in Asia Pacific Region in 2019 and expected data in 2020
(Statista, 2020)

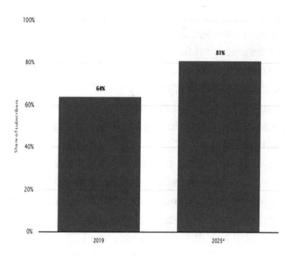

helping them make purchase decisions accurately. However, AR only provides customers visual support without smelling, hindering its function from delivering a satisfactory and helpful shopping experience.

Similarly, customers sometimes need to touch and feel the materials of the clothes to get information regarding whether it was in good quality, helping them make the right purchase decisions. AR lacking this function can also impede its delivery of a satisfactory and helpful shopping experience to customers. From this perspective, online retailers must select proper and suitable goods (only to be sensed by visualization) to sell, to realize AR's function.

Further study regarding how to adopt more advanced technology like mixed reality (MR), which combines AR and virtual reality (VR) smartly in eCommerce to sell a wider range of products, rather than being constrained in goods that can only be compared visualization is suggested to be conducted. Applying MR in eCommerce, customers are provided a more holistic feeling towards products as they can visualize, smell, and even touch them through other more complex technologies. In this way, not only can customers access and interact with more categories of products online, but they can also obtain a more satisfactory and compelling shopping experience, enhancing their willingness to buy the goods. Ultimately, eCommerce businesses earn more money to contribute to the social economy.

CONCLUSION

Based on the research, this article finds that: 1) By integrating AR in the apps of mobile devices, customers can interact with virtual products online, satisfying their need to try them before purchase; 2) By designing and developing the interactivity and virtuality characteristics and functions of AR apps well, combined with AR's facilitating effect on customer shopping journey, customers will favor and adopt AR apps frequently, providing them a satisfactory and efficient shopping experience; 3) By predicting customers' preferences through AR apps, customized promotions are provided to them, motivating them to buy their desired products, which increases eCommerce sales ultimately.

From the application perspective, more than what AR as technology has brought to eCommerce, the way the end-users perceive the technology to use and interact for their day-to-day online shopping experience plays a crucial role in AR's adoption and success rate. Specifically, for some types of products, like those health-related products used for physical health, the users may need more convincing evidence of ease of use and convenience before any purchases are being made. In this respect, AR as technology may facilitate such convincing factors by creating more interactions between the end-user and the health products.

The findings indicated above are the solutions for the two research questions. It aims to bolster the critical position of eCommerce in the social economy by enabling it to sell products efficiently and effectively. In this way, sales generated from eCommerce will occupy the total retail market more, pushing the development of the whole human community.

REFERENCES

ANVIL. (2020). *What is Augmented Reality Marketing?* Retrieved from ANVIL website: https://www.anvilmediainc.com/blog/what-is-augmented-reality-marketing/

Apple Developer Documentation. (2021). *ARKit: Overview*. Retrieved from Apple Inc. website: https://developer.apple.com/documentation/arkit

Azuma, R. T. (1997). A survey of augmented reality. *Presence, 6*(4), 355–385. doi:10.1162/pres.1997.6.4.355

Beck, M., & Crié, D. (2018). I virtually try it … I want it! Virtual Fitting Room: A tool to increase online and offline exploratory behavior, patronage and purchase intentions. *Journal of Retailing and Consumer Services, 40*, 279–286. Advance online publication. doi:10.1016/j.jretconser.2016.08.006

Cehovin, F., & Ruban, B. (2017). *The Impact of Augmented Reality Applications on Consumer Search and Evaluation Behavior.* Master Thesis.

Chylinski, M., Heller, J., Hilken, T., Keeling, D. I., Mahr, D., & de Ruyter, K. (2020). Augmented reality marketing: A technology-enabled approach to situated customer experience. *Australasian Marketing Journal, 28*(4), 374–384. doi:10.1016/j.ausmj.2020.04.004

citrusbits. (n.d.). *How Augmented Reality is being Used in Ecommerce.* Retrieved from citrusbits website: https://www.citrusbits.com/how-augmented-reality-is-being-used-in-ecommerce/

Collins, A. (2020). *The Ultimate Guide to Augmented Reality.* Retrieved from HubSpot website: https://blog.hubspot.com/marketing/augmented-reality-ar

Coppola, D. (2021). *E-commerce share of total global retail sales from 2015 to 2024.* Retrieved from statista website: https://www.statista.com/statistics/534123/e-commerce-share-of-retail-sales-worldwide/

Dacko, S. G. (2017). Enabling smart retail settings via mobile augmented reality shopping apps. *Technological Forecasting and Social Change*, 124. doi:10.1016/j.techfore.2016.09.032

Daglar, C. (2020). *Intangible Assets vs Tangible Assets: Which To Invest In?* Retrieved from daglar-cizmeci website: https://daglar-cizmeci.com/intangible-assets-vs-tangible-assets/

Eha, P. B. (2013). *An Accelerated History of Internet Speed* (Infographic). Retrieved from Entrepreneur: Technology website: https://www.entrepreneur.com/article/228489

Fan, X., Chai, Z., Deng, N., & Dong, X. (2020). Adoption of augmented reality in online retailing and consumers' product attitude: A cognitive perspective. *Journal of Retailing and Consumer Services, 53*(February), 101986. doi:10.1016/j.jretconser.2019.101986

Ferreira, N. M. (2019). *20 Ecommerce Advantages And Disadvantages You Need To Know.* Retrieved from OBERLO website: https://www.oberlo.com/blog/20-ecommerce-advantages-and-disadvantages

Filed. (2020). *An Introduction to AR in Marketing.* Retrieved from Filed website: https://www.filed.com/resources/blog/an-introduction-to-ar-in-marketing/

Garaus, M., Wagner, U., & Kummer, C. (2015). Cognitive fit, retail shopper confusion, and shopping value: Empirical investigation. *Journal of Business Research*, *68*(5). https://doi.org/10.1016/j.jbusres.2014.10.002

Google ARCore. (2020). *Developers ARCore Overview*. Retrieved from Google website: https://developers.google.com/ar/discover/

Halan, D. (2020). *How AR And VR Can Be Applied To Marketing*. Retrieved from electronicsforu website: https://www.electronicsforu.com/technology-trends/must-read/ar-vr-applied-marketing

Hasa, M. (2020). *How to Use AR In Campaigns: The Ultimate Guide to Augmented Reality Marketing*. Retrieved from pixelfield website: https://pixelfield.co.uk/blog/how-to-use-ar-in-campaigns-the-ultimate-guide-to-augmented-reality-marketing/

Heller, J., Chylinski, M., de Ruyter, K., Mahr, D., & Keeling, D. I. (2019). Let Me Imagine That for You: Transforming the Retail Frontline Through Augmenting Customer Mental Imagery Ability. *Journal of Retailing*, *95*(2). https://doi.org/10.1016/j.jretai.2019.03.005

Hilken, T., de Ruyter, K., Chylinski, M., Mahr, D., & Keeling, D. I. (2017). Augmenting the eye of the beholder: Exploring the strategic potential of augmented reality to enhance online service experiences. *Journal of the Academy of Marketing Science*, *45*(6), 884–905. https://doi.org/10.1007/s11747-017-0541-x

Hoyer, W. D., Kroschke, M., Schmitt, B., Kraume, K., & Shankar, V. (2020). Transforming the Customer Experience Through New Technologies. *Journal of Interactive Marketing, 51*. doi:10.1016/j.intmar.2020.04.001

Huang, T. L., & Liao, S. (2015). A model of acceptance of augmented-reality interactive technology: The moderating role of cognitive innovativeness. *Electronic Commerce Research*, *15*(2). https://doi.org/10.1007/s10660-014-9163-2

Huang, T. L., & Liu, F. H. (2014). Formation of augmented-reality interactive technology's persuasive effects from the perspective of experiential value. *Internet Research*, *24*(1). https://doi.org/10.1108/IntR-07-2012-0133

Interactive Advertising Bureau. (2019). *Augmented Reality for Marketing: An IAB Playbook*. Retrieved from https://books.google.co.uk/books/about/Augmented_Reality_for_Developers.html?id=8xhKDwAAQBAJ&printsec=frontcover&source=kp_read_button&redir_esc=y#v=onepage&q&f=false%0Ahttps://mediatum.ub.tum.de/1286695

Internet Advertising Bureau. (2017). *IAB New Standard Ad Unit Portofolio*. Retrieved from www.iab.com/newadportfolio

Javornik, A. (2016). *The Mainstreaming of Augmented Reality: A Brief History*. Retrieved from Harvard Business Review website: https://hbr.org/2016/10/the-mainstreaming-of-augmented-reality-a-brief-history#

Jones, M. A., Reynolds, K. E., & Arnold, M. J. (2006). Hedonic and utilitarian shopping value: Investigating differential effects on retail outcomes. *Journal of Business Research*, *59*(9). https://doi.org/10.1016/j.jbusres.2006.03.006

Khurana, A. (2019). *Disadvantages of E-commerce*. Retrieved from the balancesmall business website: https://www.thebalancesmb.com/disadvantages-of-e-commerce-1141571

Kim, J., & Forsythe, S. (2008). Adoption of virtual try-on technology for online apparel shopping. *Journal of Interactive Marketing*, *22*(2). https://doi.org/10.1002/dir.20113

Lamantia, J. (2009). *Inside Out: Interaction Design for Augmented Reality*. Retrieved from UXmatters website: https://www.uxmatters.com/mt/archives/2009/08/inside-out-interaction-design-for-augmented-reality.php

Lightspeed. (2021). *Exploring the Advantages and Disadvantages of Ecommerce*. Retrieved from Lightspeed website: https://www.lightspeedhq.com/blog/advantages-and-disadvantages-of-ecommerce/

M., D. (2020). *What are Ecommerce Advantages and Disadvantages?* Retrieved from BELVG website: https://belvg.com/blog/what-is-advantage-and-disadvantage-of-e-commerce.html

Makarov, A. (2020). *Augmented reality development: Guide for business owners and managers*. Retrieved from mobidev website: https://mobidev.biz/blog/augmented-reality-development-guide

Makarov, A. (2021). *6 ideas to leverage augmented reality for marketing & sales*. Retrieved from mobidev website: https://mobidev.biz/blog/augmented-reality-marketing-sales

Marr, B. (2018). *Facebook And Apple Are Serious About Augmented Reality*. Retrieved from Forbes website: https://www.forbes.com/sites/bernardmarr/2018/08/08/facebook-and-apple-are-serious-about-augmented-reality/?sh=5ef31ee6b4bc

McLean, G., & Wilson, A. (2019). *Customer Engagement with Augmented Reality Mobile Apps*. Paper presented at the 2019 Academy of Marketing Science Annual Conference. doi:10.1007/978-3-030-39165-2_89

Mehrabian, A., & Russell, J. A. (1974). *An Approach to Environmental Psychology*. MIT Press.

O'Farrell, J. (2019). *Augmented Reality and the Network*. Retrieved from spearline website: https://www.spearline.com/blog/post/augmented-reality-and-the-network/

Oh, H., Yoon, S. Y., & Shyu, C. R. (2008). How can Virtual Reality reshape furniture retailing? *Clothing & Textiles Research Journal, 26*(2). https://doi.org/10.1177/0887302X08314789

Ozturkcan, S. (2020). Service innovation: Using augmented reality in the IKEA Place app. *Journal of Information Technology Teaching Cases*. doi:10.1177/2043886920947110

Paine, J. (2018). *10 Brands Already Leveraging the Power of Augmented Reality: AR is changing the marketing game*. Retrieved from Inc. This Morning website: https://www.inc.com/james-paine/10-brands-already-leveraging-power-of-augmented-reality.html

Panetta, K. (2018). *5 Trends Emerge in the Gartner Hype Cycle for Emerging Technologies, 2018*. Retrieved from Smarter With Gartner website: https://www.gartner.com/smarterwithgartner/5-trends-emerge-in-gartner-hype-cycle-for-emerging-technologies-2018/

Pantano, E., & Gandini, A. (2017). Exploring the forms of sociality mediated by innovative technologies in retail settings. *Computers in Human Behavior, 77*. doi:10.1016/j.chb.2017.02.036

Pantano, E., & Servidio, R. (2012). Modeling innovative points of sales through virtual and immersive technologies. *Journal of Retailing and Consumer Services, 19*(3), 279–286. https://doi.org/10.1016/j.jretconser.2012.02.002

Petrock, V. (2019). *Virtual and Augmented Reality Users 2019*. Retrieved from eMarketer website: https://www.emarketer.com/content/virtual-and-augmented-reality-users-2019

Poushneh, A., & Vasquez-Parraga, A. Z. (2017). Discernible impact of augmented reality on retail customer's experience, satisfaction and willingness to buy. *Journal of Retailing and Consumer Services, 34*. doi:10.1016/j.jretconser.2016.10.005

Qin, H., Peak, D. A., & Prybutok, V. (2021). A virtual market in your pocket: How does mobile augmented reality (MAR) influence consumer decision making? *Journal of Retailing and Consumer Services, 58*(November), 102337. doi:10.1016/j. jretconser.2020.102337

Qiu, X. (2020). *Application of Balanced Scorecard in E-Commerce Enterprise Performance Management–Taking Alibaba Group as an Example.* doi:10.2991/ aebmr.k.200402.006

Ramella, B. (2018). *The Biggest AR/VR Trends in 2019.* Retrieved from G2 website: https://www.g2.com/articles/2019-ar-vr-trends

Rese, A., Baier, D., Geyer-Schulz, A., & Schreiber, S. (2017). How augmented reality apps are accepted by consumers: A comparative analysis using scales and opinions. *Technological Forecasting and Social Change, 124.* doi:10.1016/j. techfore.2016.10.010

Romano, B., Sands, S., & Pallant, J. I. (2020). Augmented reality and the customer journey: An exploratory study. *Australasian Marketing Journal.* doi:10.1016/j. ausmj.2020.06.010

Sabanoglu, T. (2021). *Retail e-commerce sales worldwide from 2014 to 2024.* Retrieved from statista website: https://www.statista.com/statistics/379046/worldwide-retail-e-commerce-sales/

Sabetzadeh, F. (2021). *3D Printing, Autonomous Vehicles, Augmented and Virtual Reality.* City University of Macau.

Schilling, M. A. (2020). Strategic Management of Technological Innovation (6th ed.). McGraw-Hill Education.

servreality. (2020). *Pros and cons of augmented reality apps development.* Retrieved from servreality website: https://servreality.com/blog/pros-and-cons-of-augmented-reality-apps-development/

Simons, R. (2018). Strategy Execution Module 9: Building a Balanced Scorecard. Harvard Business School.

Smart Insights. (2020). *5 ways to use Augmented Reality in your marketing strategy.* Retrieved from Smart Insights website: https://www.smartinsights.com/digital-marketing-platforms/augmented-reality/5-ways-to-use-augmented-reality-in-your-marketing-strategy/

Statista. (2020). *Adoption rate of smartphones in the Asia Pacific region in 2019 with a forecast for 2025*. Retrieved from Statista Research Department website: https://www.statista.com/statistics/1128693/apac-smartphone-adoption-rate/

Suh, K. S., & Lee, Y. E. (2005). The effects of virtual reality on consumer learning: An empirical investigation. MIS Quarterly: Management. *Information Systems, 29*(4). https://doi.org/10.2307/25148705

Swilley, E. (2016). *Moving Virtual Retail into Reality: Examining Metaverse and Augmented Reality in the Online Shopping Experience*. doi:10.1007/978-3-319-24184-5_163

van Esch, P., Arli, D., Gheshlaghi, M. H., Andonopoulos, V., von der Heidt, T., & Northey, G. (2019). Anthropomorphism and augmented reality in the retail environment. *Journal of Retailing and Consumer Services, 49*, 35–42. https://doi.org/10.1016/j.jretconser.2019.03.002

Zhang, Y. (2019). *How is Augmented Reality marketing related to your business?* Retrieved from hapticmedia website: https://hapticmedia.com/blog/augmented-reality-marketing/

Zhao, Y., Wang, A., & Sun, Y. (2020). Technological environment, virtual experience, and MOOC continuance: A stimulus–organism–response perspective. *Computers and Education, 144*. doi:10.1016/j.compedu.2019.103721

Zibreg, C. (2019). *The iOS 12 software is now powering 75 percent of all devices*. Retrieved from idownloadblog website: https://www.idownloadblog.com/2019/01/02/ios-12-adoption-rate-75-percent/

Compilation of References

Abidine, B. M. h., Fergani, B., Oussalah, M., & Fergani, L. J. K. (2014). *A new classification strategy for human activity recognition using cost sensitive support vector machines for imbalanced data.* Academic Press.

Adriaans & Zantinge. (1999). *Data Mining.* Addison Wesley Longman.

Ahir, K., Govani, K., Gajera, R., & Shah, M. (2020). Application on virtual reality for enhanced education learning, military training and sports. *Augmented Human Research*, 5(1), 1–9. doi:10.100741133-019-0025-2

Ahmad, N., Ali, Q., Crowley, H., & Pinho, R. (2014). Earthquake loss estimation of residential buildings in Pakistan. *Natural Hazards*, 73(3), 1889–1955. doi:10.100711069-014-1174-8

Alexander, G. (2003). Patient-physician communication about out-of-pocket costs. *Journal of the American Medical Association*, 290(7), 953–958. doi:10.1001/jama.290.7.953 PMID:12928475

Alhalabi, W., & Lytras, M. D. (2019). Editorial for special issue on Virtual Reality and Augmented Reality. *Virtual Reality (Waltham Cross)*, 23(3), 215–216. doi:10.100710055-019-00398-6

Allard, P., Stokes, I. A. F., & Blanchi, J. P. (1995). *Three-dimensional analysis of human movement.* Human Kinetics.

Al-Qaness, M. A., Abd Elaziz, M., Kim, S., Ewees, A. A., Abbasi, A. A., Alhaj, Y. A., & Hawbani, A. J. S. (2019). Channel state information from pure communication to sense and track human motion. *Survey (London, England)*, 19(15), 3329. doi:10.339019153329 PMID:31362425

Alwidyan, M. T., Trainor, J. E., & Bissell, R. A. (2020). Responding to natural disasters vs. disease outbreaks: Do emergency medical service providers have different views? *International Journal of Disaster Risk Reduction, 44*, 101440. doi:10.1016/j.ijdrr.2019.101440 PMID:32363141

Anahory, S., & Hurray, D. (2011). *Data Ware Housing in the Real World.* New Delhi: Pearson.

Antoniou, P. E., Chondrokostas, E., Bratsas, C., Filippidis, P. M., & Bamidis, P. D. (2021). A Medical Ontology Informed User Experience Taxonomy to Support Co-creative Workflows for Authoring Mixed Reality Medical Education Spaces. *7th International Conference of the Immersive Learning Research Network*, 1-9.

ANVIL. (2020). *What is Augmented Reality Marketing?* Retrieved from ANVIL website: https://www.anvilmediainc.com/blog/what-is-augmented-reality-marketing/

Apple Developer Documentation. (2021). *ARKit: Overview*. Retrieved from Apple Inc. website: https://developer.apple.com/documentation/arkit

Arnaldi, B., Guitton, P., & Moreau, G. (2018). *Virtual reality and augmented reality: myths and realities*. Wiley. doi:10.1002/9781119341031

Arriany, A. A., & Musbah, M. S. (2016). *Applying voice recognition technology for smart home networks*. Paper presented at the 2016 International Conference on Engineering & MIS (ICEMIS). 10.1109/ICEMIS.2016.7745292

Arun, K. P. (2003). Data Mining Techniques. Universities Press (India) Private Limited.

Asgary, A. (2017). Holodisaster: Leveraging Microsoft HoloLens in Disaster and Emergency Management. *IAEM Bulletin*, 20-21.

Asgary, A., Bonadonna, C., & Frischknecht, C. (2019). Simulation and Visualization of Volcanic Phenomena Using Microsoft Hololens: Case of Vulcano Island (Italy). *IEEE Transactions on Engineering Management*, 1–9. doi:10.1109/TEM.2019.2932291

Attwood, T. K., & Parry-Smith, D. J. (2005). *Introduction to Bioinformatics; New Delhi: Pearson Education*. Private Limited.

Aytar, Y., Vondrick, C., & Torralba, A. (2017). *See, hear, and read: Deep aligned representations*. Academic Press.

Aziz, H. A. (2018). Virtual reality programs applications in healthcare. *Journal of Health & Medical Informatics*, 9(1), 305. doi:10.4172/2157-7420.1000305

Azuma, R. T. (1997). A Survey of Augmented Reality. *Presence*, 6(4), 355–385. doi:10.1162/pres.1997.6.4.355

Bakar, U., Ghayvat, H., Hasanm, S., & Mukhopadhyay, S. C. J. N. G. S. (2016). Activity and anomaly detection in smart home. *Survey (London, England)*, 16, 191–220. doi:10.1007/978-3-319-21671-3_9

Balint, E. (1969). The possibilities of patient-centered medicine. *The Journal of the Royal College of General Practitioners*, (17), 269–276. PMID:5770926

Banakou, D., Groten, R., & Slater, M. (2013). Illusory ownership of a virtual child body causes overestimation of object sizes and implicit attitude changes. *Proceedings of the National Academy of Sciences of the United States of America*, 110(31), 110. doi:10.1073/pnas.1306779110 PMID:23858436

Banakou, D., Pd, H., & Slater, M. (2016). Virtual embodiment of white people in a black virtual body leads to a sustained reduction in their implicit racial bias. *Frontiers in Human Neuroscience*, 10, 601. doi:10.3389/fnhum.2016.00601 PMID:27965555

Bandopadhyay. (2013). A Technology Lead Business Model for Pharma – Collaborative Patient Care. *CSI Communications Journal, 37*(9), 12-13, 26.

Bao, J., Guo, D., Li, J., & Zhang, J. (2019). The modelling and operations for the digital twin in the context of manufacturing. *Enterprise Information Systems, 13*(4), 534–556. doi:10.1080/17517575.2018.1526324

Barcsay, J. (1973). *Anatomy for the artist.* Octopus Books.

Baron, R. J., & Berinsky, A. J. (2019). Mistrust in science— A threat to the patient–physician relationship. *The New England Journal of Medicine, 381*(2), 182–185. doi:10.1056/NEJMms1813043 PMID:31291524

Baukal, C. E., Ausburn, F. B., & Ausburn, L. J. (2013). A Proposed Multimedia Cone of Abstraction: Updating a Classic Instructional Design Theory. *Journal of Educational Technology, 9*(4), 15–24.

BBC. (2014, March 26). *Facebook buys virtual reality headset start-up for $2 billion.* https://www.bbc.com/news/business-26742625

BBC. (2016, April 14). *Cancer surgery broadcast live in virtual reality.* https://www.bbc.com/news/av/technology-36046948

Beck, A. (2004). The Flexner report and the standardization of American medical education. *Journal of the American Medical Association, 291*(17), 2139–2140. doi:10.1001/jama.291.17.2139 PMID:15126445

Beck, M., & Crié, D. (2018). I virtually try it … I want it! Virtual Fitting Room: A tool to increase online and offline exploratory behavior, patronage and purchase intentions. *Journal of Retailing and Consumer Services, 40*, 279–286. Advance online publication. doi:10.1016/j.jretconser.2016.08.006

Benferdia, Y., Ahmad, M. N., Mustapha, M., Baharin, H., & Bajuri, M. Y. (2018). Critical success factors for virtual reality-based training in ophthalmology domain. *Journal of Health & Medical Informatics, 9*(3), 1–14. doi:10.4172/2157-7420.1000318

Berger, J., & Lo, N. (2015). An innovative multi-agent search-and-rescue path planning approach. *Computers & Operations Research, 53*, 24–31. doi:10.1016/j.cor.2014.06.016

Bernhardt, J., Hayward, K., Kwakkel, G., Ward, N., Wolf, S., Borschmann, K., Krakauer, J. W., Boyd, L. A., Carmichael, S. T., Corbett, D., & Cramer, S. (2017). Agreed definitions and a shared vision for new standards in stroke recovery research: The Stroke Recovery and Rehabilitation Roundtable taskforce. *International Journal of Stroke, 12*(5), 444–450. doi:10.1177/1747493017711816 PMID:28697708

Beroggi, G. E. G., Waisel, L., & Wallace, W. A. (1995). Employing virtual reality to support decision making in emergency management. *Safety Science, 20*(1), 79–88. doi:10.1016/0925-7535(94)00068-E

Bhagat, K. K., Liou, W.-K., & Chang, C.-Y. (2016). A cost-effective interactive 3D virtual reality system applied to military live firing training. *Virtual Reality (Waltham Cross), 20*(2), 127–140. doi:10.100710055-016-0284-x

Blemker, S. S., & Delp, S. L. (2005). Three-dimensional representation of complex muscle architectures and geometries. *Annals of Biomedical Engineering, 33*(5), 661–673. doi:10.100710439-005-1433-7 PMID:15981866

Boorsma, M., Frijters, D. H. K., Knol, D. L., Ribbe, M. E., Nijpels, G., & van Hout, H. P. J. (2011). Effects of multidisciplinary integrated care on quality of care in residential care facilities for elderly people: A cluster randomized trial. *Canadian Medical Association Journal, 183*(11), E724–E732. doi:10.1503/cmaj.101498 PMID:21708967

Boslaugh, S. E. (2013). *Healthcare Systems around the world A Comparative Guide.* Sage Publishing. doi:10.4135/9781452276212

Bourquin, C., Stiefel, F., Mast, M., Bonvin, R., & Berney, A. (2015). Well, you have hepatic metastases: Use of technical language by medical students in simulated patient interviews. *Patient Education and Counseling, 98*(3), 323–330. doi:10.1016/j.pec.2014.11.017 PMID:25535013

Bro-Nielsen, M., & Cotin, S. (1996). Real-time volumetric deformable models for surgery simulation using finite elements and condensation. *Computer Graphics Forum, 15*(3), 57–66. doi:10.1111/1467-8659.1530057

Brooks, F. P. (1999). What's real about virtual reality? *IEEE Computer Graphics and Applications, 19*(6), 16–27. doi:10.1109/38.799723

Buchem, I., Vorwerg, S., Stamm, O., Hildebrand, K., & Bialek, Y. (2021). Gamification in Mixed-Reality Exergames for Older Adult Patients in a Mobile Immersive Diagnostic Center: A Pilot Study in the BewARe Project. *7th International Conference of the Immersive Learning Research Network (iLRN)*, 1-9.

Bujalski, P., Martins, J., & Stirling, L. (2018). A Monte Carlo analysis of muscle force estimation sensitivity to muscle-tendon properties using a Hill-based muscle model. *Journal of Biomechanics, 79*, 67–77. doi:10.1016/j.jbiomech.2018.07.045 PMID:30146173

Burdea, G., & Langrana, N. (1992). Virtual force feedback: Lessons, challenges, future applications. *Winter Annual Meeting of the American Society of Mechanical Engineers.*

Buyya, Vecchiola, & Selvi. (2013). *Mastering Cloud Computing.* McGraw Hill Education (India) Private Limited.

Byrne, P., & Long, B. (1976). *Doctors talking to patients.* HMSO.

Caba Heilbron, F., Escorcia, V., Ghanem, B., & Carlos Niebles, J. (2015). Activitynet: A large-scale video benchmark for human activity understanding. *Proceedings of the ieee conference on computer vision and pattern recognition.* 10.1109/CVPR.2015.7298698

Carter, N., Bryant-Lukosius, D., DiCenso, A., Blythe, J., & Neville, A. J. (2014). The use of triangulation in qualitative research. *Oncology Nursing Forum, 41*(5), 545–547. doi:10.1188/14. ONF.545-547 PMID:25158659

Cavalcante, W. Q. F., Coelho, A., & Bairrada, C. M. (2021). Sustainability and Tourism Marketing: A Bibliometric Analysis of Publications between 1997 and 2020 Using VOSviewer Software. *Sustainability, 13*(9), 4987. doi:10.3390u13094987

Cehovin, F., & Ruban, B. (2017). *The Impact of Augmented Reality Applications on Consumer Search and Evaluation Behavior.* Master Thesis.

Celinder, D., & Peoples, H. (2012). Stroke patients' experiences with Wii Sports® during inpatient rehabilitation. *Scandinavian Journal of Occupational Therapy, 19*(5), 457–463. doi:10.3109/11 038128.2012.655307 PMID:22339207

Centre for Health Protection, Department of Health, HKSAR. (2021). Available at https://www. chp.gov.hk/en/statistics/data/10/27/380.html

Chaka, C. (2013). *Virtualization and Cloud Computing Business Models in the Virtual Cloud.* IGI Global.

Chan, K. H., Chan, H. H., Wong, C. W., & Lau, Y. Y. (2019). Strengthening STEM and Arduino to foster integrated cares in Hong Kong. *CPCE Health Conference 2019.*

Charles, C., Gafni, A., & Whelan, T. (1997). Shared decision-making in the medical encounter: What does it mean? (or it takes at least two to tango). *Social Science & Medicine, 44*(5), 681–692. doi:10.1016/S0277-9536(96)00221-3 PMID:9032835

Charles, J. P., Grant, B., D'Août, K., & Bates, K. T. (2021). Foot anatomy, walking energetics, and the evolution of human bipedalism. *Journal of Human Evolution, 156*, 103014. doi:10.1016/j. jhevol.2021.103014 PMID:34023575

Charon, R. (2001). Narrative medicine. *Journal of the American Medical Association, 286*(15), 1897–1902. doi:10.1001/jama.286.15.1897 PMID:11597295

Che Mat, R., Shariff, A. R. M., Nasir Zulkifli, A., Shafry Mohd Rahim, M., & Hafiz Mahayudin, M. (2014). Using game engine for 3D terrain visualisation of GIS data: A review. *IOP Conference Series. Earth and Environmental Science, 20*, 1. doi:10.1088/1755-1315/20/1/012037

Chen, H., Zou, Q., & Wang, Q. (2021). Clinical manifestations of ultrasonic virtual reality in the diagnosis and treatment of cardiovascular diseases. *Journal of Healthcare Engineering*, ●●●, 2021. PMID:34257848

Cheung, K. S. L., & Yip, P. S. F. (2010). Trends in healthy life expectancy in Hong Kong SAR 1996-2008. *European Journal of Ageing, 7*(4), 257–269. doi:10.100710433-010-0171-3 PMID:21212818

Chhetri, M. B., Krishnaswamy, S., & Loke, S. W. (2004). Smart Virtual Counterparts for Learning Communities. In C. Bussler, S.-k. Hong, W. Jun, R. Kaschek, Kinshuk, S. Krishnaswamy, S. W. Loke, D. Oberle, D. Richards, A. Sharma, Y. Sure, & B. Thalheim (Eds.), Web Information Systems – WISE 2004 Workshops. Berlin: Academic Press.

Choi, Y. K., Hui, K. C., & Tang, Y. M. (2007). Fitting a Polygon Mesh Through a Set of Curves. *Lecture Notes in Computer Science*, 4469.

Chorafas & Steinmann. (1995). *Virtual Reality Practical Applications in Business and Industry.* Prentice Hall.

Cho, S., Ku, J., Cho, Y. K., Kim, I. Y., Kang, Y. J., Jang, D. P., & Kim, S. I. (2014). Development of virtual reality proprioceptive rehabilitation system for stroke patients. *Computer Methods and Programs in Biomedicine*, *113*(1), 258–265. doi:10.1016/j.cmpb.2013.09.006 PMID:24183070

Christensen, C. M., Grossman, J. H., & Hwang, J. (2008). *The Innovator's Prescription: A Disruptive Solution for Healthcare.* McGraw Hill.

Chylinski, M., Heller, J., Hilken, T., Keeling, D. I., Mahr, D., & de Ruyter, K. (2020). Augmented reality marketing: A technology-enabled approach to situated customer experience. *Australasian Marketing Journal*, *28*(4), 374–384. doi:10.1016/j.ausmj.2020.04.004

Cieślik, B., Mazurek, J., Rutkowski, S., Kiper, P., Turolla, A., & Szczepańska-Gieracha, J. (2020). Virtual reality in psychiatric disorders: A systematic review of reviews. *Complementary Therapies in Medicine*, *52*, 102480. doi:10.1016/j.ctim.2020.102480 PMID:32951730

citrusbits. (n.d.). *How Augmented Reality is being Used in Ecommerce.* Retrieved from citrusbits website: https://www.citrusbits.com/how-augmented-reality-is-being-used-in-ecommerce/

Claverie & Notredame. (2011). *Bioinformatics for Dummies.* John Wiley & Sons.

Collins, A. (2020). *The Ultimate Guide to Augmented Reality.* Retrieved from HubSpot website: https://blog.hubspot.com/marketing/augmented-reality-ar

Cook, D. J., & Schmitter-Edgecombe, M. (2009). *Assessing the quality of activities in a smart environment.* Academic Press.

Coombs, W. T., & Laufer, D. (2018). Global Crisis Management – Current Research and Future Directions. *Journal of International Management*, *24*(3), 199–203. doi:10.1016/j.intman.2017.12.003

Cooper, R. A., Fitzgerald, S. G., Boninger, M. L., Brienza, D. M., Shapcott, N., Cooper, R., & Flood, K. (2001). Telerehabilitation: Expanding access to rehabilitation expertise. *Proceedings of the IEEE*, *89*(8), 1174–1193. doi:10.1109/5.940286

Coppola, D. (2021). *E-commerce share of total global retail sales from 2015 to 2024.* Retrieved from statista website: https://www.statista.com/statistics/534123/e-commerce-share-of-retail-sales-worldwide/

Cotin, S., Delingette, H., & Ayache, N. (1999). Real-time elastic deformations of soft tissues for surgery simulation. *IEEE Transactions on Visualization and Computer Graphics*, *5*(1), 62–73. doi:10.1109/2945.764872

Cotin, S., Delingette, H., Bro-Nielsen, M., Ayache, N., Clement, J., Tassetti, V., & Marescaux, J. (1996). Geometric and physical representations for a simulator of hepatic surgery. *Studies in Health Technology and Informatics*, *1*(29), 139–151. PMID:10163746

Creek, J., & Bullock, A. (2008). Assessment and outcome measurement. *Occupational Therapy in Mental Health*, 83–114.

Crichton, M. T., & Flin, R. (2004). Identifying and training non-technical skills of nuclear emergency response teams. *Annals of Nuclear Energy*, *31*(12), 1317–1330. doi:10.1016/j.anucene.2004.03.011

Cronin, P., Ryan, F., & Coughlan, M. (2008). Undertaking a literature review: A step-by-step approach. *British Journal of Nursing (Mark Allen Publishing)*, *17*(1), 38–43. doi:10.12968/bjon.2008.17.1.28059 PMID:18399395

Cruz, E., Orts-Escolano, S., Gomez-Donoso, F., Rizo, C., Rangel, J. C., Mora, H., & Cazorla, M. (2019). An augmented reality application for improving shopping experience in large retail stores. *Virtual Reality (Waltham Cross)*, *23*(3), 281–291. doi:10.100710055-018-0338-3

CUHK. (2021). *Why Hong Kong has the Longest Life Expectancy in the World.* Available at https://www.oal.cuhk.edu.hk/cuhkenews_202101_life_expectancy/

Dacko, S. G. (2017). Enabling smart retail settings via mobile augmented reality shopping apps. *Technological Forecasting and Social Change*, *124*, 243–256. doi:10.1016/j.techfore.2016.09.032

Daglar, C. (2020). *Intangible Assets vs Tangible Assets: Which To Invest In?* Retrieved from daglar-cizmeci website: https://daglar-cizmeci.com/intangible-assets-vs-tangible-assets/

Davies, C., Miller, A., & Allison, C. (2013). Mobile Cross Reality for cultural heritage. *2013 Digital Heritage International Congress (DigitalHeritage).*

Davis, S., Nesbitt, K., & Nalivaiko, E. (2015). Comparing the onset of cybersickness using the Oculus Rift and two virtual roller coasters. *Proceedings of the 11th Australasian Conference on Interactive Entertainment*, 3-14.

De Mauro, A. (2011). Virtual reality based rehabilitation and game technology. *CEUR Workshop Proceedings*, *727*, 48–52.

Delaney, B. (2016). *Virtual Reality 1.0–The 90's: The Birth of VR in the pages of CyberEdge Journal.* CyberEdge Information Services.

Delp, S. L., & Loan, J. P. (1995). A Graphics-based Software System to Develop and Analyze Models of Musculoskeletal Structures. *Computers in Biology and Medicine*, *25*(1), 21–34. doi:10.1016/0010-4825(95)98882-E PMID:7600758

Delp, S. L., Loan, J. P., Hoy, M. G., Zajac, F. E., Topp, E. L., & Rosen, J. M. (1990). An interactive graphics-based model of the lower extremity to study orthopaedic surgical procedures. *IEEE Transactions on Biomedical Engineering, 37*(8), 757–767. doi:10.1109/10.102791 PMID:2210784

Desmyttere, G., Leteneur, S., Hajizadeh, M., Bleau, J., & Begon, M. (2020). Effect of 3D printed foot orthoses stiffness and design on foot kinematics and plantar pressures in healthy people. *Gait & Posture, 81*, 247–253. doi:10.1016/j.gaitpost.2020.07.146 PMID:32818861

Desselle, M. R., Brown, R. A., James, A. R., Midwinter, M. J., Powell, S. K., & Woodruff, M. A. (2020). Augmented and virtual reality in surgery. *Computing in Science & Engineering, 22*(3), 18–26. doi:10.1109/MCSE.2020.2972822

Dewi, C., & Chen, R.-C. (2019). *Human activity recognition based on evolution of features selection and random Forest.* Paper presented at the 2019 IEEE international conference on systems, man and cybernetics (SMC). 10.1109/SMC.2019.8913868

Dickey, P. J., Eger, T., Frayne, R., Delgado, G., & Ji, X. (2013). Research Using Virtual Reality: Mobile Machinery Safety in the 21st Century. *Minerals (Basel), 3*(2), 145–164. doi:10.3390/min3020145

Djukic, T., Mandic, V., & Filipovic, N. (2013). Virtual reality aided visualization of fluid flow simulations with application in medical education and diagnostics. *Computers in Biology and Medicine, 43*(12), 2046–2052. doi:10.1016/j.compbiomed.2013.10.004 PMID:24290920

Do, H. M., Pham, M., Sheng, W., Yang, D., & Liu, M. (2018). *RiSH: A robot-integrated smart home for elderly care.* Academic Press.

Doyle, C., Lennox, L., & Bell, D. (2013). A systematic review of evidence on the links between patient experience and clinical safety and effectiveness. *BMJ Open, 3*(1), e001570. Advance online publication. doi:10.1136/bmjopen-2012-001570 PMID:23293244

Ebert, L., Flach, P., Thali, M., & Ross, S. (2014). Out of touch – A plugin for controlling OsiriX with gestures using the leap controller. *Journal of Forensic Radiology and Imaging, 2*(3), 126–128. doi:10.1016/j.jofri.2014.05.006

Edwards, B. I., Bielawski, K. S., Prada, R., & Cheok, A. D. (2019). Haptic virtual reality and immersive learning for enhanced organic chemistry instruction. *Virtual Reality (Waltham Cross), 23*(4), 363–373.

Eha, P. B. (2013). *An Accelerated History of Internet Speed* (Infographic). Retrieved from Entrepreneur: Technology website: https://www.entrepreneur.com/article/228489

Eisenhardt, K. (1989). Building theories from case study research. *Academy of Management Review, 14*(4), 532–550. doi:10.5465/amr.1989.4308385

El Ammari, K., & Hammad, A. (2019). Remote interactive collaboration in facilities management using BIM-based mixed reality. *Automation in Construction*, *107*, 102940. doi:10.1016/j.autcon.2019.102940

El-Basioni, B. M. M., El-Kader, S., & Abdelmonim, M. (2013). *Smart home design using wireless sensor network and biometric technologies*. Academic Press.

Elgammal, A., Duraiswami, R., Harwood, D., & Davis, L. (2002). *Background and foreground modeling using nonparametric kernel density estimation for visual surveillance*. Academic Press.

Emanuel, E., & Dubler, N. (1995). Preserving the physician-patient relationship in the era of managed care. *Journal of the American Medical Association*, *273*(4), 323–329. doi:10.1001/jama.1995.03520280069043 PMID:7815662

Emanuel, E., & Emanuel, L. (1992). Four models of the physician-patient relationship. *Journal of the American Medical Association*, *267*(16), 2221–2226. doi:10.1001/jama.1992.03480160079038 PMID:1556799

Espíndola, D. B., Fumagalli, L., Garetti, M., Pereira, C. E., Botelho, S. S. C., & Ventura Henriques, R. (2013). A model-based approach for data integration to improve maintenance management by mixed reality. *Computers in Industry*, *64*(4), 376–391. doi:10.1016/j.compind.2013.01.002

Fahad, L. G., Tahir, S. F., & Rajarajan, M. (2014). *Activity recognition in smart homes using clustering based classification*. Paper presented at the 2014 22nd International Conference on Pattern Recognition. 10.1109/ICPR.2014.241

Fahad, L. G., Tahir, S. F., & Rajarajan, M. (2015). *Feature selection and data balancing for activity recognition in smart homes*. Paper presented at the 2015 IEEE International Conference on Communications (ICC). 10.1109/ICC.2015.7248373

Faisal, A. (2017). Computer science: Visionary of virtual reality. *Nature*, *551*(7680), 298–299. doi:10.1038/551298a

Fan, X., Chai, Z., Deng, N., & Dong, X. (2020). Adoption of augmented reality in online retailing and consumers' product attitude: A cognitive perspective. *Journal of Retailing and Consumer Services*, *53*(February), 101986. doi:10.1016/j.jretconser.2019.101986

Fan, X., Yang, R., Wu, D., & Ma, D. (2011). Virtual Assembly Environment for Product Design Evaluation and Workplace Planning. In D. Ma, X. Fan, J. Gausemeier, & M. Grafe (Eds.), *Virtual Reality & Augmented Reality in Industry*. Springer. doi:10.1007/978-3-642-17376-9_9

Farra, S. L., Gneuhs, M., Hodgson, E., Kawosa, B., Miller, E. T., Simon, A., Timm, N., & Hausfeld, J. (2019). Comparative cost of virtual reality training and live exercises for training hospital workers for evacuation. *Computers, Informatics, Nursing*, *37*(9), 446–454. doi:10.1097/CIN.0000000000000540 PMID:31166203

Fergani, L., Fergani, B., & Fleury, A. (2015). *Improving human activity recognition in smart homes*. Academic Press.

Ferguson, C., van den Broek, E. L., & van Oostendorp, H. (2020). On the role of interaction mode and story structure in virtual reality serious games. *Computers & Education, 143*, 103671. doi:10.1016/j.compedu.2019.103671

Ferreira, N. M. (2019). *20 Ecommerce Advantages And Disadvantages You Need To Know*. Retrieved from OBERLO website: https://www.oberlo.com/blog/20-ecommerce-advantages-and-disadvantages

Fertleman, C., Aubugeau-Williams, P., Sher, C., Lim, A.-N., Lumley, S., Delacroix, S., & Pan, X. (2018). A discussion of virtual reality as a new tool for training healthcare professionals. *Frontiers in Public Health, 6*, 44. doi:10.3389/fpubh.2018.00044 PMID:29535997

Fidopiastis, C., Stapleton, C., Whiteside, J., Hughes, C., Fiore, S., Martin, G., Rolland, J. P., & Smith, E. (2006). Human Experience Modeler: Context-Driven Cognitive Retraining to Facilitate Transfer of Learning. *Cyberpsychology & Behavior, 9*(2), 183–187. doi:10.1089/cpb.2006.9.183 PMID:16640476

Filed. (2020). *An Introduction to AR in Marketing*. Retrieved from Filed website: https://www.filed.com/resources/blog/an-introduction-to-ar-in-marketing/

Flickinger, T., Saha, S., Moore, R., & Beach, M. (2013). Higher quality communication and relationships are associated with improved patient engagement in HIV care. *JAIDS Journal of Acquired Immune Deficiency Syndromes, 63*(3), 362–366. doi:10.1097/QAI.0b013e318295b86a PMID:23591637

Flower, C. (2015). Virtual reality and learning: Where is the pedagogy? *British Journal of Educational Technology, 46*(2), 412–422. doi:10.1111/bjet.12135

Flynn. (2019). *The Cure That Works: How to have the World Best Healthcare*. Regnery Publishing.

Fong, N. K. N., Tang, Y. M., Sie, K., Yu, A. K. H., Lo, C. C. W., & Ma, Y. W. T. (2021). Task-specific virtual reality training on hemiparetic upper extremity in patients with stroke. *Virtual Reality (Waltham Cross)*. Advance online publication. doi:10.100710055-021-00583-6

Food and Environmental Hygiene Department. HKSAR. (2021). Available at https://www.fehd.gov.hk/english/

Freeman, D., Reeve, S., Robinson, A., Ehlers, A., Clark, D., Spanlang, B., & Slater, M. (2017). Virtual reality in the assessment, understanding, and treatment of mental health disorders. *Psychological Medicine, 47*(14), 2393–2400. doi:10.1017/S003329171700040X PMID:28325167

Freitas, V., Carlos de Abreu Mol, A., & Shirru, R. (2014). Virtual reality for operational procedures in radioactive waste deposits. *Progress in Nuclear Energy, 71*, 225–231. doi:10.1016/j.pnucene.2013.11.003

Galea. (2019). *Well What We Need to Talk about When We talk about Health*. Oxford University Press.

Galinina, O., Mikhaylov, K., Andreev, S., Turlikov, A., & Koucheryavy, Y. (2015). *Smart home gateway system over Bluetooth low energy with wireless energy transfer capability*. Academic Press.

Gamito, P., Oliveira, J., Coelho, C., Morais, D., Lopes, P., Pacheco, J., Brito, R., Soares, F., Santos, N., & Barata, A. F. (2017). Cognitive training on stroke patients via virtual reality-based serious games. *Disability and Rehabilitation*, *39*(4), 385–388. doi:10.3109/09638288.2014.93 4925 PMID:25739412

Gao, Z., Zhang, H., Xu, G., & Xue, Y. (2015). *Multi-perspective and multi-modality joint representation and recognition model for 3D action recognition*. Academic Press.

Garaus, M., Wagner, U., & Kummer, C. (2015). Cognitive fit, retail shopper confusion, and shopping value: Empirical investigation. *Journal of Business Research*, *68*(5). https://doi.org/10.1016/j.jbusres.2014.10.002

Gefen, A., Megido-Ravid, M., Itzchak, Y., & Arcan, M. (2000). Biomechanical Analysis of the Three-Dimensional Foot Structure During Gait - A Basic Tool for Clinical Applications. *Journal of Biomechanical Engineering*, *122*(6), 630–639. doi:10.1115/1.1318904 PMID:11192385

Gershon, J., Zimand, E., Pickering, M., Rothbaum, B. O., & Hodges, L. (2004). A pilot and feasibility study of virtual reality as a distraction for children with cancer. *Journal of the American Academy of Child and Adolescent Psychiatry*, *43*(10), 1243–1249. doi:10.1097/01.chi.0000135621.23145.05 PMID:15381891

Goldfinger, E. (1991). *Human anatomy for artists: the elements of form*. Oxford University Press.

Golomb, M. R., McDonald, B. C., Warden, S. J., Yonkman, J., Saykin, A. J., Shirley, B., Huber, M., Rabin, B., AbdelBaky, M., Nwosu, M. E., Barkat-Masih, M., & Burdea, G. C. (2010). In-home virtual reality videogame telerehabilitation in adolescents with hemiplegic cerebral palsy. *Archives of Physical Medicine and Rehabilitation*, *91*(1), 1–8. doi:10.1016/j.apmr.2009.08.153 PMID:20103390

Gombrich, E. H. (1999). *The Image and the Eye*. Phaidon Press Ltd.

Gombrich, E. H. (2001). *Art and Illusion*. Princeton Univ. Press.

Goodale, M. A., & Milner, A. (1992). *Separate visual pathways for perception and action*. Academic Press.

Google ARCore. (2020). *Developers ARCore Overview*. Retrieved from Google website: https://developers.google.com/ar/discover/

Goold, S., & Lipkin, M. (1999). The doctor-patient relationship. *Journal of General Internal Medicine*, *14*(S1), S26–S33. Advance online publication. doi:10.1046/j.1525-1497.1999.00267.x PMID:9933492

Govil, D., & Purohit, N. (2011). Healthcare Systems in India. In H. S. Rout (Ed.), *Healthcare Systems –A Global Survey*. New Century Publications.

Graf, L., Liszio, S., & Masuch, M. (2020). Playing in virtual nature: improving mood of elderly people using VR technology. In *Proceedings of the Conference on Mensch und Computer (MuC '20)*. Association for Computing Machinery. 10.1145/3404983.3405507

Grajewski, D., Górski, F., Zawadzki, P., & Hamrol, A. (2013). Application of Virtual Reality Techniques in Design of Ergonomic Manufacturing Workplaces. *Procedia Computer Science*, *25*, 289–301. doi:10.1016/j.procs.2013.11.035

Gupta, A., & Davis, L. S. (2007). *Objects in action: An approach for combining action understanding and object perception*. Paper presented at the 2007 IEEE Conference on Computer Vision and Pattern Recognition. 10.1109/CVPR.2007.383331

Gupta, S., Bagga, S., & Sharma, D. K. (2020). Hand Gesture Recognition for Human Computer Interaction and Its Applications in Virtual Reality. In *Advanced Computational Intelligence Techniques for Virtual Reality in Healthcare* (pp. 85–105). Springer. doi:10.1007/978-3-030-35252-3_5

Guzsvinecz, T., Szucs, V., & Sik-Lanyi, C. (2019). Suitability of the kinect sensor and leap motion controller-A literature review. *Sensors (Basel)*, *19*(5), 1072. doi:10.3390190510721072 PMID:30832385

Halan, D. (2020). *How AR And VR Can Be Applied To Marketing*. Retrieved from electronicsforu website: https://www.electronicsforu.com/technology-trends/must-read/ar-vr-applied-marketing

Hamilton-Giachritsis, C., Banakou, D., Garcia Quiroga, M., Giachritsis, C., & Slater, M. (2018). Reducing risk and improving maternal perspective-taking and empathy using virtual embodiment. *Scientific Reports*, *8*(1), 2975. doi:10.103841598-018-21036-2 PMID:29445183

Hart, T. (2009). Treatment definition in complex rehabilitation interventions. *Neuropsychological Rehabilitation*, *19*(6), 824–840. doi:10.1080/09602010902995945 PMID:19544183

Hasa, M. (2020). *How to Use AR In Campaigns: The Ultimate Guide to Augmented Reality Marketing*. Retrieved from pixelfield website: https://pixelfield.co.uk/blog/how-to-use-ar-in-campaigns-the-ultimate-guide-to-augmented-reality-marketing/

Hashizume, M. (2021). Perspective for Future Medicine: Multidisciplinary Computational Anatomy-Based Medicine with Artificial Intelligence. *Cyborg and Bionic Systems*.

He, Z., & Jin, L. (2009). *Activity recognition from acceleration data based on discrete consine transform and SVM*. Paper presented at the 2009 IEEE International Conference on Systems, Man and Cybernetics. 10.1109/ICSMC.2009.5346042

He, Z.-Y., & Jin, L.-W. (2008). *Activity recognition from acceleration data using AR model representation and SVM*. Paper presented at the 2008 international conference on machine learning and cybernetics.

He, A. J., & Tang, V. F. Y. (2021). Integration of health services for the elderly in Asia: A scoping review of Hong Kong, Singapore, Malaysia, Indonesia. *Health Policy (Amsterdam)*, *125*(3), 351–362. doi:10.1016/j.healthpol.2020.12.020 PMID:33422336

Heller, J., Chylinski, M., de Ruyter, K., Mahr, D., & Keeling, D. I. (2019). Let Me Imagine That for You: Transforming the Retail Frontline Through Augmenting Customer Mental Imagery Ability. *Journal of Retailing*, *95*(2). https://doi.org/10.1016/j.jretai.2019.03.005

Hemanth, J. D., Kose, U., Deperlioglu, O., & de Albuquerque, V. H. C. (2020). An augmented reality-supported mobile application for diagnosis of heart diseases. *The Journal of Supercomputing*, *76*(2), 1242–1267. doi:10.100711227-018-2483-6

Hendriyani, Y., & Amrizal, V. A. (2019, November). The Comparison Between 3D Studio Max and Blender Based on Software Qualities. *Journal of Physics: Conference Series*, *1387*(1), 012030. doi:10.1088/1742-6596/1387/1/012030

Hilken, T., de Ruyter, K., Chylinski, M., Mahr, D., & Keeling, D. I. (2017). Augmenting the eye of the beholder: Exploring the strategic potential of augmented reality to enhance online service experiences. *Journal of the Academy of Marketing Science*, *45*(6), 884–905. https://doi.org/10.1007/s11747-017-0541-x

Hill, A. V. (1938). The heat of shortening and the dynamic constants of muscle. *Proceedings of the Royal Society of London. Series B, Biological Sciences*, *126*(843), 136–195. doi:10.1098/rspb.1938.0050

Hodges, L. (2001). Treating Psychological and Physical Disorders with VR. *IEEE Computer Graphics and Applications*, 25–33.

Holowka, N. B., & Lieberman, D. E. (2018). Rethinking the evolution of the human foot: Insights from experimental research. *The Journal of Experimental Biology*, *221*(17), jeb174425. doi:10.1242/jeb.174425 PMID:30190415

Ho, T. S. G., Tang, Y. M., Tsang, K. Y., Tang, V., & Chau, K. Y. (2021). A blockchain-based system to enhance aircraft parts traceability and trackability for inventory management. *Expert Systems with Applications*, *179*, 115101. doi:10.1016/j.eswa.2021.115101

Howard, M. C. (2017). A meta-analysis and systematic literature review of virtual reality rehabilitation programs. *Computers in Human Behavior*, *70*, 317–327. doi:10.1016/j.chb.2017.01.013

Howe, K. (2019). *Green Burials Benefit the Environment, But They Also Provide Opportunities for Fraud.* Retrieved on 2 July 2021 from https://absolutetrustcounsel.com/green-burials-benefit-the-environment-but-they-also-provide-opportunities-for-fraud/

Hoyer, W. D., Kroschke, M., Schmitt, B., Kraume, K., & Shankar, V. (2020). Transforming the Customer Experience Through New Technologies. *Journal of Interactive Marketing, 51.* doi:10.1016/j.intmar.2020.04.001

Hoy, M. G., Zajac, F. E., & Gordon, M. E. (1990). A musculoskeletal model of the human lower extremity: The effect of muscle, tendon, and moment arm on the moment-angle relationship of musculotendon actuators at the hip, knee, and ankle. *Journal of Biomechanics, 23*(2), 157–169. doi:10.1016/0021-9290(90)90349-8 PMID:2312520

Hsieh, H.-F., & Shannon, S. E. (2005). Three approaches to qualitative content analysis. *Qualitative Health Research, 15*(9), 1277–1288. doi:10.1177/1049732305276687 PMID:16204405

Hsu, E. B., Li, Y., Bayram, J. D., Levinson, D., Yang, S., & Monahan, C. (2013). State of virtual reality based disaster preparedness and response training. *PLoS Currents, 5*.

Huang, T. L., & Liao, S. (2015). A model of acceptance of augmented-reality interactive technology: The moderating role of cognitive innovativeness. *Electronic Commerce Research, 15*(2). https://doi.org/10.1007/s10660-014-9163-2

Huang, T. L., & Liu, F. H. (2014). Formation of augmented-reality interactive technology's persuasive effects from the perspective of experiential value. *Internet Research, 24*(1). https://doi.org/10.1108/IntR-07-2012-0133

Hui, K. C., & Leung, H. C. (2002). Virtual Sculpting and Deformable Volume Modelling. Proceedings of Information Visualisation, 664-669. doi:10.1109/IV.2002.1028846

Hui, K. C., & Wong, N. N. (2002). Hands on a virtually elastic object. *The Visual Computer, 18*(3), 150–163. doi:10.1007003710100120

Iconaru, E. (2014). Similarities and Differences between Evaluation Protocols in Physical Therapy and Occupational Therapy – A Case Study. *Procedia: Social and Behavioral Sciences, 116*, 3142–3146. doi:10.1016/j.sbspro.2014.01.723

Ignacimuthu, S. (2005). *Basic Informatics*. New Delhi: Narosa Publishing House.

Interactive Advertising Bureau. (2019). *Augmented Reality for Marketing: An IAB Playbook*. Retrieved from https://books.google.co.uk/books/about/Augmented_Reality_for_Developers.html?id=8xhKDwAAQBAJ&printsec=frontcover&source=kp_read_button&redir_esc=y#v=onepage&q&f=false%0Ahttps://mediatum.ub.tum.de/1286695

Internet Advertising Bureau. (2017). *IAB New Standard Ad Unit Portofolio*. Retrieved from www.iab.com/newadportfolio

Itamiya, T., Tohara, H., & Nasuda, Y. (2019). Augmented Reality Floods and Smoke Smartphone App Disaster Scope utilizing Real-time Occlusion. *2019 IEEE Conference on Virtual Reality and 3D User Interfaces (VR)*.

Jaeger, B. K., & Mourant, R. R. (2001). Comparison of simulator sickness using static and dynamic walking simulators. *Proceedings of the Human Factors and Ergonomics Society Annual Meeting, 45*(27), 1896–1900. doi:10.1177/154193120104502709

James, D. L., & Pai, D. K. (1999). ArtDefo: Accurate Real Time Deformable Objects. *Proceedings of Computer Graphics*, 65-72.

Javaid, M., & Haleem, A. (2020). Virtual reality applications toward medical field. *Clinical Epidemiology and Global Health, 8*(2), 600–605. doi:10.1016/j.cegh.2019.12.010

Javornik, A. (2016). *The Mainstreaming of Augmented Reality: A Brief History*. Retrieved from Harvard Business Review website: https://hbr.org/2016/10/the-mainstreaming-of-augmented-reality-a-brief-history#

Jiang, L., Liu, D.-Y., & Yang, B. (2004). Smart home research. *Proceedings of 2004 international conference on machine learning and cybernetics* (IEEE Cat. No. 04EX826). 10.1109/ICMLC.2004.1382266

Jie, Y., Pei, J. Y., Jun, L., Yun, G., & Wei, X. (2013). *Smart home system based on iot technologies*. Paper presented at the 2013 International conference on computational and information sciences. 10.1109/ICCIS.2013.468

Jones, M. A., Reynolds, K. E., & Arnold, M. J. (2006). Hedonic and utilitarian shopping value: Investigating differential effects on retail outcomes. *Journal of Business Research, 59*(9). https://doi.org/10.1016/j.jbusres.2006.03.006

Joyce, K. (2018). *AR, VR, MR, RR, XR: A Glossary To The Acronyms Of The Future*. Retrieved 28 Dec 2019 from https://www.vrfocus.com/2017/05/ar-vr-mr-rr-xr-a-glossary-to-the-acronyms-of-the-future/

Kabir, M. H., Hoque, M. R., Thapa, K., & Yang, S.-H. (2016). *Two-layer hidden Markov model for human activity recognition in home environments*. Academic Press.

Kaiser, L., Gomez, A. N., Shazeer, N., Vaswani, A., Parmar, N., Jones, L., & Uszkoreit, J. J. a. (2017). One model to learn them all. In Improving Supervised Classification of Daily Activities Living Using New Cost Sensitive Criterion For C-SVM. Academic Press.

Kamińska, M. S., Miller, A., Rotter, I., Szylińska, A., & Grochans, E. (2018). The effectiveness of virtual reality training in reducing the risk of falls among elderly people. *Clinical Interventions in Aging, 13*, 2329–2338. doi:10.2147/CIA.S183502 PMID:30532523

Kanade, T., Rander, P., & Narayanan, P. J. (1997). Virtualized reality: Constructing virtual worlds from real scenes. *IEEE MultiMedia, 4*(1), 34–47. doi:10.1109/93.580394

Karras, T. (2018). *A Style-Based Generator Architecture for Generative Adversarial Network, Neural and Evolutionary Computing*. Cornell University.

Katsikadelis, J. T. (2002). *Boundary elements: theory and applications*. Elsevier.

Kenngott, H. G., Pfeiffer, M., Preukschas, A. A., Bettscheider, L., Wise, P. A., Wagner, M., Speidel, S., Huber, M., Nickel, F., Mehrabi, A., & Müller-Stich, B. P. (2021). IMHOTEP: Cross-professional evaluation of a three-dimensional virtual reality system for interactive surgical operation planning, tumor board discussion and immersive training for complex liver surgery in a head-mounted display. *Surgical Endoscopy*. Advance online publication. doi:10.100700464-020-08246-4 PMID:33475848

Kerttula, M., & Tokkonen, T. (2001). Virtual design of multiengineering electronics systems. *Computer*, *34*(11), 71–79. doi:10.1109/2.963447

Khanra, S., Dhir, A., Islam, A., & Mäntymäki, M. (2020). Big Data Analytics in Healthcare: A systematic literature review. *Enterprise Information Systems*, *14*(7), 878–912. doi:10.1080/175 17575.2020.1812005

Khon & Skarulis. (2012). IBM Watson Delivers New Insights for Treatment and Diagnosis. *Digital Health Conference*.

Khurana, A. (2019). *Disadvantages of E-commerce*. Retrieved from the balancesmall business website: https://www.thebalancesmb.com/disadvantages-of-e-commerce-1141571

Kilbride, M., & Joffe, S. (2018). The new age of patient autonomy. *Journal of the American Medical Association*, *320*(19), 1973–1974. doi:10.1001/jama.2018.14382 PMID:30326026

Kim, J., & Forsythe, S. (2008). Adoption of virtual try-on technology for online apparel shopping. *Journal of Interactive Marketing*, *22*(2). https://doi.org/10.1002/dir.20113

Kim, M., Jeon, C., & Kim, J. (2017). A study on immersion and presence of a portable hand haptic system for immersive virtual reality. *Sensors (Basel)*, *17*(5), 1141. doi:10.339017051141 PMID:28513545

Kim, Y., Hong, S., & Kim, G. J. (2018). Augmented reality-based remote coaching for fast-paced physical task. *Virtual Reality (Waltham Cross)*, *22*(1), 25–36. doi:10.100710055-017-0315-2

Kingdon, K. S., Stanney, K. M., & Kennedy, R. S. (2001). Extreme responses to virtual environment exposure. *Proceedings of the Human Factors and Ergonomics Society Annual Meeting*, *45*(27), 1906–1910. doi:10.1177/154193120104502711

Kit, P., Rasid, S., Ismail, W., & Mokhber, M. (2017). Can managed care really improve doctor–patient relationship? *Journal of Health Management*, *19*(1), 192–202. doi:10.1177/0972063416682895

Kizil, M. S., & Joy, J. (2001). *What can virtual reality do for safety?* St University of Queensland.

Knudson, D. (2003). *Fundamentals of biomechanics*. Kluwer Academic/Plenum. doi:10.1007/978-1-4757-5298-4

Kobatake, H., & Masutani, Y. (2017). *Computational anatomy based on whole body imaging*. Springer. doi:10.1007/978-4-431-55976-4

Koroliov, P., & Lapko, O. (2021). *Virtual Reality*. *Waltham Cross*.

Kraynak. (2017). *Cloud Data Warehousing Dummies*. John Willey & Sons.

Krupitzer, C., Müller, S., Lesch, V., Züfle, M., Edinger, J., Lemken, A., . . . Becker, C. (2020). *A Survey on Human Machine Interaction in Industry 4.0*. arXiv preprint arXiv.01025.

Kumar & Joy. (2013). Application of Zigbee Wireless Frequency for Patient Monitoring System. *CSI Communications Journal*, *37*(9), 17–18.

Kwok, P. K., Yan, M., Chan, B. K. P., & Lau, H. Y. K. (2019). Crisis management training using discrete-event simulation and virtual reality techniques. *Computers & Industrial Engineering*, *135*, 711–722. doi:10.1016/j.cie.2019.06.035

Kwok, P. K., Yan, M., Qu, T., & Lau, H. Y. K. (2020). User acceptance of virtual reality technology for practicing digital twin-based crisis management. *International Journal of Computer Integrated Manufacturing*, 1–14. doi:10.1080/0951192X.2020.1803502

Laclé, F., & Pronost, N. (2017). A scalable geometrical model for musculotendon units. *Computer Animation and Virtual Worlds*, *28*(1), e1684. doi:10.1002/cav.1684

Lals. (2018). *Public Health Management Principles*. CBS Publishers & Distributors.

Lamantia, J. (2009). *Inside Out: Interaction Design for Augmented Reality*. Retrieved from UXmatters website: https://www.uxmatters.com/mt/archives/2009/08/inside-out-interaction-design-for-augmented-reality.php

Lam, H. Y., Ho, G. T. S., Mo, D. Y., & Tang, V. (2021). Enhancing data-driven elderly appointment services in domestic care communities under COVID-19. *Industrial Management & Data Systems*, *121*(7), 1552–1576. doi:10.1108/IMDS-07-2020-0392

Lan, C., Chen, S. Y., & Lai, J. S. (2012). *Exercise training for patients after coronary artery bypass grafting surgery*. In M. Brizzio (Ed.), *Acute Coronary Syndromes* (pp. 117–128). IntechOpen.

Lanier, J. (2006). *Homuncular flexibility. In Edge*. The World Question Center.

Lau, Y. Y., Chiu, W. K., & Chan, G. H. H. (2017). Procurement management in the private elderly home. *CPCE Health Conference 2017*.

Lau, Y. Y., & Keung, K. L. (2018). An application of balanced scorecard in the private elderly home: A case study of Hong Kong. *CPCE Health Conference 2018*.

Lau, Y. Y., Tang, Y. M., Chan, I., Ng, A. K. Y., & Leung, A. (2020). The deployment of virtual reality (VR) to promote green burial. *Asia-Pacific Journal of Health Management*, *15*(2), 53–60. doi:10.24083/apjhm.v15i2.403

Lau, Y. Y., Tang, Y. M., Chau, K. Y., & Hui, H. Y. (2021). Pilot Study of Heartbeat Sensors for Data Streaming in Virtual Reality (VR) Training. *International Journal of Innovation. Creativity and Change*, *15*(3), 30–41.

Laver, K., George, S., Thomas, S., Deutsch, J., & Crotty, M. (2015). Virtual reality for stroke rehabilitation. *Cochrane Database of Systematic Reviews*, *2015*(2), CD008349. PMID:25927099

Lee, H. (2019). Real-time manufacturing modeling and simulation framework using augmented reality and stochastic network analysis. *Virtual Reality (Waltham Cross)*, *23*(1), 85–99. doi:10.100710055-018-0343-6

Legislative Council Panel on Manpower. (2013, Dec.). *Occupational Diseases in Hong Kong*. Government of the Hong Kong Special Administrative Region. https://www.legco.gov.hk/yr13-14/english/panels/mp/papers/mp1217cb2-491-12-e.pdf

Levac, D. E., & Galvin, J. (2013). When is virtual reality "therapy"? *Archives of Physical Medicine and Rehabilitation*, *94*(4), 795–798. doi:10.1016/j.apmr.2012.10.021 PMID:23124132

Levin, M. F., Weiss, P. L., & Keshner, E. A. (2015). Emergence of virtual reality as a tool for upper limb rehabilitation: Incorporation of motor control and motor learning principles. *Physical Therapy*, *95*(3), 415–425. doi:10.2522/ptj.20130579 PMID:25212522

Lewis-Evans, B. (2018). A short guide to user testing for simulation sickness in Virtual Reality. In *Games User Research*. Oxford University Press.

Li, L., Zhang, M., Xu, F., & Liu, S. (2005) ERT-VR: An immersive virtual reality system for emergency rescue. Virtual Reality, 194–197. doi:10.100710055-004-0149-6

Li, D. (2019). 5G and intelligence medicine – how the next generation of wireless technology will reconstruct healthcare? *Precision Clinical Medicine*, *2*(4), 205–208. doi:10.1093/pcmedi/pbz020 PMID:31886033

Lifton, J., Laibowitz, M., Harry, D., Gong, N., Mittal, M., & Paradiso, J. A. (2009). Metaphor and Manifestation Cross-Reality with Ubiquitous Sensor/Actuator Networks. *IEEE Pervasive Computing*, *8*(3), 24–33. doi:10.1109/MPRV.2009.49

Lightspeed. (2021). *Exploring the Advantages and Disadvantages of Ecommerce*. Retrieved from Lightspeed website: https://www.lightspeedhq.com/blog/advantages-and-disadvantages-of-ecommerce/

Li, J., & Zuo, M. (2021). Emergency Rescue Training System for Earthquakes Based on Immersive Technology. *2021 IEEE 5th Advanced Information Technology, Electronic and Automation Control Conference (IAEAC)*.

Linowes. (2015). *Virtual Reality Projects*. Pack7.

Li, Q., Huang, C., Lv, S., Li, Z., Chen, Y., & Ma, L. (2017). An Human-Computer Interactive Augmented Reality System for Coronary Artery Diagnosis Planning and Training. [PubMed]. *Journal of Medical Systems*, *41*(10), 159. doi:10.100710916-017-0805-5

Liu, J., & Yang, T. (2021). *Word Frequency Data Analysis in Virtual Reality Technology Industrialization*. Paper presented at the Journal of Physics: Conference Series.

Liu, C., Yip, K., & Chiang, H. (2020). Investigating the optimal handle diameters and thumb orthoses for individuals with chronic de Quervain's tenosynovitis - a pilot study. *Disability and Rehabilitation*, *42*(9), 1247–1253. doi:10.1080/09638288.2018.1522548 PMID:30689463

Liu, D., Bhagat, K. K., Gao, Y., Chang, T.-W., & Huang, R. (2017). The Potentials and Trends of Virtual Reality in Education. In D. Liu, C. Dede, R. Huang, & J. Richards (Eds.), *Virtual, Augmented, and Mixed Realities in Education* (pp. 105–130). Springer Singapore. doi:10.1007/978-981-10-5490-7_7

Llorens, R., Colomer-Font, C., Alcañiz, M., & Noé-Sebastián, E. (2013). BioTrak virtual reality system: Effectiveness and satisfaction analysis for balance rehabilitation in patients with brain injury. *Neurologia (Barcelona, Spain)*, *28*(5), 268–275. PMID:22727272

Loucks, L., Yasinski, C., Norrholm, S. D., Maples-Keller, J., Post, L., Zwiebach, L., ... Rizzo, A. A. (2019). You can do that?!: Feasibility of virtual reality exposure therapy in the treatment of PTSD due to military sexual trauma. *Journal of Anxiety Disorders*, *61*, 55–63. doi:10.1016/j.janxdis.2018.06.004 PMID:30005843

M., D. (2020). *What are Ecommerce Advantages and Disadvantages?* Retrieved from BELVG website: https://belvg.com/blog/what-is-advantage-and-disadvantage-of-e-commerce.html

MacDorman, K., & Ishiguro, H. (2006). The uncanny advantage of using androids in social and cognitive science research. *Interaction Studies: Social Behaviour and Communication in Biological and Artificial Systems*, *7*(3), 297–337. doi:10.1075/is.7.3.03mac

Madison, N. (2014). *Health Information Systems, Opportunities, and Challenges.* Http//commons.nmu.edu/facwork book chapters/14

Maganaris, C. N., Baltzopoulos, V., Ball, D., & Sargeant, A. J. (2001). In vivo specific tension of human skeletal muscle. *Journal of Applied Physiology*, *90*(3), 865–872. doi:10.1152/jappl.2001.90.3.865 PMID:11181594

Maier-Hein, L., Vedula, S. S., Speidel, S., Navab, N., Kikinis, R., Park, A., Eisenmann, M., Feussner, H., Forestier, G., Giannarou, S., Hashizume, M., Katic, D., Kenngott, H., Kranzfelder, M., Malpani, A., März, K., Neumuth, T., Padoy, N., Pugh, C., ... Jannin, P. (2017). Surgical data science for next-generation interventions. *Nature Biomedical Engineering*, *1*(9), 691–696. doi:10.103841551-017-0132-7 PMID:31015666

Maister, L., Slater, M., Sanchez-Vives, M. V., & Tsakiris, M. (2015). Changing bodies changes minds: Owning another body affects social cognition. *Trends in Cognitive Sciences*, *19*(1), 6–12. doi:10.1016/j.tics.2014.11.001 PMID:25524273

Makarov, A. (2020). *Augmented reality development: Guide for business owners and managers.* Retrieved from mobidev website: https://mobidev.biz/blog/augmented-reality-development-guide

Makarov, A. (2021). *6 ideas to leverage augmented reality for marketing & sales.* Retrieved from mobidev website: https://mobidev.biz/blog/augmented-reality-marketing-sales

Mäkinen, H., Haavisto, E., Havola, S., & Koivisto, J.-M. (2020). User experiences of virtual reality technologies for healthcare in learning: An integrative review. *Behaviour & Information Technology*, 1–17. doi:10.1080/0144929X.2020.1788162

Malarvani, T., Ganesh, E., Nirmala, P., Kumar, A., & Singh, M. K. (2014). WhatsAppitis: Recent Study on SMS Syndrome. *Scholars Journal of Applied Medical Sciences*, 2(6B), 2026–2033.

Malche, T., & Maheshwary, P. (2017). *Internet of Things (IoT) for building smart home system.* Paper presented at the 2017 International Conference on I-SMAC (IoT in Social, Mobile, Analytics and Cloud)(I-SMAC).

Malloy, K. M., & Milling, L. S. (2010). The effectiveness of virtual reality distraction for pain reduction: A systematic review. *Clinical Psychology Review*, 30(8), 1011–1018. doi:10.1016/j.cpr.2010.07.001 PMID:20691523

Manalastas, G., Noble, L., Viney, R., & Griffin, A. E. (2021). What does the structure of a medical consultation look like? A new method for visualizing doctor-patient communication. *Patient Education and Counseling*, 104(6), 1387–1397. doi:10.1016/j.pec.2020.11.026 PMID:33272747

Mandal, S. (2013). Brief introduction of virtual reality & its challenges. *International Journal of Scientific and Engineering Research*, 4(4), 304–309.

Mann, S., Furness, T., Yuan, Y., Iorio, J., & Wang, Z. (2018). *All Reality: Virtual, Augmented, Mixed (X), Mediated (X,Y), and Multimediated Reality.* CoRR. abs/1804.08386.

Maples-Keller, J. L., Yasinski, C., Manjin, N., & Rothbaum, B. O. (2017). Virtual reality-enhanced extinction of phobias and post-traumatic stress. *Neurotherapeutics; the Journal of the American Society for Experimental NeuroTherapeutics*, 14(3), 554–563. doi:10.100713311-017-0534-y PMID:28512692

Marini, D., Folgieri, R., Gadia, D., & Rizzi, A. (2012). Virtual reality as a communication process. *Virtual Reality (Waltham Cross)*, 16(3), 233–241. doi:10.100710055-011-0200-3

Marr, B. (2018). *Facebook And Apple Are Serious About Augmented Reality.* Retrieved from Forbes website: https://www.forbes.com/sites/bernardmarr/2018/08/08/facebook-and-apple-are-serious-about-augmented-reality/?sh=5ef31ee6b4bc

Martínez, H., Skournetou, D., Hyppölä, J., Laukkanen, S., & Heikkilä, A. (2014). Drivers and bottlenecks in the adoption of augmented reality applications. *Journal ISSN*, 2368, 5956. doi:10.11159/jmta.2014.004

Mascret, N., Delbes, L., Voron, A., Temprado, J., & Montagne, G. (2020). Acceptance of a Virtual Reality Headset Designed for Fall Prevention in Older Adults: Questionnaire Study. *Journal of Medical Internet Research*, 22(12), e20691. Advance online publication. doi:10.2196/20691 PMID:33315019

Matamala-Gomez, M., Donegan, T., Bottiroli, S., Sandrini, G., Sanchez-Vives, M. V., & Tassorelli, C. (2019). Immersive virtual reality and virtual embodiment for pain relief. *Frontiers in Human Neuroscience*, 13, 279. doi:10.3389/fnhum.2019.00279 PMID:31551731

McConnell, C. R. (2020). *Hospitals and Healthcare Systems: What they are and how they work.* Jones & Bartlett Learning.

Compilation of References

McCue, M., Fairman, A., & Pramuka, M. (2010). Enhancing quality of life through telerehabilitation. *Physical Medicine and Rehabilitation Clinics of North America*, *21*(1), 195–205. doi:10.1016/j.pmr.2009.07.005 PMID:19951786

McGinnis, P. (1999). *Biomechanics of sport and exercise*. Human Kinetics.

McLean, G., & Wilson, A. (2019). *Customer Engagement with Augmented Reality Mobile Apps*. Paper presented at the 2019 Academy of Marketing Science Annual Conference. doi:10.1007/978-3-030-39165-2_89

McMahon, T. A. (1984). *Muscles, reflexes, and locomotion*. Princeton University Press. doi:10.1515/9780691221540

McNutt, E. J., Zipfel, B., & DeSilva, J. M. (2018). The evolution of the human foot. *Evolutionary Anthropology*, *27*(5), 197–217. doi:10.1002/evan.21713 PMID:30242943

Mead, N., & Bower, P. (2000). Patient-centredness: A conceptual framework and review of the empirical literature. *Social Science & Medicine*, *51*(7), 1087–1110. doi:10.1016/S0277-9536(00)00098-8 PMID:11005395

Mechanic, D., & Schlesinger, M. (1996). The impact of managed care on Patients' trust in medical care and their physicians. *Journal of the American Medical Association*, *275*(21), 1693–1697. doi:10.1001/jama.1996.03530450083048 PMID:8637148

Medeiros, D. M., & Martini, T. F. (2018). Chronic effect of different types of stretching on ankle dorsiflexion range of motion: Systematic review and meta-analysis. *The Foot*, *34*, 28–35. doi:10.1016/j.foot.2017.09.006 PMID:29223884

Mehrabian, A., & Russell, J. A. (1974). *An Approach to Environmental Psychology*. MIT Press.

Messinger, P. R., Stroulia, E., Lyons, K., Bone, M., Niu, R. H., Smirnov, K., & Perelgut, S. (2009). Virtual worlds—past, present, and future: New directions in social computing. *Decision Support Systems*, *47*(3), 204–228. doi:10.1016/j.dss.2009.02.014

Miao, S., Shen, C., Feng, X., Zhu, Q., Shorfuzzaman, M., & Lv, Z. (2021). Upper limb rehabilitation system for stroke survivors based on multi-modal sensors and machine learning. *IEEE Access: Practical Innovations, Open Solutions*, *9*, 30283–30291. doi:10.1109/ACCESS.2021.3055960

Milgram, P., & Kishino, F. (1994). A taxonomy of mixed reality visual displays. *IEICE Transactions on Information and Systems*, *77*(12), 1321–1329.

Milgram, P., Takemura, H., Utsumi, A., & Kishino, F. (1995). *Augmented reality: A class of displays on the reality-virtuality continuum*. Telemanipulator and Telepresence Technologies.

Miniwatts Marketing Group. (2014). *Internet Usage Statistic*. The Internet Big Picture. https://www.internetworldstats.com/stats.htm

MitchellB. (2019). https://medium.com/@bryanmitchell_67448/there-is-a-second-valley-past-the-uncanny-valley-22d2ea193e0

Mo. (2015). How to Build an Ideal Health Care Information System. In *The World Book of Family Medicine*. Academic Press.

Mohamed, R., Perumal, T., Sulaiman, M. N., Mustapha, N., & Manaf, S. (2017). *Tracking and recognizing the activity of multi resident in smart home environments*. Academic Press.

Mosadeghi, S., Reid, M. W., Martinez, B., Rosen, B. T., & Spiegel, B. M. R. (2016). Feasibility of an Immersive Virtual Reality Intervention for Hospitalized Patients: An Observational Cohort Study. *JMIR Mental Health*, *3*(2), e28. doi:10.2196/mental.5801 PMID:27349654

Moskaliuk, J., Kimmerle, J., & Cress, U. (2010). Virtual Reality 2.0 and its Application in Knowledge building. In Handbook of research on Web 2.0, 3.0, and X. 0: Technologies, business, and social applications (pp. 573-592). IGI Global.

Mujber, T., Szecsi, T., & Hashmi, M. (2004). Virtual reality applications in manufacturing process simulation. *Journal of Materials Processing Technology*, *155-156*(1-3), 1834–1838. doi:10.1016/j.jmatprotec.2004.04.401

Mukund, K., & Subramaniam, S. (2020). Skeletal muscle: A review of molecular structure and function, in health and disease. *Wiley Interdisciplinary Reviews. Systems Biology and Medicine*, *12*(1), e1462. doi:10.1002/wsbm.1462 PMID:31407867

Mullen, G., & Davidenko, N. (2021, May). Time Compression in Virtual Reality. *Timing & Time Perception (Leiden, Netherlands)*, *9*(4), 377–392. doi:10.1163/22134468-bja10034

Mumtaz, A., Zhang, W., & Chan, A. B. (2014). Joint motion segmentation and background estimation in dynamic scenes. *Proceedings of the IEEE Conference on Computer Vision and Pattern Recognition*. 10.1109/CVPR.2014.54

Munir, A., Ehsan, S. K., Raza, S. M., & Mudassir, M. (2019). *Face and speech recognition based smart home*. Paper presented at the 2019 International Conference on Engineering and Emerging Technologies (ICEET). 10.1109/CEET1.2019.8711849

Mütterlein, J., & Hess, T. (2017). *Immersion, presence, interactivity: Towards a joint understanding of factors influencing virtual reality acceptance and use*. Paper presented at the Twenty-third Americas Conference on Information Systems, Boston, MA.

Mütterlein, J. (2018). The three pillars of virtual reality? Investigating the roles of immersion, presence, and interactivity. *Proceedings of the 51st Hawaii international conference on system sciences*. 10.24251/HICSS.2018.174

Naderifar, M., Goli, H., & Ghaljaei, F. (2017). Snowball Sampling: A Purposeful Method of Sampling in Qualitative Research. *Strides in Development of Medical Education*, *14*(3).

Naser, A., Lotfi, A., & Zhong, J. (2020). *Adaptive thermal sensor array placement for human segmentation and occupancy estimation*. Academic Press.

Naser, A., Lotfi, A., Zhong, J. (2021). *Towards human distance estimation using a thermal sensor array*. Academic Press.

Nazerfard, E., Das, B., Holder, L. B., & Cook, D. J. (2010). Conditional random fields for activity recognition in smart environments. *Proceedings of the 1st ACM International Health Informatics Symposium*. 10.1145/1882992.1883032

Negrillo-Cárdenas, J., Jiménez-Pérez, J.-R., & Feito, F. R. (2020). The role of virtual and augmented reality in orthopedic trauma surgery: From diagnosis to rehabilitation. *Computer Methods and Programs in Biomedicine, 191*, 105407. doi:10.1016/j.cmpb.2020.105407 PMID:32120088

Neogi, S., & Dauwels, J. (2021). *Factored latent-dynamic conditional random fields for single and multi-label sequence modeling*. Academic Press.

Noghabaei, M., Heydarian, A., Balali, V., & Han, K. (2020). Trend analysis on adoption of virtual and augmented reality in the architecture, engineering, and construction industry. *Data, 5*(1), 26–43. doi:10.3390/data5010026

Normand, J. M., Giannopoulos, E., Spanlang, B., & Slater, M. (2011). Multisensory stimulation can induce an illusion of larger belly size in immersive virtual reality. *PLoS One, 6*(1), e16128. doi:10.1371/journal.pone.0016128 PMID:21283823

O'Farrell, J. (2019). *Augmented Reality and the Network*. Retrieved from spearline website: https://www.spearline.com/blog/post/augmented-reality-and-the-network/

Occupational Safety and Health Branch. Labour Department. (2020, September). *Occupational Safety and Health Statistics 2019*. https://www.labour.gov.hk/eng/osh/pdf/archive/statistics/OSH_Statistics_2019_eng.pdf

Office of National Statistics UK. (2021). *Dataset — Coronavirus and depression in adults in Great Britain*. https://www.ons.gov.uk/peoplepopulationandcommunity/wellbeing/datasets/coronavirusanddepressioninadultsingreatbritain

Oh, H., Yoon, S. Y., & Shyu, C. R. (2008). How can Virtual Reality reshape furniture retailing? *Clothing & Textiles Research Journal, 26*(2). https://doi.org/10.1177/0887302X08314789

Olasky, J., Sankaranarayanan, G., Seymour, N., Magee, J., Enquobahrie, A., Lin, M., Aggarwal, R., Brunt, L. M., Schwaitzberg, S. D., Cao, C. G. L., De, S., & Jones, D. (2015). Identifying Opportunities for Virtual Reality Simulation in Surgical Education. *Surgical Innovation, 22*(5), 514–521. doi:10.1177/1553350615583559 PMID:25925424

Omura, M., Stone, T. E., Petrini, M. A., & Cao, R. (2020). Nurses' health beliefs about paper face masks in Japan, Australia and China: A qualitative descriptive study. *International Nursing Review, 67*(3), 341–351. doi:10.1111/inr.12607 PMID:32686094

Otani, K., Waterman, B., & Dunagan, W. (2012). Patient satisfaction: How patient health conditions influence their satisfaction. *Journal of Healthcare Management, 57*(4), 276–293. doi:10.1097/00115514-201207000-00009 PMID:22905606

Ozturkcan, S. (2020). Service innovation: Using augmented reality in the IKEA Place app. *Journal of Information Technology Teaching Cases*. doi:10.1177/2043886920947110

Padrao, G., Gonzalez-Franco, M., Sanchez-Vives, M. V., Slater, M., & Rodriguez-Fornells, A. (2016). Violating body movement semantics: neural signatures of self-generated and external-generated errors. *Neuroimage, 124*(Pt A), 174–156.

Paine, J. (2018). *10 Brands Already Leveraging the Power of Augmented Reality: AR is changing the marketing game*. Retrieved from Inc. This Morning website: https://www.inc.com/james-paine/10-brands-already-leveraging-power-of-augmented-reality.html

Panetta, K. (2018). *5 Trends Emerge in the Gartner Hype Cycle for Emerging Technologies, 2018*. Retrieved from Smarter With Gartner website: https://www.gartner.com/smarterwithgartner/5-trends-emerge-in-gartner-hype-cycle-for-emerging-technologies-2018/

Pantano, E., & Gandini, A. (2017). Exploring the forms of sociality mediated by innovative technologies in retail settings. *Computers in Human Behavior, 77*. doi:10.1016/j.chb.2017.02.036

Pantano, E., & Servidio, R. (2012). Modeling innovative points of sales through virtual and immersive technologies. *Journal of Retailing and Consumer Services, 19*(3), 279–286. https://doi.org/10.1016/j.jretconser.2012.02.002

Pan, X., & Hamilton, A. F. C. (2018). Understanding dual realities and more in VR. *British Journal of Psychology, 109*(3), 437–441. doi:10.1111/bjop.12315 PMID:29851023

Paradiso, J. A., & Landay, J. A. (2009). Guest Editors' Introduction: Cross-Reality Environments. *IEEE Pervasive Computing, 8*(3), 14–15. doi:10.1109/MPRV.2009.47

Park, J. (2018). Emotional reactions to the 3D virtual body and future willingness: The effects of self-esteem and social physique anxiety. *Virtual Reality (Waltham Cross), 22*(1), 1–11. doi:10.100710055-017-0314-3

Peck, T. C., Seinfeld, S., Aglioti, S. M., & Slater, M. (2013). Putting yourself in the skin of a black avatar reduces implicit racial bias. *Consciousness and Cognition, 22*(3), 779–787. doi:10.1016/j.concog.2013.04.016 PMID:23727712

Persaud, R. (2005). How to improve communication with patients. *BMJ (Clinical Research Ed.), 330*(7494), s136–s137. Advance online publication. doi:10.1136/bmj.330.7494.s136

Petrock, V. (2019). *Virtual and Augmented Reality Users 2019*. Retrieved from eMarketer website: https://www.emarketer.com/content/virtual-and-augmented-reality-users-2019

Pincock, S. (2003). Patients put their relationship with their doctors as second only to that with their families. *BMJ (Clinical Research Ed.), 327*(7415), 581-c–581. Advance online publication. doi:10.1136/bmj.327.7415.581-c PMID:12969915

Pirsiavash, H., & Ramanan, D. (2012). *Detecting activities of daily living in first-person camera views*. Paper presented at the 2012 IEEE conference on computer vision and pattern recognition. 10.1109/CVPR.2012.6248010

Piryankova, I. V., Wong, H. Y., Linkenauger, S. A., Stinson, C., Longo, M. R., Bülthoff, H. H., & Mohler, B. J. (2014). Owning an overweight or underweight body: Distinguishing the physical, experienced and virtual body. *PLoS One, 9*(8), e103428. doi:10.1371/journal.pone.0103428 PMID:25083784

Pop, C., Cioara, T., Antal, M., Anghel, I., Salomie, I., & Bertoncini, M. J. S. (2018). *Blockchain based decentralized management of demand response programs in smart energy grids.* Academic Press.

Post-Acute Advisor. (2021). *Why Customer Service is the Key to Success for Assisted Living Facilities.* Available at https://postacuteadvisor.blr.com/2017/03/08/why-customer-service-is-the-key-to-success-for-assisted-living-facilities/

Pourmand, A., Davis, S., Lee, D., Barber, S., & Sikka, N. (2017). Emerging utility of virtual reality as a multidisciplinary tool in clinical medicine. *Games for Health Journal, 6*(5), 263–270. doi:10.1089/g4h.2017.0046 PMID:28759254

Poushneh, A., & Vasquez-Parraga, A. Z. (2017). Discernible impact of augmented reality on retail customer's experience, satisfaction and willingness to buy. *Journal of Retailing and Consumer Services, 34.* doi:10.1016/j.jretconser.2016.10.005

Prasolova-Førland, E., Molka-Danielsen, J., Fominykh, M., & Lamb, K. (2017). Active learning modules for multi-professional emergency management training in virtual reality. *2017 IEEE 6th International Conference on Teaching, Assessment, and Learning for Engineering (TALE).*

Puljiz, D., Stöhr, E., Riesterer, K. S., Hein, B., & Kröger, T. (2019). *General Hand Guidance Framework using Microsoft HoloLens.* arXiv preprint arXiv:1908.04692.

Qin, H., Peak, D. A., & Prybutok, V. (2021). A virtual market in your pocket: How does mobile augmented reality (MAR) influence consumer decision making? *Journal of Retailing and Consumer Services, 58*(November), 102337. doi:10.1016/j.jretconser.2020.102337

Qiu, X. (2020). *Application of Balanced Scorecard in E-Commerce Enterprise Performance Management–Taking Alibaba Group as an Example.* doi:10.2991/aebmr.k.200402.006

Rachel, T. (2010). *How I Do Treat My De Quervain's Tenosynovitis?* https://ecfamilyclinic.wordpress.com/2010/10/13/how-i-do-treat-my-de-quervains-tenosynovitis/

Ramella, B. (2018). *The Biggest AR/VR Trends in 2019.* Retrieved from G2 website: https://www.g2.com/articles/2019-ar-vr-trends

Rao. (Ed.). (2011). *Virtual Technologies for Business and Industrial Applications: Innovative and Synergistic Approaches.* IGI Global.

Rasimah, C. M. Y., Ahmad, A., & Zaman, H. B. (2011). Evaluation of user acceptance of mixed reality technology. *Australasian Journal of Educational Technology, 27*(8). Advance online publication. doi:10.14742/ajet.899

Rassier, D. E., MacIntosh, B. R., & Herzog, W. (1999). The length dependence of active force production in skeletal muscle. *Journal of Applied Physiology, 86*(5), 1445–1457. doi:10.1152/jappl.1999.86.5.1445 PMID:10233103

Refai, M. I. M., Van Beijnum, B. J. F., Buurke, J. H., Saes, M., Bussmann, J. B., Meskers, C. G., . . . Veltink, P. H. (2019, July). Portable gait lab: Zero moment point for minimal sensing of gait. In *2019 41st Annual International Conference of the IEEE Engineering in Medicine and Biology Society (EMBC)* (pp. 2077-2081). IEEE.

Reid, D. (2004). The influence of virtual reality on playfulness in children with cerebral palsy: A pilot study. *Occupational Therapy International, 11*(3), 131–144. doi:10.1002/oti.202 PMID:15297894

Reilly, D. F., Rouzati, H., Wu, A., Hwang, J. Y., Brudvik, J., & Edwards, W. K. (2010). TwinSpace: an infrastructure for cross-reality team spaces. *Proceedings of the 23nd annual ACM symposium on User interface software and technology.* 10.1145/1866029.1866050

Rese, A., Baier, D., Geyer-Schulz, A., & Schreiber, S. (2017). How augmented reality apps are accepted by consumers: A comparative analysis using scales and opinions. *Technological Forecasting and Social Change, 124.* doi:10.1016/j.techfore.2016.10.010

Reski, N., & Alissandrakis, A. (2020). Open data exploration in virtual reality: A comparative study of input technology. *Virtual Reality, 24*(1), 1–22. doi:10.100710055-019-00378-w

Reur, J., Arino, J., & Olk, P. (2011). *Entrepreneurial Alliances* (Vol. 1). Boston: Pearson Higher Education.

Rizzo, A., & Kim, G. (2005). A SWOT Analysis of the Field of Virtual Reality Rehabilitation and Therapy. *Presence (Cambridge, Mass.), 14*(2), 119–146. doi:10.1162/1054746053967094

Rizzo, A., & Koenig, S. T. (2017). Is clinical virtual reality ready for primetime? *Neuropsychology, 31*(8), 877–899. doi:10.1037/neu0000405 PMID:29376669

Robert, B., & Lajtha, C. (2002). A New Approach to Crisis Management. *Journal of Contingencies and Crisis Management, 10*(4), 181–191. doi:10.1111/1468-5973.00195

Roggen, D., Calatroni, A., Rossi, M., Holleczek, T., Förster, K., Tröster, G., . . . Ferscha, A. (2010). *Collecting complex activity datasets in highly rich networked sensor environments.* Paper presented at the 2010 Seventh international conference on networked sensing systems (INSS). 10.1109/INSS.2010.5573462

Romano, B., Sands, S., & Pallant, J. I. (2020). Augmented reality and the customer journey: An exploratory study. *Australasian Marketing Journal.* doi:10.1016/j.ausmj.2020.06.010

Roter, D., & Hall, J. (2004). Physician gender and patient-centered communication: A critical review of empirical research. *Annual Review of Public Health, 25*(1), 497–519. doi:10.1146/annurev.publhealth.25.101802.123134 PMID:15015932

Rouse, W. B., Cannon-Bowers, J. A., & Salas, E. (1992). The role of mental models in team performance in complex systems. *IEEE Transactions on Systems, Man, and Cybernetics*, *22*(6), 1296–1308. doi:10.1109/21.199457

Rousseaux, F., Bicego, A., Ledoux, D., Massion, P., Nyssen, A.-S., Faymonville, M.-E., Laureys, S., & Vanhaudenhuyse, A. (2020). Hypnosis associated with 3D immersive virtual reality technology in the management of pain: A review of the literature. *Journal of Pain Research*, *13*, 1129–1138. doi:10.2147/JPR.S231737 PMID:32547176

Rus-Calafell, M., Garety, P., Sason, E., Craig, T. J., & Valmaggia, L. R. (2018). Virtual reality in the assessment and treatment of psychosis: A systematic review of its utility, acceptability and effectiveness. *Psychological Medicine*, *48*(3), 362–391. doi:10.1017/S0033291717001945 PMID:28735593

Ruthenbeck, G. S., Hobson, J., Carney, A. S., Sloan, S., Sacks, R., & Reynolds, K. J. (2013). Toward photorealism in endoscopic sinus surgery simulation. *American Journal of Rhinology & Allergy*, *27*(2), 138–143. doi:10.2500/ajra.2013.27.3861 PMID:23562204

Ruyter, K. D., Wetzels, M., Lemmink, J., & Mattsson, J. (1997). The dynamics of the service delivery process: A value-based approach. *International Journal of Research in Marketing*, *14*(3), 231–243. doi:10.1016/S0167-8116(97)00004-9

Sabanoglu, T. (2021). *Retail e-commerce sales worldwide from 2014 to 2024*. Retrieved from statista website: https://www.statista.com/statistics/379046/worldwide-retail-e-commerce-sales/

Sabetzadeh, F. (2021). *3D Printing, Autonomous Vehicles, Augmented and Virtual Reality*. City University of Macau.

Saddik, A. E. (2018). Digital Twins: The Convergence of Multimedia Technologies. *IEEE MultiMedia*, *25*(2), 87–92. doi:10.1109/MMUL.2018.023121167

Safikhani, S., Pirker, J., & Wriessnegger, S. C. (2021). Virtual Reality Applications for the Treatment of Anxiety and Mental Disorders. *2021 7th International Conference of the Immersive Learning Research Network (iLRN)*, 1-8.

Salathea, E. P., & Arangio, G. A. (2002). A Biomechanical Model of the Foot: The Role of Muscles, Tendons, and Ligaments. *Journal of Biomechanical Engineering*, *124*(3), 281–287. doi:10.1115/1.1468865 PMID:12071262

Sarkar, A. J., Lee, Y.-K., & Lee, S. (2010). *A smoothed naive bayes-based classifier for activity recognition*. Academic Press.

Sarver, D. C., Kharaz, Y. A., Sugg, K. B., Gumucio, J. P., Comerford, E., & Mendias, C. L. (2017). Sex differences in tendon structure and function. *Journal of Orthopaedic Research*, *35*(10), 2117–2126. doi:10.1002/jor.23516 PMID:28071813

Sathia Bhama, P. R. K., Hariharasubramanian, V., Mythili, O. P., & Ramachandran, M. (2020). Users' domain knowledge prediction in e-learning with speech-interfaced augmented and virtual reality contents. *Virtual Reality (Waltham Cross)*, *24*(1), 163–173. doi:10.100710055-017-0321-4

Schäfer, A., Reis, G., & Stricker, D. (2021). *Investigating the Sense of Presence Between Handcrafted and Panorama Based Virtual Environments.* arXiv preprint arXiv.03823.

Schilling, M. A. (2020). Strategic Management of Technological Innovation (6th ed.). McGraw-Hill Education.

Schoenfeld, B. J., Ogborn, D. I., Vigotsky, A. D., Franchi, M. V., & Krieger, J. W. (2017). Hypertrophic effects of concentric vs. eccentric muscle actions: A systematic review and meta-analysis. *Journal of Strength and Conditioning Research*, *31*(9), 2599–2608. doi:10.1519/JSC.0000000000001983 PMID:28486337

Schulteis, M. T., & Rothbaum, B. O. (2002). *Ethical issues for the use of virtual reality in the psychological sciences. Ethical issues in clinical neuropsychology*. Swets & Zeitlinger.

Schultheis, M., & Rizzo, A. (2001). The Application of Virtual Reality Technology in Rehabilitation. *Rehabilitation Psychology*, *46*(3), 296–311. doi:10.1037/0090-5550.46.3.296

Schulz, G. (2012). *Cloud and Virtual Data Storage, Networking*. Taylor & Francis Group.

Sebillo, M., Vitiello, G., Paolino, L., & Ginige, A. (2016). Training emergency responders through augmented reality mobile interfaces. *Multimedia Tools and Applications*, *75*(16), 9609–9622. doi:10.100711042-015-2955-0

Seifert, A., & Schlomann, A. (2021). The Use of Virtual and Augmented Reality by Older Adults: Potentials and Challenges. *Frontiers in Virtual Reality*, *2*, 1–5. doi:10.3389/frvir.2021.639718

Seinfeld, S., Arroyo-Palacios, J., Iruretagoyena, G., Hortensius, R., Zapata, L. E., Borland, D., de Gelder, B., Slater, M., & Sanchez-Vives, M. V. (2018). Offenders become the victim in virtual reality: Impact of changing perspective in domestic violence. *Scientific Reports*, *8*(1), 2692. doi:10.103841598-018-19987-7 PMID:29426819

Semolic & Baisya. (2013). *Globalization and Innovative Business Models*. New Delhi: Ane Books Private Limited.

Servotte, J.-C., Goosse, M., Campbell, S. H., Dardenne, N., Pilote, B., Simoneau, I. L., Guillaume, M., Bragard, I., & Ghuysen, A. (2020). Virtual reality experience: Immersion, sense of presence, and cybersickness. *Clinical Simulation in Nursing*, *38*, 35–43. doi:10.1016/j.ecns.2019.09.006

servreality. (2020). *Pros and cons of augmented reality apps development.* Retrieved from servreality website: https://servreality.com/blog/pros-and-cons-of-augmented-reality-apps-development/

Shah, M., Siebert-Evenstone, A., Eagan, B., & Holthaus, R. (2021). Modeling Educator Use of Virtual Reality Simulations in Nursing Education Using Epistemic Network Analysis. *2021 7th International Conference of the Immersive Learning Research Network (iLRN)*, 1-8.

Shah, P. R., Grewal, U. S., & Hamad, H. (2021). *Informed Consent*. StatPearls.

Shao, D., & Lee, I. J. (2020). Acceptance and Influencing Factors of Social Virtual Reality in the Urban Elderly. *Sustainability*, *12*(22), 9345–9363. doi:10.3390u12229345

Shao, X., Yuan, Q., Qian, D., Ye, Z., Chen, G., le Zhuang, K., Jiang, X., Jin, Y., & Qiang, D. (2020). Virtual reality technology for teaching neurosurgery of skull base tumor. *BMC Medical Education*, *20*(1), 1–7. doi:10.118612909-019-1911-5 PMID:31900135

Sharma, S., Bodempudi, S. T., Scribner, D., Grynovicki, J., & Grazaitis, P. (2019). Emergency Response Using HoloLens for Building Evacuation. In Virtual, Augmented and Mixed Reality. Multimodal Interaction. doi:10.1007/978-3-030-21607-8_23

Sheppard, J. (1992). *Anatomy: a complete guide for artists*. Dover.

Sherman, W., & Craig, A. (2019). Understanding virtual reality: Interface, application, and design (2nd ed.). Morgan Kaufmann.

Shim, K.-C., Park, J.-S., Kim, H.-S., Kim, J.-H., Park, Y.-C., & Ryu, H.-I. (2003). Application of virtual reality technology in biology education. *Journal of Biological Education*, *37*(2), 71–74. doi:10.1080/00219266.2003.9655854

Shin, C., Kim, H., Kang, C., Jang, Y., Choi, A., & Woo, W. (2010). Unified Context-Aware Augmented Reality Application Framework for User-Driven Tour Guides. *2010 International Symposium on Ubiquitous Virtual Reality*.

Shi, S. L., Tong, C. M., & Marcus, C. C. (2019). What makes a garden in the elderly care facility well used. *Landscape Research*, *44*(2), 256–269. doi:10.1080/01426397.2018.1457143

Simons, R. (2018). Strategy Execution Module 9: Building a Balanced Scorecard. Harvard Business School.

Simonyan, K., & Zisserman, A. (2014). *Two-stream convolutional networks for action recognition in videos*. Academic Press.

Sirkkunen, E., Väätäjä, H., Uskali, T., & Rezaei, P. P. (2016). Journalism in virtual reality: Opportunities and future research challenges. *Proceedings of the 20th international academic mindtrek conference*. 10.1145/2994310.2994353

Slater, M., Spanlang, B., Sanchez-Vives, M. V., & Blanke, O. (2010). First person experience of body transfer in virtual reality. *PLoS One*, *5*(5), 5. doi:10.1371/journal.pone.0010564 PMID:20485681

Smart Insights. (2020). *5 ways to use Augmented Reality in your marketing strategy*. Retrieved from Smart Insights website: https://www.smartinsights.com/digital-marketing-platforms/augmented-reality/5-ways-to-use-augmented-reality-in-your-marketing-strategy/

Smith, S. P., & Trenholme, D. (2009). Rapid prototyping a virtual fire drill environment using computer game technology. *Fire Safety Journal*, *44*(4), 559–569.

Smith, S., & Ericson, E. (2009). Using immersive game-based virtual reality to teach fire-safety skills to children. *Virtual Reality (Waltham Cross)*, *13*(2), 87–99. doi:10.100710055-009-0113-6

Smolentsev, A., Cornick, J. E., & Blascovich, J. (2017). Using a preamble to increase presence in digital virtual environments. *Virtual Reality*, *21*(3), 153–164. doi:10.100710055-017-0305-4

Snoswell, A. J., & Snoswell, C. L. (2019). Immersive virtual reality in health care: Systematic review of technology and disease states. *JMIR Biomedical Engineering, 4*(1), e15025. doi:10.2196/15025

Snow, R., Humphrey, C., & Sandall, J. (2013). What happens when patients know more than their doctors? Experiences of health interactions after diabetes patient education: A qualitative patient-led study: Table 1. *BMJ Open, 3*(11), e003583. Advance online publication. doi:10.1136/bmjopen-2013-003583 PMID:24231459

Social Welfare Department. HKSAR. (2021). Available at https://www.swd.gov.hk/en/index/site_pubsvc/page_elderly/sub_residentia/id_overviewon/

Spiegel, J. S. (2018). The ethics of virtual reality technology: Social hazards and public policy recommendations. *Science and Engineering Ethics, 24*(5), 1537–1550. doi:10.100711948-017-9979-y PMID:28942536

Stanford Medicine. (2017, July 11). *Virtual reality system helps surgeons, reassures patients.* https://med.stanford.edu/news/all-news/2017/07/virtual-reality-system-helps-surgeons-reassures-patients.html

Stansfield, S., Shawver, D., Rogers, D., & Hightower, R. (2005). Mission visualization for planning and training. *IEEE Computer Graphics and Applications*, 12–14.

Statista. (2020). *Adoption rate of smartphones in the Asia Pacific region in 2019 with a forecast for 2025.* Retrieved from Statista Research Department website: https://www.statista.com/statistics/1128693/apac-smartphone-adoption-rate/

Steinicke, F., Ropinski, T., & Hinrichs, K. (2005). A generic virtual reality software system's architecture and application. *Proceedings of the 2005 International Conference on Augmented Tele-Existence, 157*, 220-227. 10.1145/1152399.1152440

Stewart, M., & Roter, D. (1990). Communicating with medical patients. *Sage (Atlanta, Ga.).*

Stigall, J., Bodempudi, S. T., Sharma, S., Scribner, D., Grynovicki, J., & Grazaitis, P. (2018). *Building Evacuation using Microsoft HoloLens.* Academic Press.

Stojkoska, B. L. R., & Trivodaliev, K. (2017). *A review of Internet of Things for smart home: Challenges and solutions.* Academic Press.

Suh, K. S., & Lee, Y. E. (2005). The effects of virtual reality on consumer learning: An empirical investigation. MIS Quarterly: Management. *Information Systems, 29*(4). https://doi.org/10.2307/25148705

Sulbaran, T., & Baker, N. C. (2000). Enhancing engineering education through distributed virtual reality. ASEE/IEEE frontiers in education conference, 3–18. doi:10.1109/FIE.2000.896621

Sung-Hyun, Y., Thapa, K., Kabir, M. H., & Hee-Chan, L. (2018). *Log-Viterbi algorithm applied on second-order hidden Markov model for human activity recognition.* Academic Press.

Sunitha, Kokilam, & Preethi. (2013). Medical Informatics-Perk up Health Care through Information. *CSI Communications Journal, 37*(9), 7-8.

Swilley, E. (2016). *Moving Virtual Retail into Reality: Examining Metaverse and Augmented Reality in the Online Shopping Experience.* doi:10.1007/978-3-319-24184-5_163

Syed-Abdul, S., Malwade, S., Nursetyo, A. A., Sood, M., Bhatia, M., Barsasella, D., Liu, M. F., Chang, C.-C., Srinivasan, K., Raja, M., & Li, Y.-C. J. (2019). Virtual reality among the elderly: A usefulness and acceptance study from Taiwan. *BMC Geriatrics, 19*(1), 223–232. doi:10.118612877-019-1218-8 PMID:31426766

Szasz, T., & Hollender, M. (1956). A contribution to the philosophy of medicine. *A.M.A. Archives of Internal Medicine, 97*(5), 585–592. doi:10.1001/archinte.1956.00250230079008 PMID:13312700

Taneja, C. (2014). The psychology of excessive cellular phone use. *Delhi Psychiatry Journal, 17*(2), 448–451.

Tang, Y. M., Ng, G. W. Y., Chia, N. H., So, E. H. K., Wu, C. H., & Ip, W. (2021). *Application of virtual reality (VR) technology for medical practitioners in type and screen (T&S) training.* Academic Press.

Tang, C. Y., Tsui, C. P., Tang, Y. M., Wei, L., Wong, C. T., Lam, K. W., Ip, W. Y., Lu, W. W., & Pang, M. Y. (2014). Voxel-based approach to generate entire human metacarpal bone with microscopic architecture for finite element analysis. *Bio-Medical Materials and Engineering, 24*(2), 1469–1484. doi:10.3233/BME-130951 PMID:24642974

Tang, Y. M. (2010). Modeling skin deformation using boundary element method. *Computer-Aided Design and Applications, 7*(1), 101–108. doi:10.3722/cadaps.2010.101-108

Tang, Y. M., & Ho, H. L. (2020). 3D Modeling and Computer Graphics in Virtual Reality. In *Mixed Reality and Three-Dimensional Computer Graphics.* Intech Open. doi:10.5772/intechopen.91443

Tang, Y. M., & Hui, K. C. (2007). The effect of tendons on foot skin deformation. *CAD Computer Aided Design, 39*(7), 583–597. doi:10.1016/j.cad.2007.01.013

Tang, Y. M., & Hui, K. C. (2009). Simulating Tendon Motion with Axial Mass-spring System. *Computers & Graphics, 33*(2), 162–172. doi:10.1016/j.cag.2009.01.002

Tang, Y. M., & Hui, K. C. (2011). Human foot modeling towards footwear design. *CAD Computer Aided Design, 43*(12), 1841–1848. doi:10.1016/j.cad.2011.08.005

Tang, Y. M., & Lau, Y. Y. (2020). Medical training with virtual reality (VR) for the aged. *CPCE Health Conference 2020.*

Tang, Y. M., Ng, G. W. Y., Chia, N. H., So, E. H. K., Wu, C. H., & Ip, W. H. (2021). Application of virtual reality (VR) technology for medical practitioners in type and screen (T&S) training. *Journal of Computer Assisted Learning, 37*(2), 359–369. doi:10.1111/jcal.12494

Tang, Y. M., Wu, Z. H., Liao, W. H., & Chan, K. M. (2010). A study of semi-rigid support on ankle supination sprain kinematics. *Scandinavian Journal of Medicine & Science in Sports, 20*(6), 822–826. doi:10.1111/j.1600-0838.2009.00991.x PMID:19765241

Tang, Y. M., Zhou, A. F., & Hui, K. C. (2005). Comparison between FEM and BEM for Real-time Simulation. *Computer-Aided Design and Applications, 2*(1-4), 421–430. doi:10.1080/16864360.2005.10738391

Tang, Y. M., Zhou, A. F., & Hui, K. C. (2006). Comparison of FEM and BEM for interactive object simulation. *CAD Computer Aided Design, 38*(8), 874–886. doi:10.1016/j.cad.2006.04.014

Tang, Y., Au, K., & Leung, Y. (2018). Comprehending products with mixed reality: Geometric relationships and creativity. *International Journal of Engineering Business Management, 10*. doi:10.1177/1847979018809599

Tang, Y.-M., Au, K. M., Lau, H. C., Ho, G. T., & Wu, C.-H. (2020). Evaluating the effectiveness of learning design with mixed reality (MR) in higher education. *Virtual Reality (Waltham Cross), 24*(4), 797–807. doi:10.100710055-020-00427-9

Tao, F., Sui, F., Liu, A., Qi, Q., Zhang, M., Song, B., Guo, Z., Lu, S. C. Y., & Nee, A. Y. C. (2019). Digital twin-driven product design framework. *International Journal of Production Research, 57*(12), 3935–3953. doi:10.1080/00207543.2018.1443229

Tate, D. L., Silbert, L., & King, T. (1997) Virtual environments for shipboard firefighting training. In *Proceedings of the IEEE 1997 virtual reality international annual symposium*. IEEE Computer Society Press. 10.1109/VRAIS.1997.583045

Tergan, S.-O., & Keller, T. (2005). *Knowledge and information visualization: Searching for synergies*. Springer. doi:10.1007/b138081

The Hong Kong Polytechnic University. (2013). Health effects of using portable electronic devices studied. *ScienceDaily*. www.sciencedaily.com/releases/2013/09/130905160452.htm

The Lancet. (2010). Chinese doctors are under threat. *The Lancet, 376*(9742), 657. doi:10.1016/S0140-6736(10)61315-3

The Lancet. (2012). Ending violence against doctors in China. *Lancet, 379*(9828), 1764. Advance online publication. doi:10.1016/S0140-6736(12)60729-6

Thomas, E. R. L. (2014). *Cloud computing Concepts, Technology, and Architecture*. Pearson.

Tieland, M., Trouwborst, I., & Clark, B. C. (2018). Skeletal muscle performance and ageing. *Journal of Cachexia, Sarcopenia and Muscle, 9*(1), 3–19. doi:10.1002/jcsm.12238 PMID:29151281

Torraco, R. J. (2016). Writing integrative literature reviews: Using the past and present to explore the future. *Human Resource Development Review, 15*(4), 404–428. doi:10.1177/1534484316671606

Compilation of References

Torres-Ruiz, M., Mata, F., Zagal, R., Guzmán, G., Quintero, R., & Moreno-Ibarra, M. (2020). A recommender system to generate museum itineraries applying augmented reality and social-sensor mining techniques. *Virtual Reality*, *24*(1), 175–189. doi:10.100710055-018-0366-z

Tran, D., Bourdev, L., Fergus, R., Torresani, L., & Paluri, M. (2015). Learning spatiotemporal features with 3d convolutional networks. *Proceedings of the IEEE international conference on computer vision*. 10.1109/ICCV.2015.510

Tsai, S.-M., Wu, S.-S., Sun, S.-S., & Yang, P.-C. (2000). *Integrated home service network on intelligent Intranet*. Academic Press.

Tsai, Y. C., Lin, G. L., & Cheng, C. C. (2021). Work-in-Progress-Development of Immersive Nursing Skills Learning System and Evaluation of Learning Effectiveness. *2021 7th International Conference of the Immersive Learning Research Network (iLRN)*, 1-3.

Tsai, M.-K., Lee, Y.-C., Lu, C.-H., Chen, M.-H., Chou, T.-Y., & Yau, N.-J. (2012). Integrating geographical information and augmented reality techniques for mobile escape guidelines on nuclear accident sites. *Journal of Environmental Radioactivity*, *109*, 36–44. doi:10.1016/j.jenvrad.2011.12.025 PMID:22260929

ud din Tahir, S. B., Jalal, A., & Batool, M. (2020). *Wearable sensors for activity analysis using SMO-based random forest over smart home and sports datasets*. Paper presented at the 2020 3rd International Conference on Advancements in Computational Sciences (ICACS).

Uddin, M. T., & Uddiny, M. A. (2015). *A guided random forest based feature selection approach for activity recognition*. Paper presented at the 2015 International Conference on Electrical Engineering and Information Communication Technology (ICEEICT).

Van De Walle, G. (2019). *9 Factors Affecting Nutrition in Older Adults*. Available at https://dakotadietitians.com/factors-affecting-nutrition/

Van Eck, N. J., & Waltman, L. (2010). Software survey: VOSviewer, a computer program for bibliometric mapping. *Scientometrics, 84*(2), 523-538.

van Esch, P., Arli, D., Gheshlaghi, M. H., Andonopoulos, V., von der Heidt, T., & Northey, G. (2019). Anthropomorphism and augmented reality in the retail environment. *Journal of Retailing and Consumer Services*, *49*, 35–42. https://doi.org/10.1016/j.jretconser.2019.03.002

van Kasteren, T., & Krose, B. (2007). *Bayesian activity recognition in residence for elders*. Paper presented at the 2007 3rd IET international conference on intelligent environments.

Van Kasteren, T., Englebienne, G., Kröse, B. (2010). *Activity recognition using semi-Markov models on real world smart home datasets*. Academic Press.

Van Kasteren, T., Noulas, A., Englebienne, G., & Kröse, B. (2008). Accurate activity recognition in a home setting. *Proceedings of the 10th international conference on Ubiquitous computing*.

Van Royen, A., Shahabpour, M., Al Jahed, D., Abid, W., Vanhoenacker, F., & De Maeseneer, M. (2020). *Injuries of the Ligaments and Tendons in Ankle and Foot*. Academic Press.

Vassallo, R., Rankin, A., Chen, E. C., & Peters, T. M. (2017). *Hologram stability evaluation for Microsoft HoloLens. Medical Imaging 2017: Image Perception*. Observer Performance, and Technology Assessment.

Vatomsky, S. (2018). Thinking About Having a 'Green' Funeral? Here's What to Know. *The New York Times*. Retrieved on 2 July 2021 from https://www.nytimes.com/2018/03/22/smarter-living/green-funeral-burial-environment.html

Vehtari, A., Simpson, D. P., Yao, Y., & Gelman, A. (2019). Limitations of bayesian leave-one-out cross-validation for model selection. *Computational Brain & Behavior, 2*(1), 22–27. doi:10.100742113-018-0020-6 PMID:30906917

Viard, K., Fanti, M. P., Faraut, G., & Lesage, J.-J. (2016). *An event-based approach for discovering activities of daily living by hidden Markov models*. Paper presented at the 2016 15th International Conference on Ubiquitous Computing and Communications and 2016 International Symposium on Cyberspace and Security (IUCC-CSS).

Vijayrani, S. (2013). Economic Health Records- An Overview. *CSI Communications Journal, 37*(9), 9-11.

Vince, J. (1995). *Virtual Reality Systems*. Wesley Publishing Company.

Vivek, J. (2020). *Review of Preventive & Social Medicine (Including Bio-Statistics)*. Jaypee Brothers Medical Publisher.

Walius, N. A. (1962). *Stereoscopy*. Russian Academy of Science. (in Russian)

Walshe. (2014). *Healthcare Management*. McGraw-Hill.

Wang, L., Gu, T., Tao, X., Chen, H., & Lu, J. (2011). *Recognizing multi-user activities using wearable sensors in a smart home*. Academic Press.

Wang, C., Li, H., & Kho, S. (2018). VR-embedded BIM immersive system for QS engineering education. *Computer Applications in Engineering Education, 26*(3), 626–641. doi:10.1002/cae.21915

Wang, Q., Li, C., Xie, Z., Bu, Z., Shi, L., Wang, C., & Jiang, F. (2020). The development and application of virtual reality animation simulation technology: Take gastroscopy simulation system as an example. *Pathology Oncology Research, 26*(2), 765–769. doi:10.100712253-019-00590-8 PMID:30809768

Wang, W., Wu, X., Chen, G., & Chen, Z. (2018). Holo3DGIS: Leveraging Microsoft HoloLens in 3D Geographic Information. *ISPRS International Journal of Geo-Information, 7*(2), 60.

Wang, X., & Kim, H. (2015). *Detecting User Activities with the Accelerometer on Android Smartphones*. Academic Press.

Watanabe, H., & Ujike, H. (2008). The activity of ISO/Study Group on "Image Safety" and three biological effects. *Proceedings of the 2008 Second International Symposium on Universal Communication*, 210– 214. 10.1109/ISUC.2008.11

Weichert, F., Bachmann, D., Rudak, B., & Fisseler, D. (2013). Analysis of the accuracy and robustness of the Leap Motion Controller. *Sensors (Basel)*, *13*(5), 6380–6393. doi:10.3390130506380 PMID:23673678

Weinbaum, S. G. (2016). *Pygmalion's spectacles*. Simon and Schuster.

Weinberger, S., Lawrence, H. III, Henley, D., Alden, E., & Hoyt, D. (2012). Legislative interference with the patient–physician relationship. *The New England Journal of Medicine*, *367*(16), 1557–1559. doi:10.1056/NEJMsb1209858 PMID:23075183

Weiss, P., Kizony, R., Feintuch, U., & Katz, N. (2006). Virtual reality in neurorehabilitation. In *Textbook of Neural Repair and Rehabilitation* (pp. 182–197). Cambridge University Press. doi:10.1017/CBO9780511545078.015

Williams-Bell, F. M., Kapralos, B., Hogue, A., Murphy, B. M., & Weckman, E. J. (2015). Using Serious Games and Virtual Simulation for Training in the Fire Service: A Review. *Fire Technology*, *51*(3), 553–584. doi:10.100710694-014-0398-1

Wilson, C., Hargreaves, T., & Hauxwell-Baldwin, R. (2017). *Benefits and risks of smart home technologies*. Academic Press.

Wilson, G. (1992). The Rise and Rise of the Computer -- The Dream Machine: Exploring the Computer Age by John Palfreman and Doron Swade. *New Scientist, 133*(1812).

Won, A. S., Bailenson, J., Lee, J., & Lanier, J. (2015). Homuncular flexibility in virtual reality. *J. Comput. Commun, 20*, 241–259.

Wong, S., Yeung, J. K. W., Lau, Y. Y., & So, J. (2021). Technical sustainability of cloud-based blockchain integrated with machine learning for supply chain management. *Sustainability*, *13*(15), 8270–8291. doi:10.3390u13158270

World Health Organization. (2020, March 3). *Shortage of personal protective equipment endangering health workers worldwide*. https://www.who.int/news/item/03-03-2020-shortage-of-personal-protective-equipment-endangering-health-workers-worldwide

Wulfovich. (2019). Digital Health Entrepreneurship. Springer.

Xiang, Y., Arora, J. S., & Abdel-Malek, K. (2010). Physics-based modeling and simulation of human walking: A review of optimization-based and other approaches. *Structural and Multidisciplinary Optimization*, *42*(1), 1–23. doi:10.100700158-010-0496-8

Xie, L., Chen, Z., Wang, H., Zheng, C., & Jiang, J. (2020). Bibliometric and visualized analysis of scientific publications on atlantoaxial spine surgery based on Web of Science and VOSviewer. *World Neurosurgery, 137*, 435-442.

Xu, H., Pan, Y., Li, J., Nie, L., & Xu, X. (2019). *Activity recognition method for home-based elderly care service based on random forest and activity similarity*. Academic Press.

Xu, Z., Lu, X. Z., Guan, H., Chen, C., & Ren, A. Z. (2014). A virtual reality based fire training simulator with smoke hazard assessment capacity. *Advances in Engineering Software, 68*, 1–8. doi:10.1016/j.advengsoft.2013.10.004

Yamamoto, M., Shimatani, K., Hasegawa, M., & Kurita, Y. (2020). Effects of Varying Plantarflexion Stiffness of Ankle-Foot Orthosis on Achilles Tendon and Propulsion Force During Gait. *IEEE Transactions on Neural Systems and Rehabilitation Engineering, 28*(10), 2194–2202. doi:10.1109/TNSRE.2020.3020564 PMID:32866100

Yan, C., Wu, T., Huang, K., He, J., Liu, H., Hong, Y., & Wang, B. (2020). The application of virtual reality in cervical spinal surgery: A review. *World Neurosurgery*. PMID:32931993

Yang, J., Lee, J., & Choi, J. (2011). *Activity recognition based on RFID object usage for smart mobile devices*. Academic Press.

Yano, H., Kasai, K., Saitou, H., & Iwata, H. (2003). Development of a gait rehabilitation system using a locomotion interface. *The Journal of Visualization and Computer Animation, 14*(5), 243–252. doi:10.1002/vis.321

Yari, A., Ardalan, A., Ostadtaghizadeh, A., Zarezadeh, Y., Boubakran, M. S., Bidarpoor, F., & Rahimiforoushani, A. (2019). Underlying factors affecting death due to flood in Iran: A qualitative content analysis. *International Journal of Disaster Risk Reduction, 40*, 101258. doi:10.1016/j.ijdrr.2019.101258

Yedidia, M. (2007). Transforming doctor-patient relationships to promote patient-centered care: Lessons from palliative care. *Journal of Pain and Symptom Management, 33*(1), 40–57. doi:10.1016/j.jpainsymman.2006.06.007 PMID:17196906

Yee, N., Bailenson, J. N., & Ducheneaut, N. (2009). The Proteus effect: Implications of transformed digital self-representation on online and offline behavior. *Communication Research, 36*(2), 285–312. doi:10.1177/0093650208330254

Yiannakopoulou, E., Nikiteas, N., Perrea, D., & Tsigris, C. (2015). Virtual reality simulators and training in laparoscopic surgery. *International Journal of Surgery, 13*, 60–64. doi:10.1016/j.ijsu.2014.11.014 PMID:25463761

Yin, R. K. (2014). Case study research: Design and methods. *Sage (Atlanta, Ga.)*.

Young, G. W., Stehle, S., Walsh, B. Y., & Tiri, E. (2020). Exploring Virtual Reality in the Higher Education Classroom: Using VR to Build Knowledge and Understanding. *Journal of Universal Computer Science, 26*(8), 904–928. doi:10.3897/jucs.2020.049

Yu, Y., Li, Y., Zhang, Z., Gu, Z., Zhong, H., Zha, Q., . . . Chen, E. (2020). *A bibliometric analysis using VOSviewer of publications on COVID-19.* Academic Press.

Zajac, F. E. (1989). Muscle and tendon: Properties, models, scaling and application to biomechanics and motor control. *Critical Reviews in Biomedical Engineering, 17,* 359–411. PMID:2676342

Zajac, F. E., Topp, E. L., & Stevenson, P. J. (1986) A dimensionless musculotendon model. *Proceedings IEEE Engineering in Medicine and Biology.*

Zarraonandia, T., Díaz, P., Santos, A., Montero, Á., & Aedo, I. (2019). A Toolkit for Creating Cross-Reality Serious Games. In M. Gentile, M. Allegra, & H. Söbke (Eds.), Games and Learning Alliance. doi:10.1007/978-3-030-11548-7_28

Zhang, Y. (2019). *How is Augmented Reality marketing related to your business?* Retrieved from hapticmedia website: https://hapticmedia.com/blog/augmented-reality-marketing/

Zhang, X., Pauel, R., Deschamps, K., Jonkers, I., & Vanwanseele, B. (2019). Differences in foot muscle morphology and foot kinematics between symptomatic and asymptomatic pronated feet. *Scandinavian Journal of Medicine & Science in Sports, 29*(11), 1766–1773. doi:10.1111ms.13512 PMID:31278774

Zhan, T., Yin, K., Xiong, J., He, Z., & Wu, S.-T. (2020). Augmented reality and virtual reality displays: Perspectives and challenges. *iScience, 23*(8), 101397. doi:10.1016/j.isci.2020.101397 PMID:32759057

Zhao, Y., Wang, A., & Sun, Y. (2020). Technological environment, virtual experience, and MOOC continuance: A stimulus–organism–response perspective. *Computers and Education, 144.* doi:10.1016/j.compedu.2019.103721

Zheng, M. (2018). *Green Burials: Why Hongkongers remain reluctant about alternative funerals.* Coconuts Hong Kong. Retrieved on 2 July 2021 from https://coconuts.co/hongkong/features/green-burials-hongkongers-remain-reluctant-alternative-funerals/

Zhong, J., Han, T., Lotfi, A., Cangelosi, A., & Liu, X. (2019). *Bridging the Gap between Robotic Applications and Computational Intelligence in Domestic Robotics.* Paper presented at the 2019 IEEE Symposium Series on Computational Intelligence (SSCI).

Zhou, A. F., Hui, K. C., Tang, Y. M., & Wang, C. C. L. (2006). An Accelerated BEM Approach for the Simulation of Deformable Objects. *Computer-Aided Design and Applications, 3*(6), 761–769. doi:10.1080/16864360.2006.10738429

Zhou, F., Duh, H. B.-L., & Billinghurst, M. (2008). Trends in augmented reality tracking, interaction and display: A review of ten years of ISMAR. *Proceedings of the 7th IEEE/ACM international symposium on mixed and augmented reality.*

Zhou, Z., Jiang, S., Yang, Z., & Zhou, L. (2019). Personalized planning and training system for brachytherapy based on virtual reality. *Virtual Reality (Waltham Cross), 23*(4), 347–361. doi:10.100710055-018-0350-7

Zhu, R., Lucas, G. M., Becerik-Gerber, B., & Southers, E. G. (2020). Building preparedness in response to active shooter incidents: Results of focus group interviews. *International Journal of Disaster Risk Reduction, 48*, 101617. doi:10.1016/j.ijdrr.2020.101617

Zhu, S., Jin, W., & He, C. (2019). On evolutionary economic geography: A literature review using bibliometric analysis. *European Planning Studies, 27*(4), 639–660. doi:10.1080/096543 13.2019.1568395

Zibreg, C. (2019). *The iOS 12 software is now powering 75 percent of all devices*. Retrieved from idownloadblog website: https://www.idownloadblog.com/2019/01/02/ios-12-adoption-rate-75-percent/

About the Contributors

Hoi Sze Chan is an BSc graduate from the Hong Kong Polytechnic University.

Ivy Chan obtained her bachelor's degree in Management (with first class honors) from The Hong Kong University of Science and Technology and her master's degree in Business Administration & Information Systems (with distinction) from the University of Central Lancashire. After graduation, she had been working in the business and marketing fields. In 2004, she received her PhD in Information Systems from The University of Hong Kong. Her research interests center around knowledge management, student learning and engagement.

Bowen Dong is an assistant professor at the Faculty of Business, City University of Macau. He received his PhD from Zhejiang University. His research interests include corporate social responsibility (CSR), employee development, and entrepreneurship.

Kenneth N. K. Fong is Associate Professor in the Department of Rehabilitation Sciences of the Hong Kong Polytechnic University. He is an occupational therapist by training. He has been the editor-in-chief of the Hong Kong Journal of Occupational Therapy (HKJOT) (5-year Impact Factor: 0.554) for more than 10 years, and honorary advisor of several self-help organizations for people with chronic diseases and disabilities in Hong Kong. He had received the Department Outstanding Teaching Award and the Faculty Team Teaching Award of the Faculty of Health and Social Sciences. He had been awarded several public competitive research grants from, among others, the General Research Fund, and Health and Medical Research Fund in order to develop innovative neurorehabilitation intervention and studies in the ageing population. In the past 10 years, he has published more than 50 journal papers and book chapters in the fields of neurorehabilitation and ageing.

Chang Gao is a research assistant in School of Intelligent Systems Science and Engineering, Jinan University, China. Her research mainly focuses on virtual technology and industrial engineering.

Ying Ting Huang is a research assistant in School of Intelligent Systems Science and Engineering, Jinan University, China. Her research mainly focuses on virtual technology, and content analysis.

Alex Pak Ki Kwok graduated from The University of Hong Kong with a Ph.D. degree in the Department of Industrial and Manufacturing Systems Engineering. He is now an assistant professor in the Department of Applied Data Science of the Hong Kong Shue Yan University. His research interests mainly include virtual reality, technology acceptance, and consumer behavior.

Yui-Yip Lau has published more than 220 research papers in international journals and professional magazines, contributed 10 book chapters, 2 books and presented numerous papers in international conferences. He has collaborated with scholars from more than 20 countries and regions spreading over five continents on research projects. He has also secured over HK$ 7 million research grants. Recently, he has been awarded a Certificate of Appreciation by the Institute of Seatransport in recognition of his outstanding performance on research and the Best Paper Award in international leading conferences. His research interests are cruise, ferry, climate change, regional studies, higher education, health logistics, and sustainability issues.

Xin Lian is currently studying for her doctorate at the School of Computer Science and Technology at Xi'an Jiaotong University. Her research mainly focuses on bioinformatics and digital health.

Haoyu Liu is an assistant professor at the Faculty of Business, City University of Macau. He received an MPhil and a PhD in Operations Management from HKUST Business School in 2017 and 2020, respectively. He serves as a reviewer for Manufacturing & Service Operations Management (MSOM), Naval Research Logistics (NRL), and International Journal of E-Business Research (IJEBR). His research interests include technology management, philanthropy management, healthcare management, and the interface of marketing and operations.

Xiaoxiao Liu is currently the DBA student of the Faculty of Business at the City University of Macau.

N Raghavendra Rao is an Advisor to FINAIT Consultancy Services India. He has a doctorate in the area of Finance. He has a rare distinction of having experience in the combined areas of Information Technology and Business applications. His rich experience in the Industry is matched with a parallel academic experience in Management & IT in Business Schools. He has over two decades of experience in the development of application software related to manufacturing, healthcare and hospitality sectors, financial institutions and business enterprises. He contributes chapters for research reference books. He presents papers related to Information Technology and Management at National and International conferences. He contributes articles on Information Technology in mainstream newspapers and journals. His area of research interest is Mobile Computing, Virtual Technology, and Commerce in Space, Ubiquitous Commerce, Cloud Computing, e-governance, Knowledge Management, and Social Media for Business Applications. He is a member of the Editorial Advisory Board for research reference books published by IGI Global USA. He is also a Review Board Member of International Research Journals. He is the editor for the four research reference books published by IGI Global USA. The books are 1- *Virtual Technologies for Business and Industrial Applications*: *Innovative and Synergistic Approaches, 2- Enterprise Strategies in the Era of Cloud Computing, 3- Social Media listening and Monitoring for Business Applications, and 4- Global Virtual Enterprises in Cloud Computing Environments. He is the author of the book titled Effective Open Innovation Strategies in Modern Business published by IGI Global USA under Research Insights Category.*

Farzad Sabetzadeh is an assistant professor of Knowledge and Innovation Management at the City University of Macau. He has more than a decade of track record in both academia and industry in developing knowledge-based innovation systems and processes. He is teaching various subjects on knowledge management, innovation, and entrepreneurship to both undergraduate and postgraduate students in Greater China and Southeast Asia. With his diverse work and academic background in different regions, his current academic focus is on teaching, research and consultancy for innovation and entrepreneurship development in the Greater Bay Area, South East Asia and projects associated with China One Belt One Road Initiative. He is also an active technology advisor to the IT industry and is involved in various academic events, talks, and seminars as well as research publications. Over the past decade, he has completed multiple projects on knowledge management, personalized learning environment, Massive Open Online Courses (MOOC), Smart City, and Internet of Things (IoT).

Cheng Yao Wang is currently a postgraduate student at the Department of Electronic Engineering of the City University of Hong Kong. Her research mainly focuses on virtual technology and electronic engineering.

Yusong Wang is an under-graduated student from City University of Macao. Major in business administration and research in application of AR in marketing, especially e-commerce.

Yan Wan is a DBA student at the Faculty of Business of the City University of Macau, Macao.

Mian Yan graduated from The University of Hong Kong with a Ph.D. degree in the Department of Industrial and Manufacturing Systems Engineering. He is now an assistant professor in School of Intelligent Systems Science and Engineering, Jinan University, China. His research interests mainly include human factors and ergonomics, consumer behavior, and health informatics.

Pi-Ying Yen is an assistant professor at the School of Business, Macau University of Science and Technology. She received her PhD in Industrial Engineering and Decision Analytics from HKUST in 2020. She serves as a reviewer for Manufacturing & Service Operations Management (MSOM) and Naval Research Logistics (NRL). Her research interests include socially responsible operations, supply chain management, and consumer behavior.

Gareth Young is a postdoctoral research fellow on the V-SENSE project. His current research focuses on the evaluation of creative uses of cross-reality (XR) technology by applying both quantitative and qualitative human-computer interaction (HCI) evaluation techniques. This includes studying the design and use of XR technology in creative practices, focusing on the interface between users and the XR platform. Gareth's role is to observe and record how users interact with XR and design new methods that allow users to interact with XR in innovative and novel ways. Topics of exploration focus on the use of XR and volumetric video (VV) in cultural heritage, such as film, theater, and performance practice from the perspectives of both practitioners and the audience. The role of immersive content creation in mediated perspective-taking experiences of creative storytelling content is also investigated, including the use of XR as an 'empathy making machine' by facilitating perspective-taking and allowing users to experience another person's circumstances. Other duties include investigating the role of XR in the delivery of educational content in the context of higher education, research, and artistic practice and the influences of immersion and presence on the overall experiences of students.

Tomasz Zawadzki is currently an Assistant Professor in the Department of Digital Game Design at ARUCAD, Cyprus. His research focuses on game design & development, VFX, and Virtual Reality using Unity and Unreal Engine game engines. He has published over 20 peer-reviewed papers in international conference proceedings, journals, and book chapters.

Can Biao Zhuang is a research assistant in School of Intelligent Systems Science and Engineering, Jinan University, China. His research mainly focuses on virtual technology.

Index

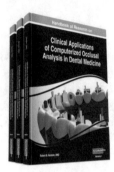
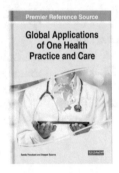
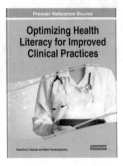
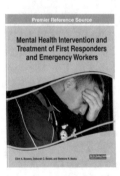
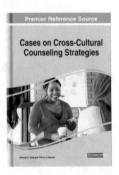
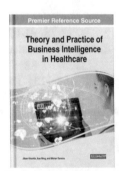
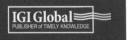

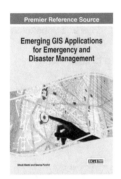
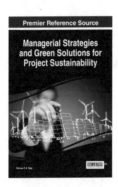
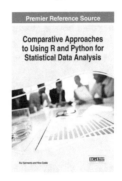
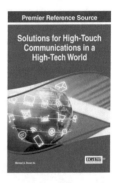

IGI Global Author Services

Providing a high-quality, affordable, and expeditious service, IGI Global's Author Services enable authors to streamline their publishing process, increase chance of acceptance, and adhere to IGI Global's publication standards.

Benefits of Author Services:

- **Professional Service:** All our editors, designers, and translators are experts in their field with years of experience and professional certifications.
- **Quality Guarantee & Certificate:** Each order is returned with a quality guarantee and certificate of professional completion.
- **Timeliness:** All editorial orders have a guaranteed return timeframe of 3-5 business days and translation orders are guaranteed in 7-10 business days.
- **Affordable Pricing:** IGI Global Author Services are competitively priced compared to other industry service providers.
- **APC Reimbursement:** IGI Global authors publishing Open Access (OA) will be able to deduct the cost of editing and other IGI Global author services from their OA APC publishing fee.

Author Services Offered:

English Language Copy Editing
Professional, native English language copy editors improve your manuscript's grammar, spelling, punctuation, terminology, semantics, consistency, flow, formatting, and more.

Scientific & Scholarly Editing
A Ph.D. level review for qualities such as originality and significance, interest to researchers, level of methodology and analysis, coverage of literature, organization, quality of writing, and strengths and weaknesses.

Figure, Table, Chart & Equation Conversions
Work with IGI Global's graphic designers before submission to enhance and design all figures and charts to IGI Global's specific standards for clarity.

Translation
Providing 70 language options, including Simplified and Traditional Chinese, Spanish, Arabic, German, French, and more.

Hear What the Experts Are Saying About IGI Global's Author Services

"Publishing with IGI Global has been **an amazing experience** for me for sharing my research. The **strong academic production** support ensures quality and timely completion." – **Prof. Margaret Niess, Oregon State University, USA**

"The service was **very fast, very thorough, and very helpful** in ensuring our chapter meets the criteria and requirements of the book's editors. I was **quite impressed and happy** with your service." – **Prof. Tom Brinthaupt, Middle Tennessee State University, USA**

Learn More or Get Started Here: For Questions, Contact IGI Global's Customer Service Team at cust@igi-global.com or 717-533-8845

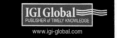

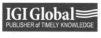

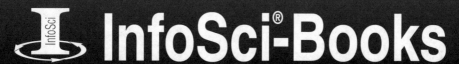
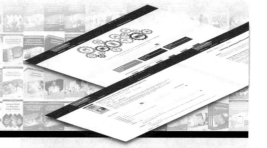

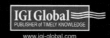

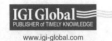

www.igi-global.com

Publisher of Peer-Reviewed, Timely, and
Innovative Academic Research Since 1988

IGI Global's Transformative Open Access (OA) Model:
How to Turn Your University Library's Database Acquisitions Into a Source of OA Funding

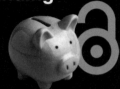

Well in advance of Plan S, IGI Global unveiled their OA Fee Waiver (Read & Publish) Initiative. Under this initiative, librarians who invest in IGI Global's InfoSci-Books and/or InfoSci-Journals databases will be able to subsidize their patrons' OA article processing charges (APCs) when their work is submitted and accepted (after the peer review process) into an IGI Global journal.

How Does it Work?

Step 1: **Library Invests in the InfoSci-Databases:** A library perpetually purchases or subscribes to the InfoSci-Books, InfoSci-Journals, or discipline/subject databases.

Step 2: **IGI Global Matches the Library Investment with OA Subsidies Fund:** IGI Global provides a fund to go towards subsidizing the OA APCs for the library's patrons.

Step 3: **Patron of the Library is Accepted into IGI Global Journal (After Peer Review):** When a patron's paper is accepted into an IGI Global journal, they option to have their paper published under a traditional publishing model or as OA.

Step 4: **IGI Global Will Deduct APC Cost from OA Subsidies Fund:** If the author decides to publish under OA, the OA APC fee will be deducted from the OA subsidies fund.

Step 5: **Author's Work Becomes Freely Available:** The patron's work will be freely available under CC BY copyright license, enabling them to share it freely with the academic community.

Note: This fund will be offered on an annual basis and will renew as the subscription is renewed for each year thereafter. IGI Global will manage the fund and award the APC waivers unless the librarian has a preference as to how the funds should be managed.

Hear From the Experts on This Initiative:

"I'm very happy to have been able to make one of my recent research contributions *freely available* along with having access to the *valuable resources* found within IGI Global's InfoSci-Journals database."

– **Prof. Stuart Palmer,**
Deakin University, Australia

"Receiving the support from IGI Global's OA Fee Waiver Initiative *encourages me to continue my research work without any hesitation*."

– **Prof. Wenlong Liu**, College of Economics and Management at Nanjing University of Aeronautics & Astronautics, China

For More Information, Scan the QR Code or Contact:
IGI Global's Digital Resources Team at eresources@igi-global.com.

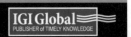

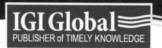
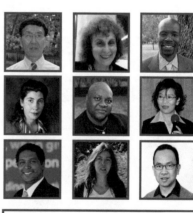

Printed in the United States
by Baker & Taylor Publisher Services